Public Behavioural Responses to Policy Making during the Pandemic

This book provides a comparative study of people's mask-wearing behaviour in response to government policies between European-Northern America and Asian countries.

Examining citizens' attitudes towards their state during the COVID-19 pandemic from the perspectives of history, linguistics, politics, economics and sociology, the contributors in this volume explore to what extent people accept the wearing of masks in countries where governments have made it mandatory as compared to countries where people wear masks voluntarily. The book thus looks at mask-wearing from a political dichotomy between authoritarianism and liberalism and posits the extent to which political divisions could have existed in public opinion over the measures taken against COVID-19.

Filled with invaluable insights through research in 13 countries, this book will appeal to readers in policy making and influencing public opinion via the Europe-Asia comparative study.

Noriko Suzuki is a professor at the Faculty of Social Sciences at Waseda University in Japan.

Xavier Mellet is an associate professor at the School of International Liberal Studies at Waseda University in Japan.

Susumu Annaka is an assistant professor at the Waseda Institute for Advanced Study in Japan.

Masahisa Endo is an associate professor at the Faculty of Social Sciences at Waseda University in Japan.

Routledge-WIAS Interdisciplinary Studies
Edited by Hideaki Miyajima and Kazuhisa Takemura
Waseda University, Japan

For more information about this series, please visit: *www.routledge.com/Routledge-WIAS-Interdisciplinary-Studies/book-series/WIAS01*

Public Behavioural Responses to Policy Making during the Pandemic

Comparative Perspectives on Mask-Wearing Policies

Edited by Noriko Suzuki,
Xavier Mellet, Susumu Annaka
and Masahisa Endo

Routledge
Taylor & Francis Group

LONDON AND NEW YORK

First published 2023
by Routledge
4 Park Square, Milton Park, Abingdon, Oxon OX14 4RN

and by Routledge
605 Third Avenue, New York, NY 10158

Routledge is an imprint of the Taylor & Francis Group, an informa business

British Library Cataloguing-in-Publication Data
A catalogue record for this book is available from the British Library

Library of Congress Cataloging-in-Publication Data
Names: Suzuki, Noriko, 1972– editor. | Mellet, Xavier, editor. |
  Annaka, Susumu, editor.
Title: Public behavioural responses to policy making during the
  pandemic : comparative perspectives on mask wearing policies /
  edited by Noriko Suzuki, Xavier Mellet, Susumu Annaka and
  Masahisa Endo.
Description: Milton Park, Abingdon, Oxon ; New York, NY :
  Routledge, 2023. | Series: Routledge-WIAS interdisciplinary studies |
  Includes bibliographical references and index. |
Identifiers: LCCN 2022025245 (print) | LCCN 2022025246
  (ebook) | ISBN 9781032154275 (hardback) | ISBN
  9781032154299 (paperback) | ISBN 9781003244127 (ebook)
Subjects: LCSH: COVID-19 (Disease)—Prevention. | Disaster
  medicine—Public opinion. | Medical policy—Citizen participation. |
  Public opinion—Health aspects.
Classification: LCC RA644.C67 P827 2023 (print) | LCC RA644.
  C67 (ebook) | DDC 362.1962/4144—dc23/eng/20220829
LC record available at https://lccn.loc.gov/2022025245
LC ebook record available at https://lccn.loc.gov/2022025246

ISBN: 9781032154275 (hbk)
ISBN: 9781032154299 (pbk)
ISBN: 9781003244127 (ebk)

DOI: 10.4324/9781003244127

Typeset in Galliard
by Apex CoVantage, LLC

Contents

Figures

Tables

Contributors

Susumu ANNAKA is an assistant professor at the Waseda Institute for Advanced Study in Japan. He received a PhD in political science from Waseda University. His main topics of interest are human development, human health and war. He published *Political Regime, Data Transparency, and COVID-19 Death Cases* (*SSM – Population Health*, 2021) and co-authored articles entitled 'Political Liberalization and Human Development: Dynamic Effects of Political Regime Change on Infant Mortality across Three Centuries (1800–2015)' (*World Development*, 2021) and 'Democracy, Conscription, and War' (SocArXiv, 2020). He also published several papers in Japanese refereed journals.

Emmanuel BRUNET-JAILLY is a professor, School of Public Administration, at the University of Victoria (Ph.D., UWO, 1999). He has been Jean Monnet Chair since 2014 (currently Jean Monnet Chair in European Union Policy and Governance (2021–24). He is the director of the Borders in Globalization research lab and director of the European Union Jean Monnet Center. Since 2001, he has published over 100 articles and book sections and 15 books and special issues of academic journals.

Athanasia CHALARI is a senior visiting fellow at Hellenic Observatory, London School of Economics and Political Science. She obtained a PhD in sociology from the University of Warwick in the United Kingdom.

CHEN Lihang is a research assistant at the Institute of Ethnology of Academia Sinica. He earned an MA in history at National Chengchi University and was an international research student at the University of Tokyo. He has published articles on the history of medicine and Taiwanese people's activities abroad during the Japanese colonial era. He is the author of *Minus 68 Degree Celsius: Taiwanese POW in Post-World War II Siberia* (Taipei: Avanguard Publishing House, 2021).

Łukasz CZARNECKI is a professor at the Institute of Law, Administration and Economics of the Pedagogical University of Krakow in Poland. Trained in sociology and law, he holds PhDs in social science from the National Autonomous University of Mexico, sociology from the University of Strasbourg (France) and law from the Jagiellonian University in Kraków (Poland), respectively. With its diverse mix of qualitative and quantitative methods, his research interest lies at the intersection of social structure, sociology and subjective well-being. He published books and articles in peer-reviewed journals in English, Spanish and Polish.

Masahisa ENDO is an associate professor at the Faculty of Social Sciences at Waseda University in Japan. His research interests cover public opinion, voting behaviour and Japanese politics. He co-authored the book entitled *The Generational Gap in Japanese Politics: A Longitudinal Study of Political Attitudes and Behavior* (Palgrave Macmillan, 2016). He obtained a PhD in political science from Waseda University.

Osamu IEDA is a professor in the Faculty of Social Sciences at Waseda University in Japan. He received his PhD in economics from the University of Tokyo. He has edited 26 books (20 in English and 6 in Japanese), including *Fukushima and Nuclear Disasters, and Beyond* (Waseda University, 2019), *Trans-Boundary Symbiosis over the Danube I, II, III* (Hokkaido University, 2014; Hokkaido University, 2015; Waseda University, 2018), *Beyond Sovereignty: From Status Law to Transnational Citizenship?* (Slavic Eurasian Studies, No. 9, SRC, Hokkaido University, 2006), *The Hungarian Status Law: Nation Building and/or Minority Protection* (SRC, Hokkaido University, 2004), *Transformation and Diversification of Rural Societies in Eastern Europe and Russia* (SRC Hokkaido University, 2002).

Gento KATO is an assistant professor at the Department of Political Science and International Relations at Nazarbayev University, Kazakhstan. His main research interest is the roles of information and identity in the mechanisms of political decision-making and attitude formation. His works have appeared in *the Journal of Theoretical Politics, Political Research Quarterly* and *Social Science Quarterly*, among other peer-reviewed journals.

Upalat KORWATANASAKUL is an associate professor at the School of Social Sciences, Waseda University and a consultant at the United Nations University Institute for the Advanced Study of Sustainability. He is an international development economist whose research interest lies in a wide range of economic and social development topics in East and Southeast Asia. He holds a PhD in international studies majoring in development economic analysis from the Graduate School of Asia-Pacific Studies, Waseda University (Tokyo, Japan).

Sivarin LERTPUSIT (PhD) is an assistant professor at the College of Interdisciplinary Studies, Thammasat University, and a lecturer and researcher in the socio-political field. She finished her doctoral degree in international studies (Southeast Asia studies) at the Graduate School of Asia Pacific Studies, Waseda University. Her studies focus on GMS and the influence of China. Her previous experiences and work include *The Chinese Transborder and Its Socioeconomic Impact to Boten People* (Laos); *The Analysis of Public Policy on Maesod Special Economic Zone (Thailand) and Mwayadee Special Economic*

Zone (Myanmar) in the Context of ASEAN Economic Community, and *The Challenges in Managing the Globalization of Migration: New Chinese Migrants in Chiang Mai and Chiang Rai.*

Hongyi LIU is a doctoral programme student at the Graduate School of Social Sciences, Waseda University, and works as research associate at the same graduate school. He majors in China's nontraditional security and international cooperation. His work includes the articles entitled 'The Role and Logic of Nontraditional Security in China's Engagement in Global Governance Mechanisms Under Xi Jinping's Regime' and 'Response of the Chinese Government to the New Coronavirus Outbreak: Announcement of "Wartime State" and Its Problems' (in Japanese).

Xavier MELLET is an associate professor at the School of International Liberal Studies in Waseda University, Japan. His research focuses on the current evolutions in French and Japanese domestic politics. He received a PhD in political science from Sciences Po Paris (France), his dissertation comparing populisms in Japan and France. His works on French politics include an article on 'The "Bayrou moment" as a mediatic bubble during the 2007 presidential election" in France" *(Mots. Les langages du politiques*, 2019).

Joachim SCHARLOTH is a professor of German Studies at the School of International Liberal Studies at Waseda University, Japan. Trained in linguistics and language sociology, his main areas of interest are language in politics and politics with language. He has published widely on social movements with a special focus on the 1968 movement in Europe. He authored the book entitled *1968: Eine Kommunikationsgeschichte* (*1968: A History from the Perspective of Communication*, Fink) and is the co-editor of *1968 in Europe* (Palgrave), *Protest Cultures. A Companion* (Berghahn Books) and the book series *Protest, Culture and Society* (Berghahn Books). His latest book, *Hässliche Wörter* (*Ugly Words. Hate Speech as a Principle of the New Right*, Metzler), was published 2021. He obtained a PhD from Heidelberg University, Germany and his Habilitation from Zurich University, Switzerland.

Tatsiana SHABAN is a non-resident fellow at the Centre for Global Studies at the University of Victoria (UVic), Canada. She has an interdisciplinary PhD with a special focus on European studies from UVic and a MA in international relations and politics from the University of Nottingham, UK. Her research focuses on the EU regional cooperation and governance of its Eastern neighbourhood, European Neighbourhood Policy and Belarus and Ukraine, in particular. Her PhD thesis analysed the benefits and actions of the EU governance and its cross-border cooperation schemes, including their impact on the transformation of national settings in the Eastern neighbourhood.

Yuko SHIMAZAKI is an associate professor at the Faculty of Social Sciences at Waseda University in Japan. She received a PhD in international studies from Waseda university and specialises in social development and human rights issues. As a researcher, she gained rich fieldwork experience in Southeast Asia. Her work has appeared in books such as *Human Trafficking and the Feminization of Poverty – Structural Violence in Cambodia* (Lexington Books: Lanham, Boulder, New York, London, 2021).

Monika SKOWROŃSKA is a deputy director and an assistant professor at the Institute of Law, Administration and Economics of the Pedagogical University of Krakow (Poland). She holds a PhD in law from Jagiellonian University, Krakow. Her research interests focus on EU law, human rights, ethics of the legal profession and administrative proceedings. For many years, she was a lecturer in EU law for various audiences, such as judges, prosecutors, trainees in the legal profession, civil service officers and businessmen. She is an attorney-at-law in the National Fiscal Administration; a member of the Krakow Bar Association of Attorneys-at-Law; and the President of the District Committee of Inspector Attorneys-at-Law.

Noriko SUZUKI is a professor in the Faculty of Social Sciences at Waseda University in Japan and specialises in political sociology, specifically, European citizenship and immigration in France. She received her PhD in political science from Keio University (Tokyo, Japan) and DEA in European studies from Sciences Po Strasbourg (France). Her recent publication is *Origins and Consequences of European Crises: Global Views on Brexit* (Birte Wassenberg and Noriko Suzuki (eds), Peter Lang, 2020). Her article on Japan under COVID-19 is included in *Et la pandémie bouleversa le monde* (Jean-Michel De Waele and Ahmet Insel (eds), Larcier, to be published in September 2022).

Madoka WATANABE is a part-time lecturer of political science at Hokkaido University of Education, Japan. Her main research theme is the comparative study of welfare states and consultative political procedures. She is on the board of directors of the Hokkaido Sweden Society. She published several treatises in Japanese including 'The Corona Measures in Sweden', which assumes people's trust asset (*Science 10*, 2020), and 'Labor Policy under COVID-19 in Sweden – Focusing on School-Related Labor Policy' [*Labor Law Bulletin 1975–76.1* (2021)].

Chino YABUNAGA is a professor of Social Policy in the Faculty of Global and Regional Studies of Toyo University. Her main research theme centres on comparative studies on welfare states and societies. She is a chair of the Japan Association for Northern European Studies and a former board member of the Japan Association of Political Sciences. She published several books in Japanese, including *Child Care Policies in the World* (2012) and *Welfare State and Tourism: A New Industrial Strategy in Nordic Countries and Japan* (2018).

Preface

The world is still suffering from a yet uncontained mutation of coronavirus disease 2019 (COVID-19) two years after the World Health Organization announced the pandemic. COVID-19 has forced the awareness of numerous phenomena on people worldwide and has exerted a profound impact on human lives. First, we now realise how globalised our lives have become. Deaths from pneumonia of unknown origin began to occur in Wuhan at the end of December 2019; soon after, a small number of people were infected in Japan, a country with robust human and economic relations with China. At the end of January 2020, the Japanese government closed its boundaries to arrivals from the infected regions of the world. In February, a mass virus outbreak occurred on a cruise ship calling at the port of Yokohama. The Japanese government did not allow the quarantined passengers to disembark for more than a fortnight. The terrified cruise passengers took to social media to ask for help, and their home countries requested the Japanese government to allow them to come ashore so they could be taken home. This situation attracted maximum worldwide attention. Western nations suspended travel to China, Japan and South Korea to prevent the spread of the disease in East Asia. Later, the United States barred travel to Europe when the COVID-19 infection spread rapidly through the continent, and European countries shut down their borders one after another in violation of the EU principle of the free movement of persons. Globalised human mobility was thus suspended.

Second, universal COVID-19 measures became noticeable. Japan closed schools, stopped the movement of people and shifted to online classes and teleworking. These measures disrupted social and economic activities. People avoided the 'Three Cs' (closed spaces with poor ventilation, crowded places with many people nearby and close-contact settings such as close-range conversations). They were recommended to disinfect their hands, wear masks and vaccinate. Similar measures were introduced across the world, and they required people to change their behaviours. Many individuals have conformed to such mandates.

Third, the public response to such universalised measures has differed from country to country, particularly with respect to wearing masks. People in Japan wore masks without a problem; surprisingly, however, many individuals in Western nations questioned the effectiveness of masks and resisted the direction to wear them. Similarly, from the Western perspective, people could question why all Japanese people wear masks.

I discussed these ideas with Jean-Michel De Waele and other participants at the POSOC19 (POwers and SOcieties facing the Covid-19 Crisis) webinar.[1] I suggested an international comparative study of mask-wearing to Jean-Michel, who subsequently organised a POSOC19 webinar titled *Le port du masque en période de COVID-19: Un regard comparatif sur les enjeux, approches, politiques, normes, pratiques et controverses à travers le monde*. I contacted my colleagues in Waseda, Masahisa Endo, Susumu Annaka and Xavier Mellet, to participate in the project and begin a comparative study of mask-wearing in pandemic circumstances in Japan and France. Ultimately, we decided to publish a book in English in addition to participating in the POSOC19 webinar and undertake an international comparative study with a wider range of Asian and European case studies.

Thus, we invited researchers with connections to Waseda University to participate in the publication project. We were successful in expanding our networks to establish an interdisciplinary team of authors of a wide variety of nationalities. It was most difficult to find Chinese authors. China was named by the world as the source of COVID-19, and the Chinese government was internationally censured for its poor initial response. The regime in China thus began to repress any criticism. For example, Fang Fang's *Wuhan Diary: Dispatches from a Quarantined City* was published in Japan and other countries but not in China, and the Chinese authorities deleted her posts on Weibo. Additionally, a person who criticised the Chinese government has disappeared.[2] Given this context, Chinese researchers refused to participate in our project. A researcher living in China informed us that writing about COVID-19 could make it impossible for him to stay in China. Therefore, we were lucky to find Liu Hongyi, a young researcher who agreed to write about the issue.

The proposed book will be published at the Waseda Institute for Advanced Study, where Annaka works as part of the Routledge-WIAS Interdisciplinary Studies book series. We are grateful for the opportunity to publish this book. The anonymous reviewers of the publication project have also advised us to include North American and minority cases along with the Asian and European investigations. In this regard, we have included the circumstances of discrimination against Asians during the COVID-19 disaster in the chapter on Canada. We could ensure that our content was more global and inclusive thanks to the advice of the reviewers. Finally, we would like to express our sincere gratitude to Waseda University for their support towards the academic publication and the release of this book.

Tokyo, March 2022, Noriko Suzuki

Notes

1 This webinar was titled *La crise et les rapports géopolitiques* and was organised by POSOC19 on 7 July 2020. POSOC19 is a network of French-speaking researchers in social and political sciences from different countries and continents. The association was created in May 2020 with the initiative of Jean-Michel De Waele

(professor of political science at Université Libre de Bruxelles) and Laurent Sermet (professor of international law at Sciences Po Aix).

2 Helen Davidson, 'Critic who called Xi a "clown" over Covid-19 crisis investigated for "serious violations"', *The Guardian*, 8 April 2020. www.theguardian.com/world/2020/apr/08/critic-xi-jinping-clown-ren-zhiqiang-covid-19-outbreak-investigated-china (Accessed 25 February 2022).

1 Introduction

Controversy in mask-wearing

Noriko Suzuki

1.1 Introduction

In January 2020, a new coronavirus (COVID-19) was discovered in China, which led to unprecedented cases of infection. Since February, this infection has spread to East Asia. In Europe and the United States (US), movements among Asians were restricted, and Asians were avoided or subjected to violence in Western countries. However, positive cases surged in northern Italy in March, and the disease spread to neighbouring countries. The World Health Organization (WHO) declared a pandemic on 11 March 2020 in response to the rapid increase in positive cases worldwide. The problem no longer originated in Asia.

Nearly two years later, and looking back at images of the world before that time, wearing face masks would have made a big difference. People in the East and West are aware that wearing face masks is critical to preventing the spread of COVID-19. Moreover, the Centers for Disease Control and Prevention (CDC) in the US recommends the universal use of face masks as one of the important public health measures for controlling the spread of COVID-19 in the community (Honein et al. 2020).

However, wearing masks during the COVID-19 pandemic has become a hot topic of debate in politics worldwide. For example, in Europe and the US, where masks were rarely used, many people resisted the obligation to wear masks. In the US, an ideological conflict divides the states between those wearing masks (mainly Democrats) and those who refuse to wear them (mainly Republicans). From the perspective of Japan, where masks were used even before COVID-19, the reactions were remarkable. In East Asia, such as Japan, South Korea and Taiwan (Chinese Taipei), wearing masks was common due to air pollution, the severe acute respiratory syndrome (SARS) outbreak, and previous experiences with infectious diseases. Thus, people's reactions to wearing masks differed in Europe, the US and Asia. Government measures against COVID-19 varied across countries, whereas people's behavioural responses to this measure also differed.

China and Taiwan deployed 'mask diplomacy' in the international scene by supplying face masks to other countries in Asia and Europe, where the number of

DOI: 10.4324/9781003244127-1

masks available was unable to meet the demand due to the widespread infection. In this manner, adaptation to face masks differed across countries and regions.

1.2 Historical and cultural background of mask-wearing in Japan

A well-known fact is that the Japanese people have been wearing surgical masks to prevent the spread of COVID-19. Historically, face masks in Japan became prevalent with the breakout of the Spanish flu one century ago. Since 1921, nearly half of Japan's population (approximately 23.89 million) have been infected with the Spanish flu, and approximately 388,000 have died. Therefore, the national and prefectural governments urged the people to wear masks in gatherings and used posters to encourage people to wear them to prevent infection (*Kochi News* 2020). As such, mask-wearing has become deeply ingrained in the lives of the Japanese concerning certain health risks.

According to Horii (2014), two turning points characterised the wearing of masks in Japan. The first is the SARS outbreak in 2003, whereas the second is the outbreak of bird flu in 2004, which greatly increased the awareness of mask-wearing within Japanese society. Furthermore, in the 2000s, as the neoliberal ideology gained strength and people began to call for *self-care* in terms of health and *self-responsibility* to draw attention to the risk of infectious diseases, *cough etiquette* became nearly equivalent to wearing masks for those who cough or sneeze. Eventually, mask-wearing became common practice to prevent hay fever and air pollution due to fine particulate matter (PM2.5). After the accident at the Fukushima Daiichi Nuclear Power Plant in 2011, masks were also worn as a measure against radiation. Thus, wearing masks has become part of daily life in Japan to protect people from health risks and for 'beauty and comfort' through 'cough etiquette' (Horii 2014).

Due to these historical and social backgrounds, many Japanese people wear masks to prevent infection during the COVID-19 pandemic even without government intervention. The percentage of people wearing face masks increased after the spread of COVID-19. According to a survey conducted in a town 100 km away from Tokyo in June-July 2020, 98% of the respondents wore masks, including 26.7% who continually used masks before COVID-19 and 71.3% who had newly started using masks.[1] Thus, many Japanese wear masks in public places, public transport, shops, schools and workplaces.

However, the sight of numerous people wearing masks in Japan was seemingly unique to people in the West, because their interpretation of mask-wearing differed. A medical professional in the United Kingdom (UK) called mask-wearing among Asians 'a false reassurance' (*Japan Times* 2009). How can we explain why mask-wearing, which the Japanese accept, is controversial in many European countries? Do these differences stem from the distinction between the East and West? Is it due to the political culture that respects the freedom to wear masks instead of being forced to wear them? Is it the difference between a liberal political system and an authoritarian one?

1.3 Resistance to mask-wearing in the West

1.3.1 Mask-wearing as a COVID-19 measure is not common in the West

According to a survey by the Max Planck Institute for Demographic Research in Germany, mask-wearing as a COVID-19 measure in the Western countries is less common compared with social distancing, regular hand-washing, avoidance of public transport and regular use of hand sanitisers. Among eight Western countries (i.e. Belgium, France, Germany, Italy, the Netherlands, Spain, the UK and the US), the prevalence of mask-wearing varies widely, which ranges from approximately 7% in the Netherlands to approximately 60% in Italy (Perotta et al. 2020).[2]

In Italy, where only 26% of people wore masks in public, the epidemic spread faster than in any other country in Europe on 10 March 2020. One week later, the rate of mask-wearing increased to 59%. By 8 April, the mask-wearing rate had reached 82% as an increasing number of people died from the infection. This rate remained within the range of 80% until the end of February 2021, which indicated a change in people's attitudes towards wearing masks. In Spain, where only 5% of people wore masks in public places, the mask-wearing rate increased to 42% at the end of March then reached 84% on 19 May. In contrast, in Asian countries, except for Singapore and Australia, the percentage of people wearing masks in public places was within the range of 50% in March and 70% in April. It remained at 80% on average until the end of February 2021 (YouGov 2020a).

Thus, the rates of mask-wearing in Italy and Spain dramatically increased from March to May 2020, when the number of positive cases rapidly increased. However, the increased proportion of people wearing masks was later and slower than in many Asian countries. In other European countries, people wore masks later and less frequently than they did in Asian countries.

1.3.2 Three types of countries regarding mask-wearing

According to the findings, a survey conducted by Pollster YouGov (2020a) demonstrated self-reported mask-wearing habits globally and the emergence of three groups. The first group comprises Asian countries with high rates of mask-wearing and increased mask-wearing habits in response to the 2003 SARS outbreak, where certain countries have mandated the wearing of masks. The second group includes Spain, France and Germany, which initially exhibited low rates of mask-wearing, which significantly increased after mandating mask-wearing. The third group consists of Scandinavian countries and the UK, where the rate of mask-wearing remains low. In Denmark, medical institutions recommend that healthy people should not wear masks if they live a normal life.

Based on this explanation, we selected the countries in our study from this survey and showed their percentage of people wearing masks in the period from 23 February when it started this survey of YouGov to 31 December 2020 and found that they fit into the three groups mentioned (see Figure 1.1).

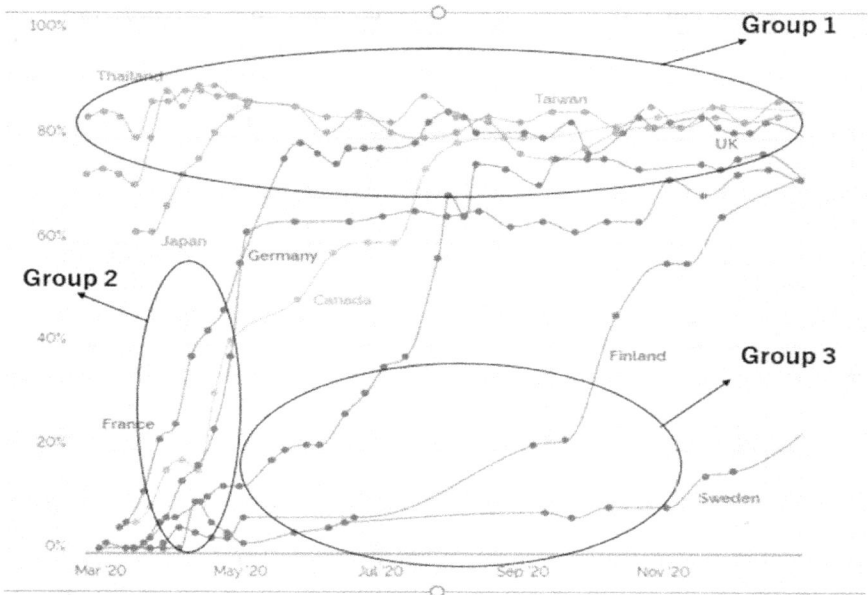

Figure 1.1 Three groups of countries that promote mask-wearing in public places

Note: YouGov (2020a) data span 23 February to 31 December 2020. % of countries promoting mask-wearing in public places, choosing Japan, China, Taiwan, Thailand, the UK, France, Germany, Sweden, Finland and Canada.

Source: Author, based on YouGov (2020a).

Many medical organisations, including the WHO, initially questioned the effectiveness of mask-wearing in preventing diseases. However, it recommended mask-wearing as a precautionary measure because covering the mouth limits the transmission of the virus and reduces the risk of infection by 85% (*Bloomberg* 2020). Thus, there was a significant increase in the number of governments that recommended and even mandated mask-wearing by the summer of 2020. In Western countries, the situation dramatically changed with clear rules that encouraged healthy people to wear masks in public places. Former British Prime Minister Boris Johnson and former US President Donald Trump, who disliked wearing masks, wore them in public, which may have positively impacted people in terms of mask-wearing (*BBC News* 2020).

1.3.3 *Why is mask-wearing compulsory in the West?*

In the UK, which has the highest number of deaths in Europe as of July 2020, 37% of the British have not worn face masks outside their homes in the past seven days. Nevertheless, most (51%) of those who never wear masks believe that masks have health benefits, and 83% would like to see their use made mandatory on public transport (YouGov 2020b). If the British government were to recommend mask-wearing in public places to prevent the spread of COVID-19, 74% of British said they would follow this advice (Ipsos MORI 2020). Therefore, England has followed Scotland in mandating masks in stores since 24 July.

The British example demonstrates that people are inclined to follow the government's requirement in terms of mask-wearing. This perspective is unique from the point of view of Japan, where the Japanese people wear masks as a preventive measure even though doing so is not obligatory due to the enhanced generalisation and diversification of mask-wearing.

1.4 The difference is not based on the distinction between the East and West

1.4.1 High rates of mask-wearing and penalties

In countries where this manner of thinking prevails, the governments introduced mandatory mask-wearing when the number of infections and deaths increased. By August 2020, more than 100 countries announced nationwide mandatory mask-wearing. In addition, even when the federal government decided to lift the mandate, certain states and cities required employees to wear masks (e.g. the US and Brazil). Therefore, many countries have made mask-wearing compulsory in the entire country or in limited areas.

In several countries, mandatory mask-wearing resulted in 90% compliance, such as Singapore (93%), the Philippines (92%) and Brazil (90%) (Council on Foreign Relations [CFR] 2020). Why are masks worn at higher rates in these countries? This notion is because these countries impose penalties on those who do not follow the rules, which greatly vary.

In Singapore, this rate reached approximately 23% in early March. However, it increased to 90% after the government distributed free masks and imposed fines. For example, monitors called Safe Distance Ambassadors in public places fined people without masks approximately 228 USD (*Asahi* 2021).[3] According to the Immigration and Checkpoints Authority (2021), the court will prosecute a Singaporean woman for putting others at risk of COVID-19 infection under the Infectious Diseases Act and for failing to wear a mask outside her place (Temporary Measures; Control Order; Regulations 2020). This woman entered the country from Cambodia and received a Notice of Stay (Stay-Home Notice [SHN]); thus, strict compliance with SHN requirements will apply. Non-compliance could lead to a fine of up to S$10,000 (7,449.76 USD) or imprisonment for up to six months.

If penalties are imposed for not wearing masks, people will naturally wear them. Following the directive of former President Duterte to arrest and detain people not wearing masks in public places, the Philippine National Police has elevated its operations against people who deviate from health and safety protocols in public places during the pandemic. As such, armed police officers have been patrolling public places and punishing and beating people without masks (*One News* 2020; Roble 2021).

In Brazil, one of the countries with the highest number of confirmed cases and deaths, the state of Sao Paulo introduced mask-wearing in public places in May 2020 and fined violators nearly 120 USD. One month later, the expansion of the policy to the entire country was considered, but President Bolsonaro opposed it. Therefore, the policy was in effect in only a few areas (Japan External Trade Organization 2020). However, the rate of mask-wearing was high (90%) due to numerous deaths.

The three cases demonstrate that the obvious burden of not wearing masks – fines, severe penalties and, in worst cases, death – is a significant factor in the high rates of mask-wearing. Other countries in Europe have also introduced fines for refusal to wear masks.

1.4.2 Countries where mask-wearing is recommended or not required

In contrast to the global trends of mandating mask-wearing and imposing penalties, a few countries neither recommended nor mandated mask-wearing. As of August 2020, 24 countries around the world (Asia: Japan, China and Cambodia; Oceania: New Zealand; Europe: Iceland, Ireland, Norway, Sweden, Finland, Lithuania, Estonia, Belarus and Slovakia; Africa: Livia, Eretria, Somalia, Tanzania, Malawi, Eswatini and Togo; the Middle East: Yemen, Syria and Afghanistan; Latin America: Nicaragua) (CFR 2020).

A common feature of these countries is that mask-wearing is not mandatory. However, certain nuances are observed. We point out three points of difference among them. Firstly, a division is noted between countries where most people wear and do not wear masks. The second is economic differences, and the last one pertains to differences in political systems.

As the first point, the percentage of people wearing masks differs across countries. In Japan, nearly 90% of the population wears them, as previously mentioned, even though the government does not mandate mask-wearing. In China, 67% of the people use masks despite the lack of mandate (CFR 2020). Alternatively, in Sweden and Finland, the infection rate was low as of the summer of 2020 (Chapter 6 of this book). Thus, mask-wearing was only recommended, whereas citizens were expected to take responsible and voluntary action to prevent infection. However, would people voluntarily wear masks in countries where this habit is not customary?

For the second point, a difference exists between economically prosperous, peaceful and politically stable countries and poor, conflict-ridden and politically unstable countries. In the first group, COVID-19 spread rapidly due to the frequent movement of people associated with active economic activities. As a result, governments established lockdowns to restrict movement. For the second group, economic activity was relatively limited to the domestic market. Movement across borders was restricted between countries in war or political unrest. These social and economic backgrounds limited the risk of infection; thus, the number of positive cases remained low as of the summer of 2020. Furthermore, the poor could not afford the high cost of medical care upon infection. Thus, they intended to protect themselves and their families even without a government mandate.

Lastly, differences were noted between regimes, such as democratic and non-democratic, in addition to political stability. Democracy is characterised by a minimum definition of elections and limited power, whereas non-democracy includes constitutionalist regimes with limited voting rights, tyranny, fascist or communist regimes, and military dictatorships (Huntington 1995, pp. 9–12). In countries such as Afghanistan, Eritrea, Syria and Yemen, where civil wars and political turmoil persist, or in failed states, issuing mandates for mask-wearing or providing free masks may be difficult.

The reasons for the lack of mandates for mask-wearing in these countries may be due to preventive habits or, conversely, the lack of habit of wearing them; small numbers of positive cases; lack of public health mandates in non-democratic countries due to political turmoil; or lack of access to masks due to poverty or turmoil.

We compared the political and social backgrounds of countries that mandated mask-wearing and those that did not. The results indicated three types of behaviour towards mask-wearing: mandatory, habit and resistance. We point out three reasons behind these types of behaviour. First, for political reasons, we assume that coercion by different regimes to wear masks elicits various reactions. That political culture may influence the attitude of people when the government mandates mask-wearing. The second reason is the habit of using masks. In several Asian countries, people began wearing masks as a preventive measure during the SARS outbreak (Fukuoka 2020). Since then, many people have worn them daily as a measure against air pollution and hay fever. In contrast, the dominant perception in Western countries is that masks are worn only by sick people. Thirdly, people may wear masks for economic reasons. In countries that mandate mask-wearing, people wear masks to protect themselves from expensive fines. In economically poorer countries, people wear masks to protect themselves and their families from medical expenses. In these countries, people typically cover their mouth and nose with cloth or masks. This chapter will further discuss political reasons.

1.5 Relationship between mask-wearing and political reasons

1.5.1 *The validity of arguments on political regime regarding mask-wearing*

The rights and freedom of people are guaranteed in a liberal democracy, such that they can resist restrictions by the government. Alternatively, in a non-democracy regime, where the government restricts rights and freedom, people follow the government's coercive policies. Therefore, authoritarian states may find it more effective to enforce mask-wearing during a pandemic than democratic states.

However, Huntington (1995) notes that whether a country is democratically governed or not is of little importance to people's lives. This is because most public policies are shaped not by the nature of the regime but by the level of economic development of the country. The difference between order and disorder is more fundamental for people than democracy and autocracy. Indeed, democracy can and has abused individual rights and freedom because political democracy is closely related to individual freedom. In contrast, a well-regulated authoritarian state can provide high degrees of stability and order for its citizens (Huntington 1995, pp. 26–27). It seems as if the arguments of Huntington also apply to the current pandemic: it has been noted that many democratic governments restrict freedom by imposing penalties on people who refuse to follow orders, while a few authoritarian countries maintain order without making masks mandatory.

How can political systems, such as democracy and authoritarianism, be beneficial to analysing whether or not people follow public policies? Considering the relevance of these political systems in this analysis seems difficult for the following reasons. Firstly, the distinction between democratic and authoritarian countries is ambiguous. Second, political systems fluctuate, such that even democracies can revert to undemocratic rule (Huntington 1995, pp. 14–15). In this regard, defining authoritarian regimes is difficult. According to Frantz (2021), a democratic regime is one in which the ruler is selected through competitive elections; however, even elected democracies can transform into authoritarianism. The recent research on democracy points to the behaviour of governments in new democracies, which endeavour to change the distribution of power and policies decided by democratic institutions using means that do not conform to democracy. This notion has been an international trend since the 2000s. Four patterns in the regression of democracy can be observed today: collapse (Thailand); erosion (Hungary and Poland); temporarily weakened but re-enforced authoritarianism (Russia); and co-existence of democracy and authoritarianism (Mexico) (Kawanaka 2018, pp. 1–13).

This regression of democracy continues. Of the countries addressed in this book, China, Cambodia and Thailand have considered *closed autocracies*, while the regression of democracy in Hungary and Poland, classified as *electoral autocracy* and *electoral democracy*, respectively, can be observed in 2020 compared to 2010 (V-Dem 2021). This tendency has been noted, especially in Eastern and Central European countries. Even Hungary and Poland, whose democracies have been considered stable since they joined the European Union (EU), have raised concerns that they may be going against the basic values of the EU. The problem is that although these countries maintained electoral democracy, freedom and constitutionalism have been eroded (Nakada 2020, p. 115).

Kawanaka (2018) pointed out this regression in democracy for three causal mechanisms. Firstly, people have come to demand a political system that allows quick decision-making by increasing the executive power of the government. Secondly, politicians and political groups have selected and emphasised the social cleavages that emerged from political and economic crises in their favour. This tendency has destabilised democracy. Third, authoritarian rule has been effective in enhancing the ability of the state to govern (Kawanaka 2018, pp. 251–257). Thus, people want strong leaders who can quickly decide and implement policies. In a crisis such as a pandemic, this case will become increasingly common. As a result, out of the countries discussed in this book, China, Greece, Cambodia and Poland were classified as *major violators* of democracy during the pandemic (V-Dem 2021) (see Table 1.1).

Table 1.1 Classification of countries with regard to democratic violations under pandemic conditions

Rank	Country	Status	PanDem Score
1	Canada	Non violation	0
2	Germany	Non violation	0
3	Finland	Non violation	0
4	Taiwan	Non violation	0
5	Japan	Minor Violation	0.1
6	France	Minor Violation	0.1
7	Sweden	Minor Violation	0.15
8	Hungary	Moderate Violation	0.3
9	Thailand	Moderate Violation	0.3
10	Poland	Major Violation	0.35
11	Cambodia	Major Violation	0.4
12	Greece	Major Violation	0.45
13	China	Major Violation	0.74

Note: The countries featured in this publication were selected from the V-Dem Institute's Pandemic Backsliding Project (V-Dem 2021, p. 10) and are listed by the author in descending order of the Pandemic Violation Index (PanDem Score) by democracy criteria.

However, the degree of authoritarianism in the discussions on Poland today does not remain consistent among researchers because the retreat of democracy indicates a deterioration in the quality of democracy, and the degree of authoritarianism is dependent on the severity of deterioration (Frantz 2021, pp. 116–117). Moreover, the interpretation of political regimes may differ between researchers of a country and those from abroad. Western researchers have classified China as an authoritarian regime with a communist dictatorship (Frantz 2021). However, Kawashima (2020) argues that Chinese-speaking scholars who imported the debate on the resilience of authoritarian regimes have developed this theme differently from Western scholars (Kawashima 2020, pp. 133–142).

As defining whether a country is democratic or authoritarian is extremely difficult, this book avoids classifying countries through political regimes, given that discussions about political regimes concerning mask-wearing may be invalid. Thus, we focus on people's attitudes towards public policies and political culture.

1.5.2 *Political culture and attitudes towards public policies*

Political culture may influence the attitudes of people when the government mandates mask-wearing. A comparative study on attitudes in Western Europe and East and Southeast Asia among 18 countries (Inoguchi and Blondel 2010), which surveyed identity, confidence in public institutions and satisfaction with daily life, assumes that people's perception of the state influences their attitude towards political institutions and policies. The result of the survey identifies six typologies, which the present study will refer to concerning the eight countries and regions discussed in this book. (1) In *happy non-citizen* countries, such as

France, Germany and Sweden, people are satisfied with their lives and confident in state authorities. (2) People from *mildly pessimistic* countries, such as Taiwan, have low levels of trust in state authorities. (3) The Japanese, classified as *hesitant citizens*, are less satisfied with their lives. (4) The Greeks are *dissatisfied patriots* and exhibit low trust in state authorities. (5) The Thai are considered *citizens satisfied with development* and display high trust in state authorities. (6) Lastly, the Chinese are *optimistic* and give high levels of trust in state authorities and exhibit satisfaction with their lives. The results demonstrate that citizens in France, Germany, Sweden, China and Thailand are highly satisfied with their lives, whereas Japanese citizens are less satisfied. In addition, citizens in France, Germany, Sweden, China and Thailand exhibit high levels of trust in state authorities, whereas those in Greece and Taiwan report low levels of trust.[4] According to Inoguchi and Blondel (2010), life satisfaction strongly influences the relationship between citizens and the state regardless of their level of trust in state authorities or how strongly they identify with the state.

Therefore, citizens' response to public policies, such as mask-wearing, which many countries implement to combat the spread of COVID-19, is important for examining the relationship between the state and its citizens. If public policies can mitigate infectious diseases, then citizens will become more satisfied with their lives, which, in turn, will increase their support for the state. Conversely, if the people are dissatisfied with their daily lives due to public policies, then the state will lose the support of the people. Certain states effectively implement their policies and endeavour to manage citizens even with penalties to avoid this scenario. The study infers that this tendency remains regardless of the political system.

How does the public react to the measures implemented by governments against infectious diseases across political systems? This book compares citizens' reactions to government policies in countries in Asia, Europe and Canada, focusing on mask-wearing as an example of public policies.

1.6 The objective of this book

This book intends to present a comparative study of people's behaviour towards the state's policymaking through mask-wearing patterns between Europe, Canada and Asia in terms of national, historical, political, economic and social characteristics. People began wearing masks more smoothly in several countries, especially in Asia. In contrast, in other regions, such as Europe, mask-wearing became common after high mortality rates due to COVID-19. Political decisions on mask-wearing differ by country, whether compulsory measures or voluntary requests. This book intends to answer one of the main questions: To what extent do people accept the encouragement to wear masks in countries where governments have mandated their use? What factors define mask-wearing in countries where it is voluntary?

For these reasons, this book considers two points. Firstly, we analyse why mask-wearing is defined differently in Europe, Canada and Asia at the individual and political levels. We examine the historical origins of mask-wearing in countries and recent reactions through public opinions on the measures taken by governments to combat the pandemic. We intend to compare Asian experiences and perceptions regarding mask-wearing with those of European countries and Canada after COVID-19. Such a comparison focuses on political meanings and roles attributed to mask-wearing in terms of cultural characteristics and recent changes at the national level. Secondly, we determine the association between patterns of mask-wearing and citizens' reactions towards the measures taken by governments. For example, the Japanese scenario demonstrates that the public was inclined to follow the government's recommendation. However, in many European countries, governments mandate mask-wearing and introduce lockdown periods. The current controversies in European countries regarding mask-wearing illustrate the tension between obedience to authority and freedom. Furthermore, we explore the extent to which political division may have existed in public opinion concerning measures taken against COVID-19.

1.7 The structure of this book

This book examines public policies, including mandatory mask-wearing, implemented in response to COVID-19, and citizens' responses to and attitudes towards these policies in more than ten countries from the West to the East via Canada during COVID-19. Firstly, this book is characterised by empirical evidence presented by researchers from the perspectives of history, politics, economics, law, sociology and linguistics. Secondly, the book is interdisciplinary in its authors and the variety of nationalities represented (i.e. Japan, France, Germany, Greece, Poland, Belarus, Canada, China, Thailand and Taiwan). This diversity contributes to the originality of insights per chapter.

This chapter presents the theoretical framework, objective and structure of this book. In Chapter 2, Susumu Annaka statistically analyses the determinants of mask-wearing in 29 countries in 2020 using more than 400,000 survey responses. The results reveal that a considerable variance exists in the awareness of mask-wearing across countries. Afterward, we present case studies conducted in different regions worldwide, from Europe to Asia, along with the historical background of COVID-19 concerning the Spanish flu, which spread from Europe to the world.

Chapter 3 focuses on Europe, where Osamu Ieda highlights the social dimension of public health policies based on epidemiology and historically analyses the case of Hungary, which introduced preventive measures against the Spanish flu to the public 100 years ago.

Although the worldwide spread of COVID-19 has changed behaviours in Europe, where mask-wearing was uncommon, the French and German cases present an analysis of media discourse. In Chapter 4, Xavier Mellet illustrates how a face mask as a countermeasure of COVID-19 was perceived as a new phenomenon in the French political context in 2020. The author employs an inductive approach that follows the concept of mask-wearing in a national newspaper, *Le Figaro*.

In Chapter 5, Joachim Scharloth reconstructs the debate on mask-wearing in Germany during COVID-19 using a linguistic approach and explains the politicisation of masks. He views the mainstream social acceptance of masks and criticisms about mask-wearing in a right-wing online discourse.

In Chapter 6, Chino Yabunaga and Madoka Watanabe focus on the choice of moderate governmental restrictions on the behaviour and compliance of citizens towards infectious disease mitigation in Sweden and Finland, where mask-wearing is uncommon. They discuss the relationship between citizens and the state in crises, such as a pandemic, by arguing whether welfare states limit the movement and freedom of citizens through power.

In contrast to these relatively democratic states, we present the cases of two countries classified as violators of democracy in Europe. In Chapter 7, Łukasz Czarnecki and Monika Skowrońska show how mask-wearing policies reproduce the mechanisms of power and inequality in Polish society by analysing the new legal framework on mask-wearing during the COVID-19 epidemic. The legal analysis reveals the restriction of human rights through government power. In Chapter 8, Athanasia Chalari sociologically explores the background of negative attitudes towards mask-wearing in Greek society by analysing the literature on mask-wearing attitudes, official government data and digital media.

Across the Atlantic, Tatsiana Shaban and Emmanuel Brunet-Jailly examine the action and policy taken by governments in response to the COVID-19 outbreak in British Columbia (BC), Canada and examine the public response to recommendations for mask-wearing in Chapter 9. They also investigate the issues of discrimination and xenophobia against Asian people that emerged in BC and across Canada to an unparalleled degree.

Although anti-mask protests in Western countries were prominently featured in international news coverage of the pandemic, the public in many Asian countries overwhelmingly supported policies that mandated mask-wearing. Moreover, we examine why governments in Asia succeeded in implementing mask-wearing policies to mitigate COVID-19 with a discussion of social contexts.

In Chapter 10, Chen Lihang demonstrates the historical reasons why people wear masks in Taiwan, where anti-COVID-19 measures have been successful. A direct reason for the positive public response in Taiwan was the SARS outbreak in 2003. In contrast, an indirect reason is that face masks have been heavily promoted alongside other projects to improve public hygiene since the Japanese colonial era. He examines the history of mask-wearing in Taiwan from the 1890s to the 1980s, focusing on the relationship between public hygiene and policies promoting mask-wearing. He reviews diaries, newspapers and magazines from the colonial and post-war eras to illustrate the public response to government policies that promoted mask-wearing.

In Japan, which forwarded the habit of mask-wearing to Taiwan in the early 20th century, most people wore masks during the COVID-19 pandemic even without government coercion. Masahisa Endo and Gento Kato analysed a web survey on COVID-19-related behaviours in Chapter 11 and identified socio-demographic groups that wore masks. Moreover, they examine the influence of social values on mask-wearing behaviours.

China reported relatively low numbers of infections and deaths compared with other countries. In Chapter 12, Liu Hongyi depicts that mask-wearing was uncommon among the Chinese in contrast to Japan and Taiwan. He analyses the mechanisms of the crisis management system of the Chinese government to understand why its countermeasures against novel coronavirus infections have been effective. He also explores the reasons underlying the success of the Chinese government in mandating mask-wearing with Shanghai City as a case study.

Alongside China, Thailand and Cambodia have been categorised as violators of democracy by V-Dem (2021). However, how did these governments address the spread of COVID-19 and the public's reaction? In Chapter 13, Upalat Korwatanasakul and Sivarin Lertpusit examine the relationship between public behaviour in response to the COVID-19 pandemic, particularly mask-wearing behaviour, and public perception of government measures against COVID-19 in Thailand. They identify factors that shape mask-waring behaviours through quantitative and quantitative analyses, including the degree of health impact; public awareness and concern; social trustworthiness; age; and activities in specific public places. The analysis demonstrates that the fundamental motivations behind mask-wearing behaviours are self-protection, social pressure and social norms reflected by different age groups.

In Chapter 14, Yuko Shimazaki explores the response of the Cambodian government, one of the most economically challenged countries in Southeast Asia, to COVID-19, the public's reaction to these measures and the extent to which these measures were effective. The author interviews to examine the interpretation of the Cambodians of the new threat posed by the disease and the extent to which they followed government measures.

Finally, we summarise the findings of the case studies in this book on the following bases: How did governments instruct citizens to wear masks as a measure for controlling the spread of COVID-19? Who wore masks in response to this policy, and who did not? What was the basis of the people's judgement regarding mask-wearing? What were the social effects of mask-wearing? In summarising these points, we endeavour to draw certain conclusions (albeit limited) for this book in Chapter 15.

Notes

1 Nawa et al. (2021). According to this survey of 645 adults in a random sample household in Utsunomiya City, Japan, from 14 June 2020 to 5 July 2020, 172 (26.7%) were consistent mask users and 460 (71.3%) were new users, while 13 (2.0%) were current non-users.
2 This survey is based on a total of 71,612 completed questionnaires, collected between 13 March and 19 April 2020.
3 According to Singapore Legal Advice (2021), Safe distancing ambassadors (SDA) do not have the same powers to enforce COVID-19 regulations, that is, compel the public to follow them, as they are not Safe distancing enforcement officers (EO) who are appointed by the Minister of Health under section 35(1) of the COVID-19 (Temporary Measures) Act 2020. SDAs instead advise the public to comply with safe distancing measures. According to the National Environment Agency, which is the leading public organisation responsible for ensuring a clean

and sustainable environment for Singapore, SDAs will be paired with EOs during their patrols.
4 Inoguchi and Blondel (2010) point out that the proportion of citizens who consider the relationship between state and nation as important is low in the first three categories, while it is high in the latter three categories. However, in this chapter, we have not given much consideration to this and have focused on the level of satisfaction with life and trust in the state for citizens. This survey was conducted in 2000, so the patterns today may be different from that time.

References

Asahi (2021, 30 January) 'Covid-19 punishments abroad', p. 2.

BBC News (2020, 14 July) 'Coronavirus: Why attitudes to masks have changed around the world'. Available at www.bbc.com/news/world-53394525 (Accessed 10 April 2022).

Bloomberg (2020, 17 July) 'The world is masking up, some are opting out'. Available at www.bloomberg.com/graphics/2020-opinion-coronavirus-global-face-mask-adoption/ (Accessed 1 March 2021).

Council on Foreign Relations [CFR] (2020, 4 August) 'Which countries are requiring face masks?'. Available at www.cfr.org/in-brief/which-countries-are-requiring-face-masks (Accessed 2 March 2021).

Frantz, E. (2021) *Authoritarianism: What Everyone Needs to Know*, trans. Uetani, N. et al. Tokyo: Hakusuisha.

Fukuoka, S. (2020) 'Taiwan's growing presence in the containment of new coronaviruses', in Contemporary China Research Base at Institute of Social Science, University of Tokyo (ed.) *East Asian Regional Dynamics after COVID-19*. Tokyo: University of Tokyo Press, pp. 141–154.

Honein, M. A., Christie, A., Rose, D. A., Brooks, J. T., Meaney-Delman, D., Cohn, A., Sauber-Schatz, E. K., Walker, A., Clifford McDonald, L., Liburd, L. C., Hall, J. E., Fry, A. M., Hall, A. J., Gupta, N., Kuhnert, W. L., Yoon, P. W., Gundlapalli, A. V., Beach, M. J., Walke, H. T. and CDC COVID-19 Response Team. (2020, 11 December) 'Summary of guidance for public health strategies to address high levels of community transmission of SARS-CoV-2 and related deaths', *MMWR (Morbidity and Mortality Weekly Report)*, Vol. 69, No. 49, pp. 1860–1867.

Horii, M. (2014) 'Why do the Japanese wear masks? A short historical review', *ejcjs*, Vol. 14, No. 2. Available at www.japanesestudies.org.uk/ejcjs/vol14/iss2/horii.html (Accessed 1 March 2021).

Huntington, S. P. (1995) *The Third Wave: Democratization in the Late Twentieth Century*, trans. Tsubogo, M., Nakamichi, H. and Yabuno, Y. Tokyo: Sanrei Shobo.

Immigration and Checkpoints Authority (2021, 30 July) 'Singaporean woman to be charged for exposing others to the risk of COVID-19 Infection and failing to wear a mask'. Available at www.ica.gov.sg/news-and-publications/newsroom/media-release/singaporean-woman-to-be-charged-for-exposing-others-to-the-risk-of-covid-19-infection-and-failing-to-wear-mask#:~:text=Individuals%20who%20are%20found%20not,of%20up%20to%20six%20months (Accessed 10 February 2022).

Inoguchi, T. and Blondel, J. (2010) *Citizens and the State: Attitudes in Western Europe and East and Southeast Asia*, trans. Inoguchi, T. Tokyo: University of Tokyo Press.

Ipsos MORI (2020, 24 April) 'Government advice could change Britons' attitudes to wearing facemasks'. Available at www.ipsos.com/ipsos-mori/en-uk/government-advice-could-change-britons-attitudes-wearing-facemasks (Accessed 2 March 2021).

Japan External Trade Organization (2020, 16 July) 'Obligation to wear masks at the national level, where to wear is at issue'. Available at www.jetro.go.jp/biznews/2020/07/7ec7e8650fbd376e.html (Accessed 8 March 2021).

Japan Times (2009, 30 April) 'Britain, Japan at odds on face mask merit'. Available at www.japantimes.co.jp/news/2009/04/30/national/britain-japan-at-odds-on-face-mask-merit/ (Accessed 10 April 2022).

Kawanaka, T. (ed.) (2018) *Democracy in Retreat, Democracy in Strength*. Kyoto: Minerva Shobo.

Kawashima, S. (2020) 'Resilience in contemporary Chinese politics: Perspectives on the Hu Jintao and Xi Jinping regimes', in Japan Association for Comparative Politics (ed.), *The Fragility of Democracy and the Resilience of Authoritarianism, Journal of Japan Association for Comparative Politics*. Kyoto: Minerva Shobo, pp. 123–142.

Kochi News (2020, 17 May) ' "Wear a mask" 100 years ago. Three outbreaks of Spanish flu in three years'. Available at www.kochinews.co.jp/article/367925 (Accessed 8 March 2021).

Nakada, M. (2020) 'The 'democratic retreat' in East Central Europe: Fragmentation and conjunction of "democracy" and constitutionalism', in Japan Association for Comparative Politics (ed.), *The Fragility of Democracy and the Resilience of Authoritarianism, Journal of Japan Association for Comparative Politics*. Kyoto: Minerva Shobo, pp. 89–120.

Nawa, N., Yamaoka, Y., Koyama, Y., Nishimura, H., Sonoda, S., Kuramochi, J., Miyazaki, Y. and Fujiwara, T. (2021) 'Association between social integration and face mask use behavior during the SARS-CoV-2 pandemic in Japan: Results from U-CORONA study', *International Journal of Environmental Research and Public Health*, Vol. 18, No. 9, 4717. Available at https://doi.org/10.3390/ijerph18094717

One News (2020, 22 July) 'Duterte: Wear face mask or face arrest; PNP to intensify operations against violators of COVID-19 protocols'. Available at www.onenews.ph/ (Accessed 4 March 2021).

Perotta, D., Grow, A., Rampazzo, F., Cimentada, J., Del Fava, E., Gil-Clavel, S. and Zagheni, E. (2020, 15 July) 'Behaviours and attitudes in response to the COVID-19 pandemic: Insights from a cross-national Facebook survey', *Max Planck Institute for Demographic Research*. Available at https://doi.org/10.1101/2020.05.09.20096388 (Accessed 1 March 2021).

Roble, A. (2021, 12 February) 'Filipinos breaking Covid-19 rules risk beatings, humiliation – unless they're rich or well-connected'. Available at www.scmp.com/week-asia/health-environment/article/3121587/filipinos-breaking-covid-19-rules-risk-beatings (Accessed 4 March 2021).

Singapore Legal Advice (2021, 1 September) 'COVID-19: Can safe distancing enforcement officers do this?' Available at https://singaporelegaladvice.com/covid-19-safe-distancing-enforcement-officers/ (Accessed 10 February 2022).

V-Dem (Varieties of Democracy) (2021) 'Autocratization Turns Viral', Democracy Report 2021. V-Dem Institutes. Available at www.v-dem.net/static/website/files/dr/dr_2021.pdf (Accessed 10 April 2022).

YouGov (2020a, 17 March) 'Personal measures taken to avoid COVID-19. COVID-19 behaviour changes tracker: Wearing a face mask when in public places'. Available at https://yougov.co.uk/topics/international/articles-reports/2020/03/17/personal-measures-taken-avoid-covid-19 (Accessed 2 March 2021).

YouGov (2020b, 15 July) 'Why won't Britons wear face masks?' Available at https://yougov.co.uk/topics/health/articles-reports/2020/07/15/why-wont-britons-wear-face-masks (Accessed 2 March 2021).

2 Public awareness of mask usage in 29 countries in 2020[1]

Susumu Annaka

2.1 Introduction

The COVID-19 pandemic – the worst pandemic since the Spanish flu – has dramatically changed the world, with a significant number of people still suffering and dying from the disease. Without vaccination and booster shots, one of the essential items to protect people from the disease is the face mask (Chu et al. 2020; Wei et al. 2021). Studies in the United States (Chernozhukov et al. 2021), Germany (Mitze et al. 2020), Hong Kong (Cheng et al. 2020) and other regions (Aravindakshan et al. 2020) have reported on the effectiveness of wearing masks. Some studies have also analysed what characteristics affect mask-wearing behaviour – for example, gender (Howard 2021), age, place of residence (Haischer et al. 2020) and social norms (Barceló and Sheen 2020). However, only one study (Badillo-Goicoechea et al. 2021) appears to have thoroughly analysed the effectiveness and determinants of mask-wearing based on cross-national data. Even Badillo-Goicoechea et al. (2021) do not consider country-level factors. This is why this chapter will analyse which populations in which countries have a higher awareness of wearing masks by using cross-national and multilevel data for more than 400,000 persons.

The main finding of this chapter is that considerable cross-country variance exists in the awareness of mask usage. Citizens of more democratic and prosperous countries are less likely to wear masks even after controlling for positive cases and other factors. The analysis also reveals that women are more likely to wear masks than men at the individual level.

2.2 Data

Figure 2.1 shows the trends in awareness of mask-wearing among more than 400,000 people in 29 countries in 2020, based on the Imperial College London YouGov COVID-19 Behaviour Tracker Data Hub (2020). The graphs measure the country-month average of the responses to the question 'Worn a face mask outside your home (e.g. when on public transport, going to a supermarket, going to a main road)' with numbers ranging from 1 (Not at all) to 5 (Always). The original order (from 1 (Always) to 5 (Not at all)) is reversed for understandability. The graphs in the figure reveal a consistently high level of awareness of wearing

DOI: 10.4324/9781003244127-2

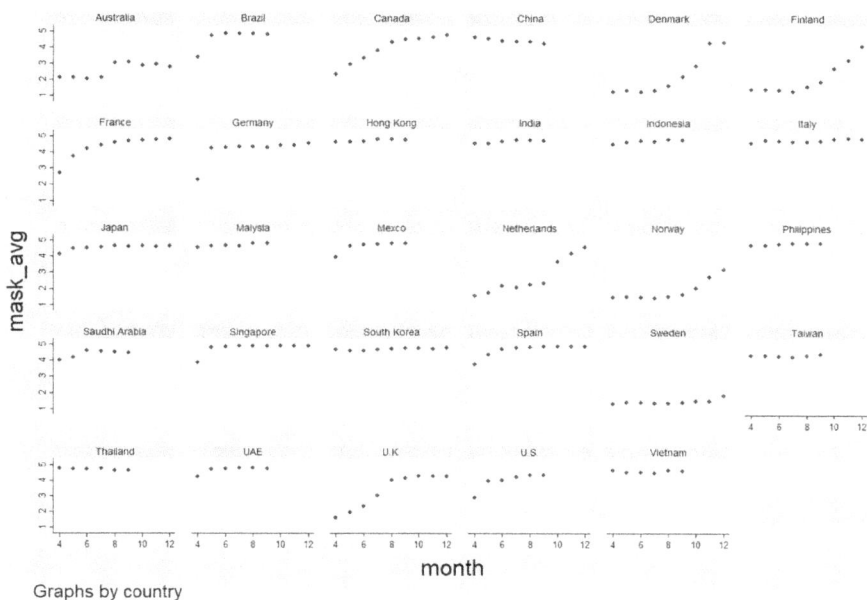

Figure 2.1 Trends of mask-wearing by country

masks throughout the year for Hong Kong, Indonesia, Malaysia, South Korea and Thailand; an increasing level of awareness for Canada, Denmark, Finland, the Netherlands, the UK and the US; and a consistently low level of awareness for Norway and Sweden. These patterns are consistent with previous research (Badillo-Goicoechea et al. 2021).

It seems that citizens of Asian countries, where fewer COVID-19 cases and deaths are reported, are more likely to wear masks in public spaces than are citizens of Scandinavian countries, where individual freedom is regarded as especially important. However, these trends do not consider the number of positive cases. In other words, people in severely (less) affected countries tend to wear masks (less often). In the next section, this chapter analyses the effects of these factors on the awareness of wearing masks.

2.3 Methods

2.3.1 Statistical model

This section explores determinants of awareness of wearing masks across countries with statistical methods and considers other factors such as political regime, living standards, and population density at the national level. Two models are estimated separately to avoid multicollinearity. The equations are as follows:

$$Mask\_avg_{it} = \beta_0 + \beta_1 \ln(COVID\,cases)_{it} + \gamma_i + e_{it} \tag{1}$$

$$Mask_{avg_{it}} = \beta_0 + \beta_1 \ln(COVID\,cases)_{it} + \beta_2\,Democracy_i + \beta_3\,\ln(GDP)_i$$
$$+ \beta_4\,\ln(Popden)_i + e_{it} \tag{2}$$

Where in equation 1, *Mask_avg* is the country-month average of the responses to the question 'Worn a face mask outside your home (e.g. when on public transport, going to a supermarket, going to a main road)' ranging from 1 (Not at all) to 5 (Always). The original order is reversed. *COVID cases* is the monthly averages of COVID-19 positive. This variable is obtained from the Oxford COVID-19 Government Response Tracker (Hale et al. 2020) and was originally collected by The Center for Systems Science and Engineering (CSSE) at Johns Hopkins University (2020). This equation does not include the number of deaths to avoid multicollinearity (the correlation coefficient between two positive cases and deaths is almost 0.9). γ is country-fixed effects that are treated as an independent variable. e_{it} is the error term of regression. i is countries, and t is months. In equation 2, Democracy is the political regime variables, Polity2 for 2018 taken from the Polity V project (Marshall et al. 2020) or Electoral democracy index for 2019 from the V-Dem institute (Coppedge et al. 2020). Polity2 codes democracy levels from −10 (most autocratic) to 10 (most democratic). Electoral democracy index codes democracy levels from 0 (most autocratic) to 1 (most democratic). *GDP* is GDP per capita for living standard, and is *Popden* population density obtained from World Development Indicators (2020). The variables except for Polity2 and Electoral democracy index are logged. This equation does not include country dummies because their inclusion omits the time-invariant independent variables to avoid multicollinearity. Ordinary Least Square is applied for both analyses. Appendix A2.1 is descriptive statistics.

Figure 2.2 shows the results of country variation (the base category is the UAE) based on equation 1. These results reveal the variation across countries after controlling for the COVID-19 positive condition. Here again, the analysis confirms the patterns that Figure 2.1 above suggested, and model 1 in Appendix A2.2 is the regression result.

Figures 2.3 (for Polity2) and 2.4 (Electoral democracy index) show the results of the analysis based on the equation 2, and models 2 and 3 in Appendix A2.2 are the regression results of each model. These figures show the positive relationship between positive cases and mask usage as expected. Polity2 and Electoral democracy index are negatively correlated with mask usage at the statistically significant level. But the effect size of the latter is much bigger than the former because the scales of the variables are different from each other – the former ranges from −10 to 10, and the latter does from 0 to 1. These results imply that people in democratic countries tend to wear masks less often than those in authoritarian countries. GDP per capita is also negatively correlated with the awareness of wearing masks. On the other hand, population density is positively correlated. These effects are expected signs. These results suggest that citizens of rich democratic countries are less likely to wear masks.

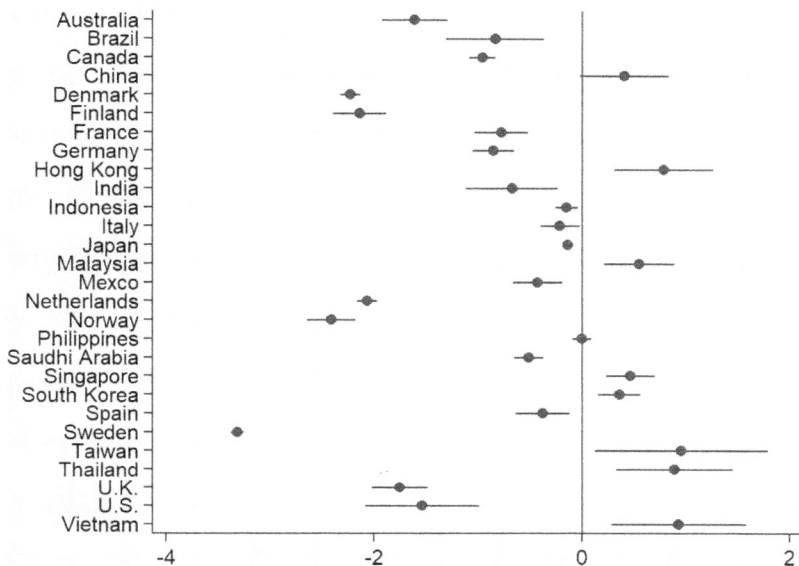

Figure 2.2 Regression result of cross-national difference of wearing masks

Note: 29 countries, $N = 219$, standard errors are clustered by country

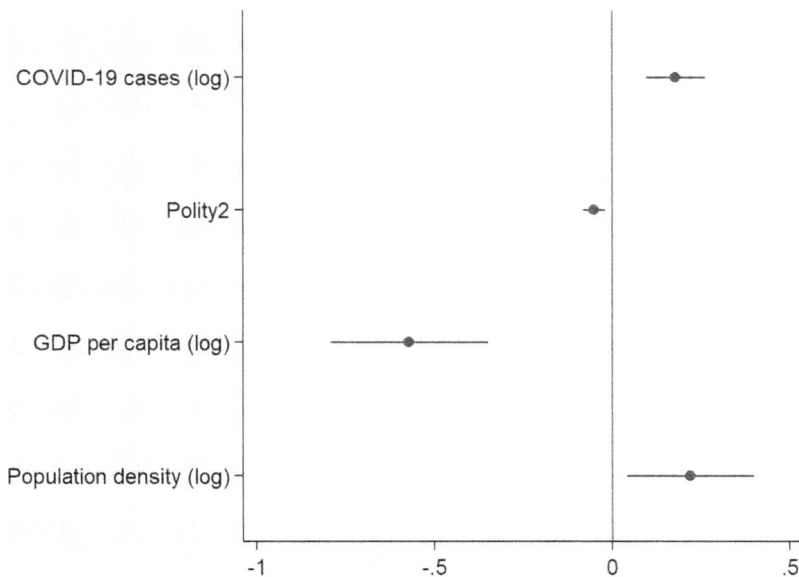

Figure 2.3 Regression result of other cross-national determinants of wearing masks (polity)

Note: 29 countries, $N = 201$, standard errors are clustered by country

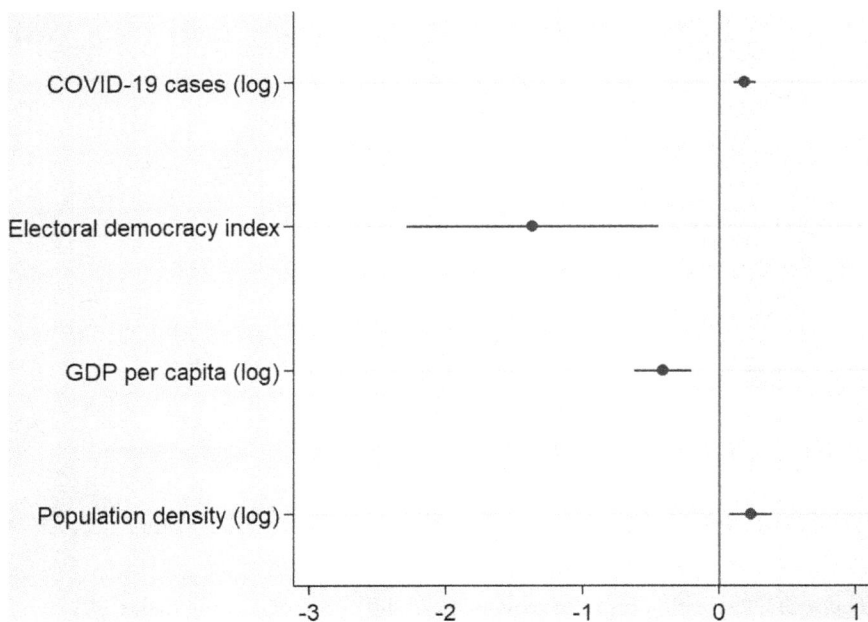

Figure 2.4 Regression result of other cross-national determinants of wearing masks (V-Dem)

Note: 29 countries, $N = 207$, standard errors are clustered by country

2.3.2 Multilevel analysis

This section conducts multilevel analysis to consider individual-level factors based on Ye and Lyu (2020). Two models are estimated because values of employment status are missing, but the base model is the same. The equation is as follows:

Level 1 (individual-level)

$$Mask_i = \beta_{oj} + \beta_{iVj}(IV)_{ij} + r_{ij}$$

Level 2 (country-level)

$$\beta_{oj} = \gamma_{00} + \gamma_{01}(P)_j + \mu_{oj}$$

$$\beta_{iVj} = \gamma_{iV0} + \mu_{iVj}$$

Where $Mask_i$ is the awareness level of mask usage in person i, and β_{oj} is the intercept of regression at country j. $(IV)_{ij}$ is the vector of independent variables (age, gender and employment status), and β_{iVj} is their regression coefficients in country i. r_{ij} is the error term of regression. Factors at the country level determine the intercept of the regression at the individual level. At Level 2, γ_{00} is the intercept at the country level, and γ_{01} is the coefficient of, $(P)_j$ which expresses logged

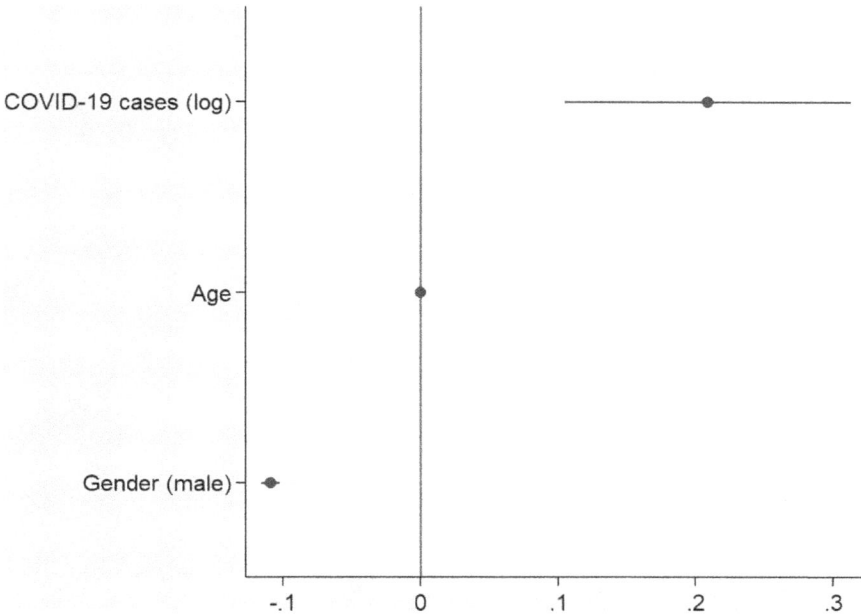

Figure 2.5 Multilevel result of other cross-national determinants of wearing masks
Note: 29 countries, $N = 413,042$

monthly average COVID-19 positive cases. μ_{0j} represents the error term of this regression. The coefficients β_{iVj} of the independent variables have intercepts γ_{iv0} and error terms μ_{ivj} at the country level because the country level also affects the regression coefficients at the individual level.

Figures 2.5 and 2.6 (including employment status) show the results of multilevel analyses based on equation 3, and models 4 and 5 in Appendix A2.3 are the regression results of each model. COVID-19 positive is positively associated with the awareness of wearing masks, as Figures 2.3 and 2.4 report. Age is not correlated with the awareness of mask usage, and men tend to wear masks less often than women in Figure 2.5. Figure 2.6 is the result of the analysis, including employment status. The variable is coded 1 if the responses are 'full-time employment', 'part-time employment' and 'full-time student' and 0 if responses are 'retired', 'unemployed', 'not working' and 'other'. A higher number means isolation from society. The inclusion of this employment status variable in the model leads to about 100,000 fewer samples due to missing values on the employment question. The coefficient of the variable suggests that people isolated from society are less likely to wear masks. And in this model, age is positively correlated with mask usage at the statistically significant level.

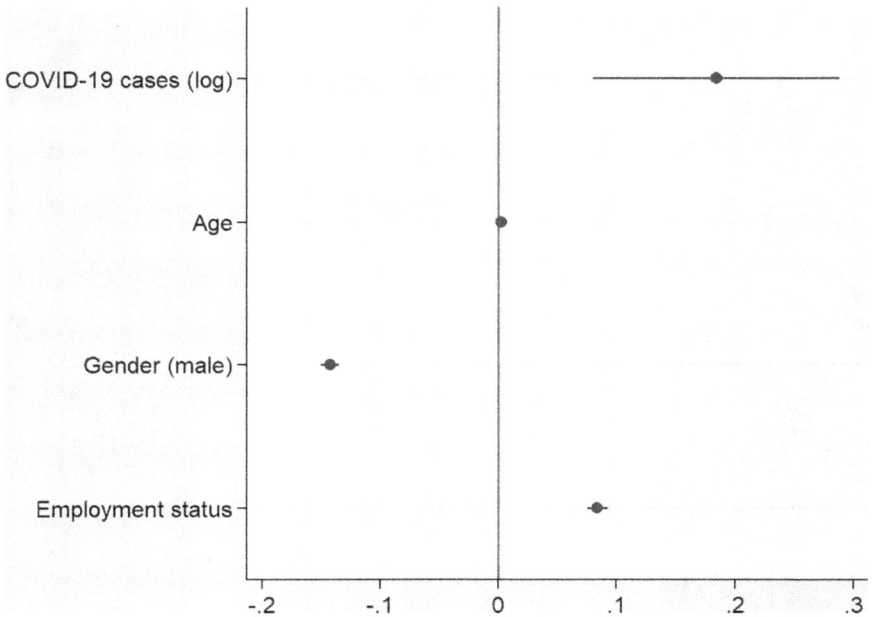

Figure 2.6 Multilevel result of other cross-national determinants of wearing masks including employment

Note: 22 countries, $N = 322{,}749$

2.4 Discussion

This chapter finds a clear difference in patterns of mask usage awareness: Figures 2.1 and 2.2 support cross-national survey analysis (Badillo-Goicoechea et al. 2021). Citizens of Asian countries are more likely to wear masks than citizens of Scandinavian countries. This study also reveals that COVID-19 confirmed cases positively affect mask usage awareness. This result may imply that people are cautious about the virus when the number of positive cases grows. However, a study in Spain reports a null result of the positive case effect (Barceló and Sheen 2020). That research shows that the respondents' region has a much stronger effect than positive cases on mask-wearing. Figures 2.3 and 2.4 report that citizens of more democratic and prosperous countries are less likely to wear masks. This result has been known anecdotally, but this chapter confirms it with statistical methods. Figures 2.5 and 2.6 also show the existence of a gender effect, as revealed by one study (Howard 2021) but not confirmed by another one (Barceló and Sheen 2020). The figures do not endorse a consistent age effect on wearing masks, which previous studies also reported (Haischer et al. 2020; Barceló and Sheen 2020). Figure 2.6 finds that employment status is associated with mask usage.

2.5 Conclusion

This chapter analysed the determinants of mask-wearing in 29 countries in 2020 using more than 400,000 survey responses. The results show considerable variance in the awareness of mask usage across countries. Citizens of Asian countries are more likely to wear masks than citizens of Scandinavian countries. This study also reports that citizens of more democratic and prosperous countries are less likely to wear masks. Women are more likely to wear masks than men. This chapter contributes to the literature by revealing citizens' attitudes towards wearing masks.

Appendix A2.1: Descriptive statistics

Variable	Obs	Mean	Std. Dev.	Min	Max
Mask usage average per month	219	3.9102	1.1916	1.2796	4.9320
Average confirmed cases per month (log)	219	5.9500	2.7957	−1.7918	11.3780
Polity2	213	6.9155	5.6043	−10	10
Electoral democracy index	219	0.6794	0.2787	0.0150	0.91
GDP per capita (log)	207	10.2826	0.9535	7.5830	11.4308
Population density (log)	213	4.7550	1.8299	1.1780	8.9813
Multilevel					
Mask usage	4,48,482	3.8072	1.6251	1	5
Average confirmed cases per month (log)	4,48,541	6.0395	2.7691	−1.7918	11.3780
Age	4,48,541	43.5066	16.3714	18	99
Gender	4,48,541	0.4988	0.5000	0	1
Employment Status	3,35,197	0.6549	0.4754	0	1

Appendix A2.2: Regression results for Figures 2.2, 2.3, 2.4

	(1)	*(2)*	*(3)*
Variables	*Mask avg*	*Mask avg*	*Mask avg*
COVID-19 cases (log)	0.196***	0.179***	0.189***
	(0.0620)	(0.0405)	(0.0407)
Polity2		−0.0508***	
		(0.0152)	
Electoral democracy index			−1.365***
			(0.447)

(Continued)

Appendix A2.2 (Continued)

Variables	(1) Mask avg	(2) Mask avg	(3) Mask avg
GDP per capita (log)		−0.572***	−0.410***
		(0.108)	(0.101)
Population density (log)		0.221**	0.233***
		(0.0870)	(0.0769)
Country dummies	Y	N	N
Constant	3.469***	7.960***	6.785***
	(0.383)	(1.075)	(0.928)
Observations	219	201	207
R-squared	0.826	0.494	0.504

Robust standard errors in parentheses

*** $p < 0.01$, ** $p < 0.05$, * $p < 0.1$

Appendix A2.3: Regression results for Figures 2.5 and 2.6

Variables	(4) Mask	(5) Mask
COVID-19 cases (log)	0.209***	0.184***
	(0.0532)	(0.0532)
Age	−0.000127	0.00253***
	(0.000115)	(0.000141)
Gender (male)	−0.109***	−0.142***
	(0.00354)	(0.00404)
Employment status		0.0837***
		(0.00458)
Constant	3.129***	3.427***
	(0.503)	(0.543)
Observations	413,042	322,749
Number of Countries	29	22

Standard errors in parentheses

*** $p < 0.01$, ** $p < 0.05$, * $p < 0.1$

Note

1 This work was supported by JSPS KAKENHI Grant Number JP20K22079, as well as the contributions of Masahisa Endo, Gento Kato and Masanori Kikuchi.

References

Aravindakshan A., Boehnke J., Gholami E. and Nayak A. (2020) 'Mask-wearing during the COVID-19 pandemic'. *medRxiv* doi:10.1101/2020.09.11.20192971

Badillo-Goicoechea E., Chang T.H., Kim E. et al. (2021) 'Global trends and predictors of face mask usage during the COVID-19 pandemic', *BMC Public Health* 21(1): 2099. doi:10.1186/s12889-021-12175-9

Barceló J. and Sheen G.C.H. (2020) 'Voluntary adoption of social welfare-enhancing behavior: Mask-wearing in Spain during the COVID-19 outbreak', *PLoS ONE* 15(12): e0242764.doi:10.1371/journal.pone.0242764

Cheng V.C., Wong S.C., Chuang V.W. et al. (2020) 'The role of community-wide wearing of face mask for control of coronavirus disease 2019 (COVID-19) epidemic due to SARS-CoV-2', *Journal of Infection* 81(1): 107–114. doi:10.1016/j.jinf.2020.04.024.

Chernozhukov V., Kasahara H. and Schrimpf P. (2021) 'Causal impact of masks, policies, behavior on early COVID-19 pandemic in the U.S.', *Journal of Econometrics* 220(1): 23–62. doi:10.1016/j.jeconom.2020.09.003.

Chu D.K., Akl E.A., Duda S. et al. (2020) 'Physical distancing, face masks, and eye protection to prevent person-to-person transmission of SARS-CoV-2 and COVID-19: a systematic review and meta-analysis', *The Lancet* 395(10242): 1973–1987. doi:10.1016/S0140-6736(20)31142-9.

Coppedge M., Gerring J., Knutsen C.H. et al. (2020) 'V-Dem [Country – Year/Country – Date] Dataset v10.' Varieties of Democracy (V-Dem) Project. doi:10.23696/vdemds21.

Haischer M.H., Beilfuss R., Hart M.R. et al. (2020) 'Who is wearing a mask? Gender-, age-, and location-related differences during the COVID-19 pandemic', *PLoS ONE* 15(10): e0240785. doi:10.1371/journal.pone.0240785.

Hale T., Webster S., Petherick A., Phillips T. and Kira B. (2020) 'Oxford COVID 19 government response tracker, Blavatnik School of Government'. Data use policy: Creative Commons Attribution CC BY standard. Available at www.bsg.ox.ac.uk/research/research projects/coronavirus government response tracker#data (Accessed 20 January 2021).

Howard M.C. (2021) 'Gender, face mask perceptions, and face mask wearing: Are men being dangerous during the COVID-19 pandemic?', *Personality and Individual Differences* 170: 110417. doi:10.1016/j.paid.2020.110417.

Imperial College London (2020) 'YouGov COVID-19 behaviour tracker data hub'. Available at https://github.com/YouGov-Data/covid-19-tracker (Accessed 20 February 2021).

Marshall M.G., Jaggers K. and Gurr T.R. (2020) 'Polity V Project, political regime characteristics and transitions, 1800–2018'. *Center for Systemic Peace.* Available at www.systemicpeace.org/inscrdata.html (Accessed 8 August 2020).

Mitze T., Kosfeld R., Rode J. and Wälde K. (2020) 'Face masks considerably reduce COVID-19 cases in Germany', *Proceedings of the National Academy of Sciences* 117(51): 32293–32301. doi:10.1073/pnas.2015954117.

The Center for Systems Science and Engineering (CSSE) at Johns Hopkins University (2020) 'COVID 19 data repository'. https://github.com/CSSEGISandData/COVID19 (Accessed 20 February 2021).

Wei J., Guo S., Long E., Zhang L., Shu B. and Guo L. (2021) 'Why does the spread of COVID-19 vary greatly in different countries? Revealing the efficacy of face masks in epidemic prevention', *Epidemiology & Infection* 149: e24. doi:10.1017/S0950268821000108.

World Development Indicators (2020) Available at http://datatopics.worldbank.org/world development indicators/ (Accessed 8 August 2020).

Ye M. and Lyu Z. (2020) 'Trust, risk perception, and COVID-19 infections: Evidence from multilevel analyses of combined original dataset in China', *Social Science & Medicine* 265: 113517.

Part I
Europe

3 Historical analysis of public health policies for preventing epidemics in Hungary

Osamu Ieda

3.1 Introduction

Humanity has experienced pandemics previously, such as the Black Death during the 14th century, cholera in the 19th century and the Spanish flu at the beginning of the 20th century. Humanity has always considered pandemics a war against an invisible enemy; the same is true for the ongoing COVID-19 pandemic in the 21st century.

Pandemics necessitate unity among humans beyond communities and nations because diseases can spread across boundaries. However, public policies against pandemics are contradictory for society because they require people to isolate themselves. Moreover, humans need to help one another fight against diseases through *social distancing*. Therefore, how can this contradiction between isolation and cooperation be solved? Social scientists need to investigate the history of pandemics and public policies to provide answers.

Wearing face masks could be a solution to this problem. However, face masks are a relatively new invention. This chapter focuses on the policies and behaviours related to the earlier pandemics and discusses public intervention. Secondly, this chapter further highlights a previous pandemic called the Spanish flu. Specifically, it will focus on the Spanish flu in Hungary and on the medical expertise related to policy-making and public health. Before World War I (WWI), the domain of public policy was very limited due to the prevailing liberalism (laissez-faire, or no state intervention into the economy). Nevertheless, public health was an exceptionally serious concern for the social and political aspects of the Middle Ages, and, especially, during the 19th century.

WWI was the first total war among the European nations. At the time, public policies were prioritised to preserve human resources and social peace. Public health became one of the most crucial issues in maintaining staffing for the European governments, especially when the Spanish flu hit the European nations during the war.

The Spanish flu began to spread during the last years of WWI, which killed tens of millions of people worldwide. When WWI began in 1914, Hungary was a kingdom located at the eastern half of the Austro-Hungarian dual monarchy under the rule of the Habsburgs. Hungary gained independence in 1918,

DOI: 10.4324/9781003244127-4

whereas the Spanish flu hit the country from 1918 to 1920. Due to the chaotic situation, the opportunity for the consistent implementation of public policies against the raging pandemic was extremely limited for the Hungarian government and its people. This scenario was called the triple crisis, namely, the ongoing war, the collapse of authorities and social disorder. Nevertheless, medical professionals formulated guidelines for public hygiene to prevent the Spanish flu from spreading throughout the country. The main section of the chapter discusses the experiences of Hungary concerning the Spanish flu. It provides suggestions on how the present governments and people can cope with a similar crisis.

3.2 Earlier pandemics

This section focuses on two earlier pandemics, namely, the Black Death and cholera, and examines changes in the public policies of the authorities.

3.2.1 *The Black Death*

The Black Death struck the world in the middle of the 14th century, when Europe lost more than one-third of its population and led to the decline of the most significant authority in the Middle Ages, the Roman Catholic Church. The working population, called serfs in the medieval manor system, sharply diminished. Consequently, the classical feudal systems ended or underwent reorganisation. With the twilight of medieval authorities, a new era emerged: the Renaissance and the Modern Age.

Recent studies (Cesana et al. 2016) give geographical routes of the spread of the Black Death during the 1340s to 1360s. The routes indicate the range where the infection spread per year. The range shows trade routes were more decisive in spreading the infection than for state territories. Particularly, the medieval states were vulnerable to infectious diseases due to the lack of strict border control. In contrast, the people could enjoy free movement beyond the state borders during the medieval period.

After the catastrophic consequences of the Black Death, the state administration introduced the quarantine system for infection control. As a result, modern authorities (e.g. absolutist monarchies), empires and nation-states have recognised borders as components that function as a boundary for the military, economic and diplomatic domains and regulate the movement of people and goods from the viewpoint of epidemic prevention. The quarantine system became the initial public health policy, which required isolating infected individuals from the community.

3.2.2 *Cholera*

The next great pandemic that hit Europe was cholera during the 19th century. Cholera originated from India and began in the 1820s. The infection spread by approximately six times in a cycle of approximately 10 to 20 years until the end of the 19th century. The cholera pandemic was a *by-product* of the globalised British economy, which made cholera, which was endemic to India, a large-scale global pandemic. Modern nations lacked other means for maintaining residents safe from the infection apart from the quarantine system against the repeated spread of cholera. However, the quarantine system did not function well because there was little knowledge of the cause of the disease.

Consequently, the fear of unknown infectious diseases emotionally strengthened prejudice, resulting in various forms of discrimination against other people, such as foreigners and individuals from different cultures and social classes. For example, the causes of the disease were identified as *under-development in Asia*, the *immorality of the lower class, punishment from God* and *poisoning by political enemies.* A rumour spread in Europe widely when Britain and France sent medical teams to Moscow and Warsaw, the first infected cities in Europe. The British and French believed they 'don't have to be afraid of being infected by the plague prevailing among non-cultured people' due to the *high level of civilization* in Western Europe' (Omori 2004, p. 75).

Meiji in Japan was not exempt. Japan was also affected by the cholera pandemic, which initiated the same prejudice among the Japanese: the Japanese people believed that cholera came from outside, especially China. Japan scorned China for being filthy and uncultured, whereas 'the Cholera epidemic triggered nationalism awakening among the Japanese people against the Chinese people' (Omori 2004, p. 75).

In Hungary, cholera outbreaks took one million lives (Rózsa 1975), which accounted for nearly 10% of the country's total population at the time. Moreover, problems overlapped between cholera, poor harvest and livestock plague (rinderpest). Thus, the impact of the epidemic became synergistically disastrous for the peasantry. Another incident worsened the situation: a medical doctor overprescribed calcium, which killed a cholera patient. This incident evolved into a rumour that 'landlords and the Jews poisoned the well', such that even a lord was assaulted (Hóman-Szekfű 1920). Alternatively, the epidemic, which caused a huge loss in the number of peasants at the national scale, boosted the support of politicians to protect the peasantry (*Deák 1882–1886*). The policies resulted in the abolition of serfdom in 1848.

3.3 The emergence of epidemiology: a new medical science

During the Middle Ages, the Black Death led to the decline of the existing authorities and eventually created a new social climate for public health in Europe. Moreover, the cholera epidemic during the 19th century played a significant role in the emergence of a new community and a nation, where the new idea of public health policy developed. However, such an idea of public policy remained less popular in general. Nevertheless, the repeated cholera infection highlighted poor public sanitation, especially in cities overcrowded due to industrialisation. Urban redevelopment, such as sewerage construction, began with the emerging concept of public health policies (Ishi 2018; Omori 2014).

The concept of public health and public sanitation became the background of new medical science, that is, epidemiology, in the middle of the 19th century. One of the pioneers of epidemiology was John Snow, who introduced the analysis of the distribution of disease clusters into medical surveys. At the time, cholera was widespread in London. Snow proposed that a new system should replace the well-water pump system. However, the city officials opposed this proposal. Nevertheless, Snow did not give up until his vision was realised (Snow 1856; Johnson 2007). The new system worked effectively, which led to the further development of epidemiology (Paneth 2004; Johnson 2007).

Another pioneer in the new medical science was Ignac Semmelweis, who worked at an obstetric hospital in Vienna, the capital of the Habsburg Empire. Semmelweis invented the same idea as Snow: the distribution of disease clusters. Among his colleagues, he proposed the concept of handwashing to prevent puerperal fever, an infectious disease whose cause has been long associated with *bad air*. Nowadays, Semmelweis's proposal of handwashing is a common sanitary behaviour, especially during the COVID-19 era. However, this simple and effective idea was unacceptable during mid-19th-century Vienna. After he moved back to his hometown, Budapest, his proposal was successfully realised in the hospitals (Chung and Case 1997).

The two scientists devised these prevention measures using a novel approach, which visualised invisible enemies using geographical and statistical data about cases of infections.

Furthermore, micro-bacteriology was significantly developed during the 19th century, although virology was still in its infancy. Nevertheless, new achievements in the medical sciences led to further concepts in modern public health policies, which initiated preventive and precautionary interventions. The Spanish flu witnessed the initial application of epidemiology in practice (Celentano et al. 2019).

3.4 The Spanish Flu

Shortly after the cholera pandemic subsided, Europe and the rest of the world faced a new infectious disease, *the Spanish flu*, which spread worldwide during and after WWI. Soldiers, war prisoners, logistics personnel and war refugees were the vehicles of infection. The subsequent sections discuss the professional intervention in public health in the case of the Spanish flu in Hungary.

In the middle of the great war, European governments feared that serious damages due to the Spanish flu would leak to enemy countries. Against this background, governments intended to conceal the real severity of the infection, even from their residents. As a result, the new virus spread easily across Europe due to a lack of governmental control over the disease. The Spanish flu crossed the continental borders to Asia and Africa from the European battlefield. The main victims of the Spanish flu were not the Europeans but the residents of non-European regions, such as India and China, from which the personnel were mobilised to the war (Ishi 2018).

Initially, the Spanish flu was reported in European countries as *a simple cold*, such that the flu slipped through the quarantine system. In addition, when the war ended, soldiers and logistics personnel returned home, and large numbers of war prisoners and refugees also headed for their home countries. These people served as intermediaries of infection to their homelands.

3.4.1 The Spanish flu in Hungary

Hungary fell into turmoil due to the loss of most of its territories after its defeat in the war. Consequently, the actual data on infection remained unknown (Vincze 2020). For the recorded year, which is 1918, the confirmed death toll was 53,201. For comparison with other countries based on figures per 1 million population, the death toll in Hungary was 2,888, which was relatively small in Europe. The worst was Italy at 7,118, followed by Spain and Switzerland at 6,907 and 5,373, respectively (Valentiny 2020).

The collapse of the Hungarian Kingdom and of the Habsburg Empire coincided with the spread of the Spanish flu. Many European empires fell, such as the Austrian, German, Russian and Ottoman empires. Alternatively, new nation-states were born in Eastern Europe, such as Czechoslovakia and Yugoslavia, following the decline of these empires. However, new state borders were not established immediately after the political changes in Europe. As a result, no quarantine system was in place for a relative period due to changes in state boundaries. For this reason, Hungary suffered the most.

The number of fatal victims in Budapest, the capital of Hungary, was 4,225 per 1 million of the population in 1918, which was the third highest among major European cities. Rome reported the largest number at 7,320 (Valentiny 2020).

3.5 Local initiatives for public health

At the time, the official media in Hungary and those in other countries do not report actual information about the infectious disease. In the autumn of 1918, when the first wave of the Spanish flu reached its peak in Hungary, the local authorities, instead of the central government, distributed handbills to the citizens. Among the local cities, the mayor of Miskolc city took initial action to provide the bills on 1 October.

The bill of the city reads as follows:

> For the prevention of Spanish influenza
> Influenza that is prevalent now has a symptom similar to a cold when it is mild and when it becomes severe, it causes a high fever of 39–40 degrees. Infected individuals suffer from fatigue, loss of appetite, or pain, and the disease may develop pneumonia.
> Large-scale and rapid infections occur in a crowded place, especially in a closed space, that is, large gatherings, theaters, cinemas, restaurants, coffee shops, taverns, waiting rooms such as train stations, social gatherings, and entertainment venues such as banquet halls. You should refrain from going there.

Do not visit homes with infected people.
Do not get on a crowded train or tram if you don't need it urgently.
When coughing, hold your mouth and nose with a handkerchief.
It is dangerous to spit.
Shaking hands causes infection.
Gargle many times every day.
Keep your body, clothes and home clean.
Enforce hand washing before meals.

(partially omitted; Reiman 2019)

The instructions given by the local government suggest that public hygiene measures against infection were developed even in those days. The only difference is wearing face masks, which were unpopular and not widely available in Hungary. Handkerchiefs, as seen in the bill, eventually substituted for face masks. The hygienic behaviour of the citizens in terms of their social and private lives was the same as they are during the COVID-19 pandemic. *The New Lifestyle*, which is currently called out in Japan, is a rehash of the preventive measures implemented 100 years ago. Despite professional guidelines, the Spanish flu further spread, similar to the case of COVID-19. The situation was critical in Hungary due to the chaos from the triple crisis. The following discussion outlines the Hungarian experience, with a special focus on the city of Budapest.

3.6 Beyond the triple crisis

On 16 June 1918, 60 soldiers were confirmed infected with the flu in a military hospital in Budapest. Two days later, 30 soldiers were further confirmed infected at another hospital, and 18 Russian prisoners of war were found infected at the end of June (Valentiny 2020). In Budapest, the infected (or sourced) Russian prisoners of war formed a small proportion of the 400,000 Russian prisoners of war held in Hungary. The latter worked together with Hungarian workers at factories in the city (Otsuru 2013).

In July, the infectious disease was named the Spanish flu. However, the tone of the newspapers was not serious, which reported the following:

The Spanish flu has now struck Germany and Austria after France and Britain, and it has finally come to Budapest. Would this dear customer avoid us?! The symptoms are very mild, and at most, they will subside in three days. It's the same as a cold.

(Vincze 2020)

Some medical doctors, however, gave a warning;

it might progress to life-threatening inflammatory pneumonia.

(Vincze 2020)

Nevertheless, the chief medical officer of the government repeatedly issued statements to counteract citizens' anxiety:

> It's just the flu that has been common. People who exaggerate the Spanish flu overstated a little.
>
> (Vincze 2020)

The *common flu* spread rapidly into rural areas; in September, the infection returned to Budapest. At this point, schools were closed one after another.

> It is none other than people who spread the disease. Especially those infected people who have no symptoms. They are free to roam the streets and get on and off the train.
>
> (Valentiny 2020)

Bálint Rezső, a military medical officer and university professor, gave this warning, suggesting that the medical officer learned about modern epidemiology and related precautionary principles. In other words, the Spanish flu was highly infectious even before the appearance of its symptoms. For this reason, people were encouraged to maintain social distancing and to avoid going to public places despite the absence of symptoms.

The distribution of the handbills in Miskolc was seemingly proposed based on the epidemiological expertise given by Rezső. The Hungarian expert-recommended precautionary guidelines that would be considered appropriate during the modern era could be a heritage given by the history of epidemiology in Hungary, which Semmelweis initiated in the middle of the 19th century. Thus, the local authorities accepted these epidemiological suggestions to formulate public health policies. Moreover, the local authority in Miskolc began the distribution of the handbills even before the central government recognised the Spanish flu as an epidemic.

3.7 Passive central government

In contrast to local initiatives, the central government hesitated to cope with the prevailing infection actively. However, the central government shifted its attitude from passive to active in terms of public health policies during the last days of September (Valentiny 2020). On 27 September, the government took several steps against the infection, such as obligatory notification for positive cases, requesting hospitals set up beds specialised for infected individuals and converting the Exhibition Hall into a temporary hospital for infectious diseases due to its large capacity in preparation for the rapidly increasing number of patients. On 28 September, positive cases of the Spanish flu were isolated for the first time.

The Public Health Committee finally recognised the Spanish flu as an epidemic by the end of September. However, the chief medical officer gave another announcement with a different nuance and said that the possible fatality rate of the flu could be 0.5% instead of the initial estimation of 4% to 5%. As such, the government committee could not reach a consensus about the main issue: what is the cause of the disease? The only fact shared within the committee was that the disease should be qualified as an epidemic (Géra 2009).

On 2 October, the government announced new rules. All schools except for universities and after-school daycare centres should be closed for two weeks. Secondly, the district medical officers were obliged to report the cases of infection. Thirdly, hospital visits were prohibited, whereas hospitalisation was limited to patients with severe infection (Vincze 2020; Valentiny 2020).

On 4 October, instruction posters were distributed in the capital with the same content as the handbills in Miskolc. The time lag between the capital and the local town suggests that the central administration did not function well due to the lack of consistent views about the disease on the one hand and the independent behaviour of the local authorities from national policy-makers on the other hand.

3.8 Twisting Budapest

The mayor of Budapest took a step to ban outdoor markets. Nevertheless, most of the restaurants and entertainment venues in the city continued their businesses at their own risk. Furthermore, schools were closed, though children lined up in a queue in front of greengrocers and butchers instead of going to school. Thus, suspending the classes was ineffective. The situation was chaotic due to the lack of cooperation among authorities and citizens.

According to a report issued by the Public Health Commission on 9 October, 90% of infected individuals were aged 14 to 35 years. They were mainly individuals in the middle classes, whereas women contracted the infection 3 times more than men. The report also stated that many women contracted the flu during social activities, such as procession in a queue for rationed goods, distribution of ration tickets and volunteer work to welcome demobilised soldiers. The reported data were informative but unreliable because the data collection was partial and biased (Géra 2009).

The central government provided 2,500 beds of the military hospitals and ambulances of the Red Cross to the capital administration. Temporary military tents were also used for the authority of the capital city. The authorities began cooperating with one another when the infection became increasingly serious in October, when thousands of people became infected and dozens of deaths were confirmed daily. The hospitals lacked beds; the citizens became overwhelmingly dissatisfied with the central government and the expert committee due to the inconsistent and lagging countermeasures. The only step that the central government took to alleviate public dissatisfaction was to publicise that the disease was not dangerous repeatedly (Valentiny 2020; Vincze 2020; Géra 2009).

The mayor of Budapest requested the central government to enforce the closure of shops, but the government issued a late response. Instead, the government only instructed restaurants 'to clean up frequently, reduce the number of seats to two-thirds, and ventilate more frequently'. In contrast, trams, the major form of transportation for the citizens, continuously operated with a limited number of passengers on the wagons. The shortage of nurses and medical doctors became increasingly serious, such that medical students were mobilised despite lacking the official qualification for clinical treatment (Valentiny 2020).

3.9 Systemic changes in the October Revolution

On 17 October, defeat in the war was officially announced. On 20 October, the mayor of Budapest announced that he would conduct considerable additional measures, including the suspension of all schools (except universities) in the city until 3 November. Moreover, standing rooms in public transport were abolished; performances in movie theatres, theatres and entertainment facilities were cancelled; meetings in public places were prohibited; gatherings and demonstrations were banned; ventilation and cleaning were required at coffee shops and restaurants; handwashing equipment was set up at official offices and factories; pharmacies were opened until 9 p.m.; the operation of the metropolitan public transportation was limited; work shifts at factories were restricted; museums and libraries were closed; lastly, events of large companies and churches were prohibited (Valentiny 2020). However, a strong possibility exists that the local authorities followed the professional guidelines but not the central administration.

The mayor of Budapest continuously implemented independent public health policies, as evidenced by the suspension of horse racing on 22 October and his request to neighbouring municipalities to take the same measures implemented by the capital. When half of the students of a technical college contracted the flu, the students required the central government to close the college. In cooperation with the students, the mayor requested the Ministry of Culture to close the university and further requested the Ministry of Justice to cease deliberations in district courts. The citizens were requested to limit the use of telephones only for constrained cases (Valentiny 2020).

Between 23 October and 1 November, a historic cataclysm occurred. Following its defeat in the war, a new administration took power. The new government of Hungary declared independence from the Habsburgs after the four-century-long rule of the dynasty. Instead of monarchy, republican Hungary was established. This event was called the October Revolution or Daisy Revolution after the symbol of the revolution, that is, the daisy flower. The political change in Hungary was a part of the dynamism of European politics after WWI. Consequently, other defeated countries, such as Austria, Germany and Turkey, were coincidentally transformed into republics.

On the streets in Budapest, the mass demonstrations of citizens, soldiers, students and workers supported political changes. Large numbers of people gathered every day in front of the parliament and in the city centre. Clashes with the police occurred during the demonstrations, and several individuals were killed. Budapest fell into chaos, such that infection control measures were neglected.

The new administration declared the abolition of censorship, and Count Mihály Károlyi was designated as the Prime Minister on 31 October. The authorities in Budapest accepted the new state administration. Immediately after taking office, Károlyi issued a statement that the new administration lifted the business restrictions for theatres, movie theatres and restaurants, among others, on the pretext of decreasing the new cases of infection. Moreover, the new prime minister requested theatres to conduct celebratory performances for the new administration. In this manner, the government 'hoped the citizens to regain their composure' (Vincze 2020; Géra 2009).

Coincidentally, the infection rate slightly decreased in November despite the loosened restriction, although the situation was far from converging. On 28 November, the Epidemic Committee (formerly the Public Health Committee) reported 464 new cases and 44 new deaths. Finally, the commission acknowledged that the main routes of infection were soldiers and war refugees.

3.10 Conclusion

Figure 3.1 depicts the citizens and soldiers in Budapest during the Daisy Revolution. Even children wore daisies, the symbol of the revolution, creating an atmosphere similar to an exciting festival. Figure 3.2, which illustrates the railway station, represents the scene of soldiers returning from the battlefields to the

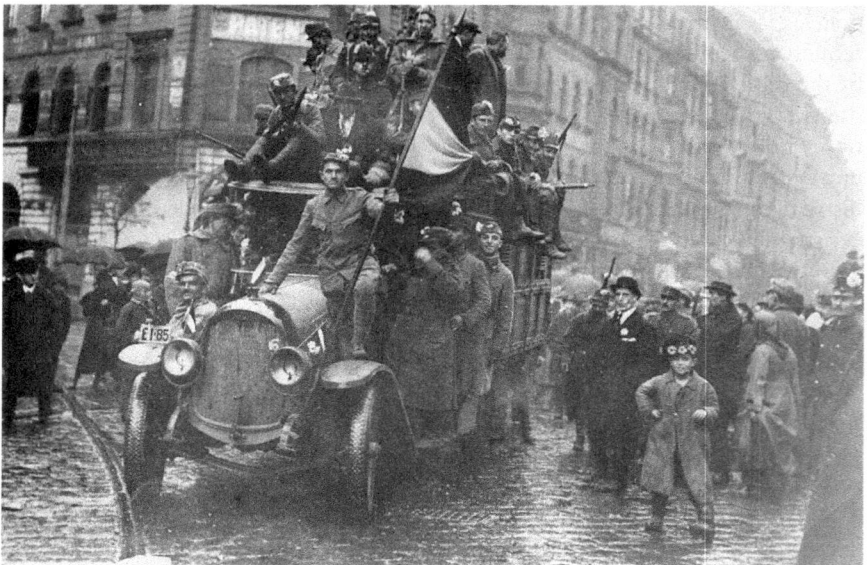

Figure 3.1 Citizen and soldiers in the October Revolution, Budapest
Source: MTI Photo, MTI/Media Service Support and Asset Management Fund

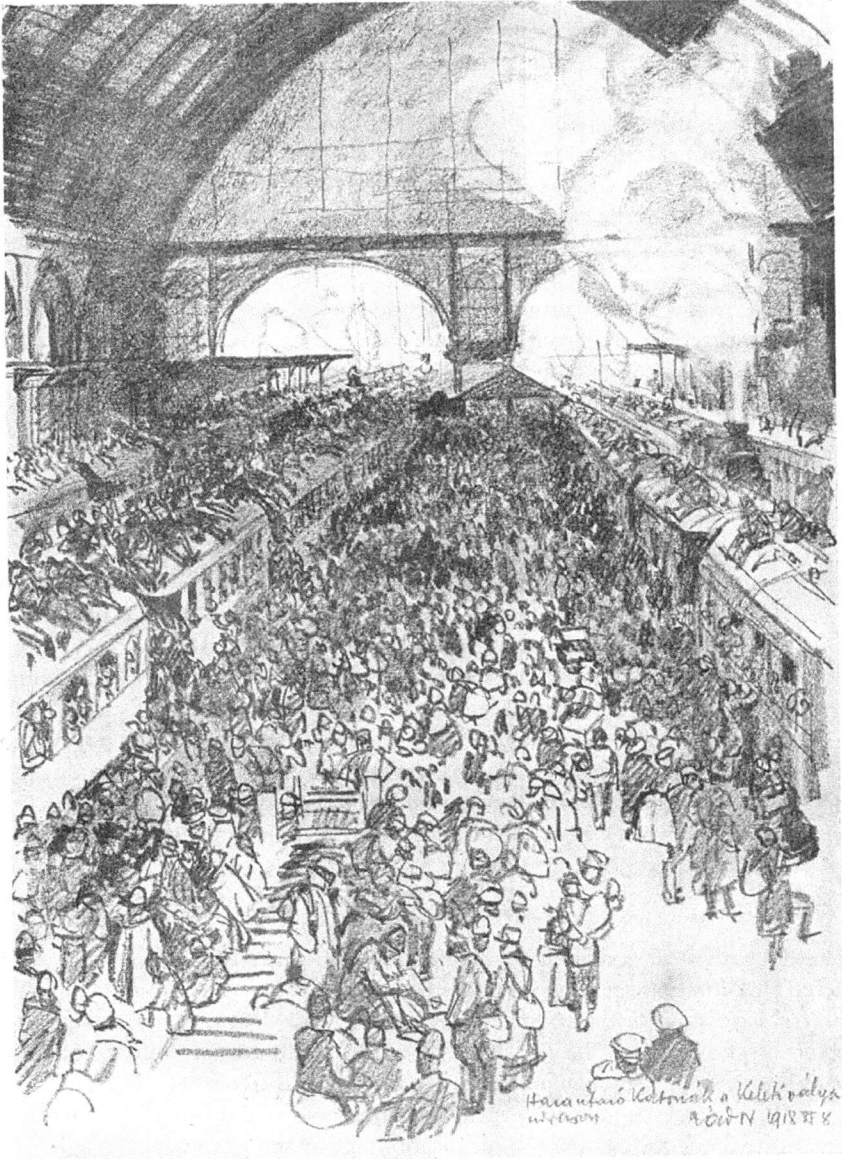

Figure 3.2 Returning soldiers arriving at Budapest Central Station

Source: http://elsovh.hu/wp-content/uploads/2018/12/katonavonatok_keletipu_vu_19181127.jpg

main station in Budapest on 27 November 1918. The train was full of soldiers, such that others even rode on the roof. The women welcomed these soldiers. Afterward, the veterans scattered across the country as they headed for their hometowns. The two figures present no concern about the pandemic or death. Due to the exciting events, the photographer and the painter may have forgotten about the flu in this fleeting moment.

Therefore, how did policy-makers in public health assess the behaviours of the people and their local initiatives? The discussion of the professional experts in the committee reveals that cooperation and separation depended on political bargaining between the government and the people. A document of the committee reads as follows:

> the extreme Nihilist group [within the committee] criticized that most of the measures were superfluous and not effective, saying that influenza had existed any time and the problems had been solved by the nature. Most of the committee members thought; many things were not clear, and the country was on the edge of bankruptcy. Therefore, the government could not conduct many things. Action could be spectacular. However, we had to create such measures that could be implemented and that should aim, first of all, to make the people relieved. The members prioritized that outside observers would believe that the situation was under control. The majority of the committee, including the Nihilist groups, shared the idea; that is, they had to take a lesson from the events in the end of October; namely, the social order would be overthrown if the people were severely constrained in their free behavior and if the separation policy was radical. All the committee members feared that if the committee would introduce ban of social gathering, many people would suspect a political intention behind the policy.[1] Any member agreed with that all measures that the city authority introduced in Budapest with a good will could not be fully successful, as far as the state government would not provide a uniformed program, which would be effective to all over the country.
>
> (Géra 2009, pp. 225–226)

The document suggests that the committee's priority was *social order* and rendered the situation seemingly *under control*. Therefore, the committee avoided *radical separation policy* and the *severe constraint of free behaviour* by 'taking a lesson from the events in the end of October', although the committee recognised 'a uniformed program would be effective to all over the country'. Eventually, the committee members took only the least consideration in terms of epidemiological effectiveness due to their self-justification: 'many things were not clear and the country was on the edge of bankruptcy'.

Epidemiology is a natural science. However, the implementation of epidemiological knowledge could be highly political because it involved the public and the administration by nature. Two pioneers of epidemiology, namely, Snow and

Semmelweis, struggled to make the authorities adapt their new knowledge during the 19th century (Johnson 2007).

In reality, the Spanish flu in Hungary receded in 1919, where the death toll per million decreased to 298 in Budapest. In 1920, however, the epidemic re-emerged, which led to a death toll per million of as many as 1,550. In 1921, surprisingly, the infection suddenly ended with 78 fatal cases in Budapest.

Why did the number of victims reduce to one-third in 1920 compared with 1918? Why did the virus disappear in 1921? The answers may be the re-established state borders, herd immunity or the end of social turmoil, such as revolutions (Valentiny 2020; Vincze 2020). Alternatively, these factors may have worked together. Eventually, the reasons remain unknown. Nevertheless, the years between 1919 and 1921 were not peaceful in Hungary because the country further experienced extreme turbulence in its political and social aspects after the October Revolution in 1918. The Communist Party came to power in spring 1919 but lasted only briefly. Meanwhile, the Romanian army invaded Hungary, where battles occurred for months involving the capital, Budapest. A civil war broke out, where the monarchists, led by admiral Miklós Horthy, restored peace in the country. Finally, the wars ended in the spring of 1920.

The residents could not expect continuous or consistent public health policies against the Spanish flu as a natural result of the long-lasting chaos. The break in the pandemic during 1919 and the infection entirely disappearing after 1921 may have been miracles. God had blessed the miserable people: 'Atoning sorrow hath weighed down sins of past and future days' (National Anthem of Hungary).[2]

In 2020, when COVID-19 began to spread, the Hungarian government powerfully introduced preventive policies one after another; in November of the same year, when the COVID-19 wave was at its peak, the government declared the wearing of face masks in public places legally mandatory. However, public opinion in Hungary did not agree with the government: 41% of the respondents in a public-opinion survey in November indicated *No* to the question: 'Do you agree with making wearing face masks obligatory in a public place?' (*Statista* 19/11/2020). The people's attitude since the beginning was against the issue of wearing face masks in public places. Specifically, more than half of the respondents (53%) stated that they did not want to wear face masks in public places, according to another public-opinion survey conducted in the spring of 2020 (*Statista* 9/4/2020). The independent attitude of the people suggests an opposition to the *authoritarian* government led by Prime Minister Viktor Orbán, whom EU leaders repeatedly criticised for his violation of the *rule of law* (*Heti Világgazdaság online* 2020). This view has remained the same since the Spanish flu, which occurred about 100 years ago.

Wearing face masks is neither a political nor a legal behaviour *per se* but a hygienic habit recommended through epidemiological knowledge. The modern history of the pandemic in Hungary and that of the world requires social scientists to investigate epidemiology more as social science and less as medical science to fight against infection and society and politics.

Notes

1 The perception of the committee members, who were dominantly scientists, suggests that they understood the October Revolution as a consequence of the severe constraining measures by the Budapest authority. The historiography of the October Revolution never mentioned correlation between the revolution and the Spanish flu.
2 National Anthem of Hungary in English: 'O, my God, the Magyar bless With Thy plenty and good cheer! With Thine aid his just cause press, Where his foes to fight appear. Fate, who for so long did'st frown, Bring him happy times and ways; Atoning sorrow hath weighed down Sins of past and future days'.

References

Celentano, D.D. Platz, E. and Mehta, H.S. (2019) 'The Centennial of the Department of Epidemiology at Johns Hopkins Bloomberg School of Public Health: A Century of Epidemiologic Discovery and Education', *American Journal of Epidemiology*, 188(12): 2043–2048. doi: 10.1093/aje/kwz176.

Cesana, D., Benedictow, O.J. and BiAnucci, R. (2016) 'The Origin and Early Spread of the Black Death in Italy: First Evidence of Plague Victims from 14th-Century Liguria (Northern Italy)', *Anthropological Science*, 125(1): 15–24.

Chung, K.-T. and Case, L.C. (1997) 'Semmelweis: A Lesson in Epidemiology', *SIM News*, 47(5): 234–237. www.researchgate.net/profile/King-Thom-Chung/publication/237209267_Semmelweis_A_Lesson_in_Epidemiology/links/56ba49c808ae0a6bc9555571/Semmelweis-A-Lesson-in-Epidemiology.pdf (Accessed 10 September 2021).

Deák (1882–1886) *Deák Ferenc Beszédei*, ed. by Manó Kónyi. https://mek.oszk.hu/02200/02213/html/ (Accessed 20 September 2020).

Géra, E. (2009) 'A Spanyolnátha Budapesten', *Budapesti Negyed*, 17(2). https://library.hungaricana.hu/hu/view/BFLV_bn_64_17_2009_2/?pg=2&layout=s. The citation is from *Főváros Közlöny*, 13 December 1918, p. 2289 and 20 December 1918, pp. 2322–2324 (Accessed 9 September 2021).

Heti Világgazdaság Online (2020) https://hvg.hu/itthon/20200403 (Accessed 20 November 2020).

Hóman-Szekfű (1920) 'Magyarország története, a 1920'. https://mek.oszk.hu/00900/00940/pdf/Homan_Szekfu_-_Magyar_tortenet_7.pdf (Accessed 28 August 2020).

Ishi, H. (2018) *Kansensho no Sekaishi (World History about Infectious Diseases)*, *Kadokawa Sophia Bunko*. Tokyo: Kadokawa.

Johnson, S. (2007) *The Ghost Map: The Story of London's Most Terrifying Epidemic – and How It Changed Science, Cities, and the Modern World (Kansen Chizu: Rekishi wo Kaeta Michi no Byogentai*, translated by Yano, M.). Tokyo: Kawade Shobo Sinsha.

Omori, H. (2004) '1832 nen Pari Korera to Fueisei Jutaku' (in Japanese) (Paris Cholera of 1832 and the 'Unsanitary House'), *Seijo Daigaku Keizai Kenkyu* (Seijo University economic papers), 164, Seijo University, pp. 69–75. www.seijo.ac.jp/pdf/faeco/kenkyu/164/164-oomori.pdf (Accessed 14 September 2020).

Omori, H. (2014) *Furansu Koshu Eiseishi: 19 Seiki Pari no Ekibyo to Jukankyo* (in Japanese) (History of Public Health in France, Epidemics and Living Conditions in 19th Century Paris). Tokyo: Gakujutsu Shuppankai.

Otsuru, A. (2013) *Horyo ga hataraku toki* (in Japanese) (When the Prisoners of War Work). Kyoto: Jimbun Shoin.

Paneth, N. (2004) 'Assessing the Contributions of John Snow to Epidemiology', *Epidemiology*, 15(5): 514–516. doi:10.1097/01.ede.0000135915.94799.00.

Reiman, Z. (2019, 23 November) 'Gyilkosabb a háborúnál – a spanyolnátha Miskolcon'. https://miskolciszemelvenyek.blog.hu/2019/11/23/spanyolnatha_ (Accessed 9 September 2021).

Rózsa, G. ed. (1975) *Magyarország Története III 1790–1849*. Budapest: Tankönyvkiadó.

Snow, J. (1856) 'Cholera and the Water Supply in the South Districts of London in 1854', *Journal of Public Health and Sanitary Review*, 2(7): 239–257. www.ncbi.nlm.nih.gov/pmc/articles/PMC6004154/ (Accessed 21 November 2021).

Statista (2020a, 9 April) 'Do You Wear a Face Mask against Coronavirus (COVID-19)?' www.statista.com/statistics/1104018/hungary-people-wearing-face masks-against-coronavirus/ (Accessed 5 September 2021).

Statista (2020b, 19 November) 'Do You Agree with Making Wearing Face Masks in Public Places Obligatory?' www.statista.com/statistics/1187802/hungary-poll-on-wearing-masks-in-public-places/ (Accessed 5 September 2021).

Valentiny, P. (2020) Spanyolnátha, Budapest, 1918, *KRTK KTI*, Közgazdaság és Regionális Tudományi Kutatóközpont, Közgazdaságtudományi Intézete. www.mtakti.hu/koronavirus/spanyolnatha-budapest-1918/13320/ (Accessed 25 September 2020).

Vincze, M. (2020, 22 March) Száz éve ért véget a Magyarországot is rettegésben tartó spanyolnáthajárvány, Kultúra. https://24.hu/kultura/2020/03/22/spanyolnatha-magyarorszag-influenza-betegseg-virus-jarvany-budapest/ (Accessed 27 September 2020).

4 The mask as a new political and symbolic issue in France in 2020

A qualitative analysis of news media controversies

Xavier Mellet

The sudden appearance of masks on the street as part of the fight against COVID-19 represented a new phenomenon in French society. Before the pandemic, masks were mostly assimilated to Asian countries and enclosed medical spaces. Used by surgeons and other medical professionals, masks were uncommon and never requested for citizen use. Wearing one in public was not a potential solution for people, who simply never did so. The novelty of mask-wearing took on a particular flavour in a national context in which the act of hiding one's face in public was already an important issue due to the controversies surrounding the interpretations of *laïcité*, French secularism. Hiding one's face in the public space has been illegal since April 2011, except for certain specific cases (motorcycle helmets, for example) or when imposed by the authorities (Ministry of Justice, Directorate of Legal and Administrative Information 2020).

In early 2020, debates and issues emerged rapidly, taking several forms, making masks a new topic of interest for political studies. Masks both raised new issues – for example, their efficiency and legitimacy at preventing contamination – and refashioned existing controversies – for example, around governmental policies. In this sense, masks operated as a 'quasi-object' tracing new social relations and framing political controversies and groups, beyond their role as medical objects (Serres 1982, pp. 146–147). Analysing the various forms of the mask – as a concept – during 2020 can reveal how its definition and characteristics were determined by (and highlighting) elements of the French context. This chapter aims at describing the diverse and changing modalities of the meanings given to masks, accompanying political and cultural evolutions provoked by the pandemic. Studying the characteristics of masks will give us a better understanding of contemporary French social and political dynamics.

To this end, this chapter will analyse the evolving meanings given to masks through examining newspaper archives from the beginning of the pandemic in February 2020 to the end of the summer, when mask-wearing became commonplace. The novelty of masks in France encouraged an inductive methodology, which consisted in starting from a 'blank sheet', with no specific pre-established questions and hypotheses, to better follow empirical phenomena. Barney Glazer and Anselm Strauss labelled this 'grounded theory', a radically inductive method that consists

DOI: 10.4324/9781003244127-5

in letting the data guide the research as much as possible to avoid being trapped by preconceived interpretations (Glaser and Strauss 1967). In line with this method, we aimed at creating good conditions for the emergence of analytical categories – codes – interpreted from the datasets rather than from the literature. Doing so required considering all the mentions of masks in the data to follow all the emerging characteristics. A second methodological inspiration for this research was the 'actor-network theory' developed by Bruno Latour, as it consists in following one acting element (*actant*) – here the concept of mask – by describing its empirical connections with other concepts, to smoothly represent its network of relations within a specific ecosystem, which ultimately determines its own conceptual identity (Latour 2005; Latour et al. 2012). This research will look at the pandemic through the meanings given to the concept of mask in a French context.

The dataset is a corpus of newspaper articles, which described the facts and issues related to the pandemic on a daily basis. The press served as a relevant medium for presenting the reader with simplified descriptions and analyses of complex controversies through an agenda-setting process determining which information deserved mention and which keywords deserved to be used (McCombs and Shaw 1972). This chapter will follow the coverage of masks in one major national conservative newspaper, *Le Figaro*, because its readership is larger than that of other similar newspapers and because of its wealth of exploitable articles. First, all articles containing at least one occurrence of '*masqu*' – the common root for the words referring to masks in French – between 21 January 2020 (first occurrence) and 14 December 2020, were extracted from the database Factiva. Second, all articles that were not relevant for the analysis were manually erased from the corpus (for example, when the word 'mask' was designated as an object used in theatre plays, an attitude or intention, etc.). Ultimately, the corpus collected 1,002 articles from *Le Figaro*.

Throughout 2020, the concept of mask metastasized in many directions. The corpus analysis revealed three main empirical modalities reflecting three major lines of inquiry inherent in the French mask experiment.

Mask as a norm. Masks existed as an object intended to protect the population, and, therefore, their use required official regulation. The areas where their use was required gradually expanded, from indoor to outdoor spaces, as governmental policies evolved. This dimension was strongly related to the high prerogatives of – and popular expectations towards – the role of the central state in guaranteeing public safety.

Mask as an issue. Masks existed as a subject of political controversy and political appropriation for opposition figures at first, then for the government and the president, in a context in which opinion polls showed strong popular support for general use. This political or conflictual dimension reflected how distrust towards political elites affected public debates.

Mask as a symbol. Masks were charged with symbolic value, related to the many changes that they provoked, as well as to the inherent characteristics of French society that they revealed. Mask use led to manifestations of anxiety, highlighting the cultural imbrication existing between aesthetics and the role of the face in the projection of the self.

After describing the significant characteristics and phases of the concept of mask in *Le Figaro*, the three modalities will be analysed in the same order, which corresponds to their quantitative importance in the data.

4.1 Five shades of masks: accompanying change

The meanings and issues attached to masks have rapidly evolved in a limited period of time (seven months). Its concept, as it appeared in *Le Figaro* in 2020, went through five phases, forming an 'M' curve, which accompanied changes in political decisions and perceptions. We will describe its main emerging characteristics for each phase – telling the story of the mask – before analysing its three modalities. The following description will avoid quoting all the newspaper articles directly to ensure better readability. Quotations are translated by the author.

1. An external object: 21 January to 20 March. Masks were first considered as a simple descriptive element within stories taking place outside France, mostly in China. They were seen as an Asian or Chinese object and practice: 'will the French end up behaving like Asians?' (20 March, *'les français vont-ils finir par faire comme les asiatiques?'*).

Masks were presented as a useful preventive tool for the first time on 1 February, but questions about their efficiency started appearing in March. They were highly recommended for sick people (4 March) or people with symptoms (14 March), even if, as explained by public health professor Antoine Flahault, 'no study has ever proven their utility for non-symptomatic people, and this option

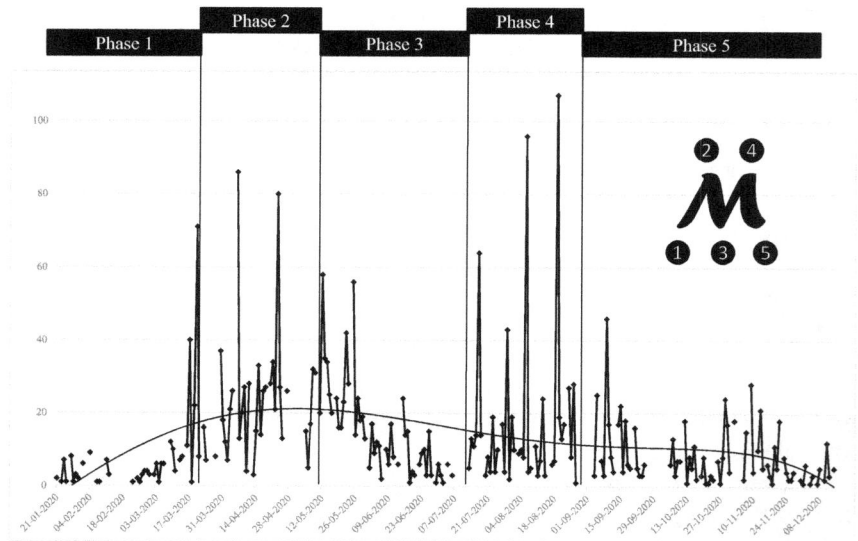

Figure 4.1 The concept of mask in 2020: number of daily occurrences in *Le Figaro*

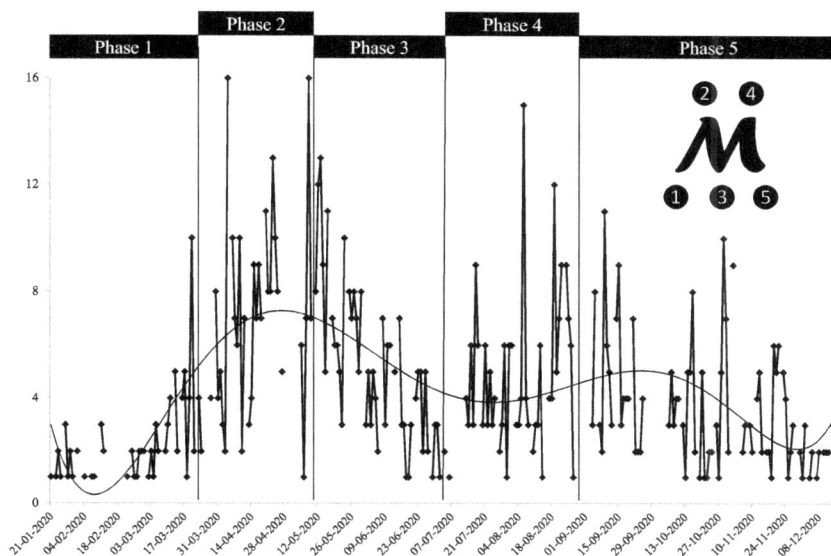

Figure 4.2 The concept of mask in 2020: number of daily articles in *Le Figaro*

[imposing the mask on citizens] is almost impossible considering the current lack of masks in the West' ('*aucune étude n'a jamais démontré leur utilité chez les non-symptomatiques et cette option est quasiment impossible au vu de la carence actuelle de masques en Occident*'). Questioning became more intense on 19 and 20 March, as mask-wearing '[did] not have unanimous support' ('*ne fait pas l'unanimité*') and was perceived as having a low impact, although *Le Figaro* criticised the minister of health, Olivier Véran, for explaining that 'masks are not useful for self-protection' ('*les masques sont inutiles pour se protéger*').

2. A central issue: 21 March to 10 May. The second phase is the one with the highest number of occurrences: masks became a central issue a few days after the beginning of the first confinement of French citizens (from 17 March to 11 May).

This trend started with questions about masks as a potential solution to the rising pandemic, even at the risk of encouraging citizen complacency (3 April). An editorial on 6 April wondered if 'the French must wear a mask to prevent coronavirus propagation?' ('*Les Français doivent-ils tous porter un masque pour freiner la propagation du coronavirus?*'). The mask was described as a precious barrier ('*précieuse barrière*'), and the Academy of Medicine argued in favour of its widespread use.

Public opinion on this topic was measured for the first time through polls showing strong popular support for making masks mandatory within cities (9 April).

A new association between masks and the word 'mandatory' (*'obligatoire'*) was established for France after being established for many foreign countries beyond China (15 April).

President Emmanuel Macron made his first statement about masks on 14 April, when he explained that 'the state will have to enable every citizen to obtain a general public mask' (*'l'État devra permettre à chaque Français de se procurer un masque grand public'*), introducing to the debate the notion of a 'general public mask' (*'masque grand public'*).

The end of this second phase corresponded to the emergence of stories on how the state was supplying masks to the population; on the places where the population was required to wear masks, such as public transportation (from 22 April) and other enclosed spaces; and on the rules to be respected, before the end of the confinement period, on 11 May.

3. Becoming commonplace: 11 May to 6 July. After the confinement period, the number of occurrences diminished, because mask usage in everyday life in France became banal.

It is at this moment that mask-wearing became a matter for political controversy, between the government and its opponents, local and national figures, who criticised a governmental failure and promoted a massive distribution of masks to a population that seemed favourable.

Simultaneously, masks began to be mentioned from an aesthetic or even anthropological perspective. For example, an article analysed their impact on the 'beauty routines' (*'routines de beauté'*, 21 May); masks are frequently described as 'suffocating' (*'suffocant'*) between 28 and 29 May; an article deals with difficulties in wearing a mask on a daily basis, especially at work (10 June).

4. Leaving enclosed spaces: 7 July to 27 August. The number of occurrences rose again in early summer, when new questions emerged about mask-wearing, this time in outdoor environments, in preparation for the back-to-school season.

The physical space where masks were required expanded throughout the two summer months: in the street, at work and on TV shows (*'plateaux télé'*, 20 August).

This expansion was reflected in the political voluntarism of the newly appointed prime minister, Jean Castex (3 July), who appeared regularly in various venues to promote mask-wearing, unlike former prime minister Edouard Philippe. This new official discourse concluded a slow appropriation process of masks by the French government.

5. Being commonplace: from 4 September. Masks appeared less frequently in newspaper articles from September on, mainly because masks were no longer an important issue. No new aspects to masks and mask-wearing are noticeable during this last phase, except for a reflection on the potential continuity of mask use in the future: 'will we have to wear masks eternally? Live in a Japanese way?' (11 September, *'Devra-t-on porter éternellement un masque? Vivre à la japonaise?'*).

4.2 Mask as a norm: the return of the state

When masks became more than a purely descriptive element, mask-wearing was mainly mentioned in *Le Figaro* as a norm to be applied or questioned and a means enforced by the public authorities in the fight against COVID-19. Aspects related to the norms associated with their use appeared during the first confinement period (second phase): masks were required only for ill and symptomatic people before they became 'mandatory' in May, when the confinement ended. Their use was later requested in other places, public transportation, shops and enclosed public spaces, until outside spaces were included in the summer. The territorial expansion of the mask concerned both people (from ill people and medical staff to the entire population) and places (from indoor to outdoor places).

This expansion illustrated the major role of the centralised state in ensuring public safety. Crisis management was centralised and bureaucratic, based on a top-down decision process with the president as the primary definer for the whole nation, explaining how and when to use masks. Nicolas Roussellier described the situation in terms of a return of the 'regalian state', as the guarantor of public safety capable of using violence or constraining its own population (Roussellier 2020). The pandemic revealed how the state is charged with the common good, which has been a common feature of French political culture since the 1789 Revolution and the Napoleonic Empire (Rosanvallon 1993), in contrast with the current perception of public authorities as being incapable of reaching objectives considered as fundamental, leading to collective anxiety, given ongoing high expectations of state action (Gauchet 2016; Bedock 2017).

The situation of crisis illustrated this national specificity in different ways, starting with a combination of popular obedience and criticism towards the implemented measures. The pandemic showed how the state managed to obtain a large degree of popular obedience to the harsh measures – confinement and mask use – despite a high level of distrust in the government and Emmanuel Macron's actions. Contrary to past circumstances, citizens had both the capacity and opportunity to engage in online daily criticism of the measures taken in their name, feeding anxiety and leading to a strange mix of obedience and criticism (Roussellier 2020). The distinction between obedience to the state and distrust towards governmental measures can be perceived in the two modalities of the concept of mask: as a norm massively followed and as an issue fed by dissatisfaction.

Masks were one of the tools at the disposal of the state to enforce its sanitary measures, reducing some individual freedoms for the greater good. Bergeron et al. (2020) highlighted the paradox of public authorities in France who dealt with the crisis by creating new institutions instead of using already-existing resources or dismantling useless ones. The most representative illustration of this bureaucratic creativity – and centrepiece to the French government's handling of the pandemic – consisted in the enforcement of three confinement periods, lasting approximately one month each (17 March to 10 May 2020, 30 October to 15 December 2020, 3 April to 3 May 2021) and applying a prohibition on movement according to different modalities. The initially extra-legal nature of this measure necessitated numerous institutional innovations (Bergeron et al. 2020). The evolution of mask use regulations in France depended on this 'stop and go', alternating between confinement and freedom, a tool for the central state to adapt society to change. It was after the first confinement period that masks became 'mandatory' and commonplace as a condition for freeing the population.

In this context, masks were a means for avoiding confinement and came to represent both freedom and constraint.

Another key feature was the way measures were adopted and presented to the public: in a centralised top-down decision-making process. The president played a major role in the enforcement of such strong measures. Emmanuel Macron himself announced confinement periods and mask use regulations to the population through 'messages to the French' (*'adresses aux français'*) on television – before public debates in the parliament – a direct top-down process reminiscent of Charles de Gaulle's political style (12 and 16 March, 13 April, 14 June; 28 October and 24 November 2020) (elysee.fr). The government's official communications were characterised by much hesitation and error, contributing to a rapid loss of popular trust, until Emmanuel Macron clarified the decisions on television, on 12 and 16 March (Le Clainche 2021). He has since adopted a strong martial tone, declaring, for example, that France was 'at war' (16 March, *'nous sommes en guerre'*) and that the executive power would protect people's health 'at any cost' (12 March, *'quoi qu'il en coûte'*). The sinologist Jean-Louis Rocca has analysed the martial discourse as being a common point between Emmanuel Macron and Chinese president Xi Jinping (Lazar et al. 2020). Unlike the then-Chancellor Angela Merkel in Germany, the French president never admitted any mistake (Le Clainche 2021, p. 436).

Measures implemented in France during the pandemic were actually not evaluated as 'illiberal' and/or 'authoritarian' (Edgell et al. 2021): for example, the parliament did not operate under any restrictions; no discriminatory measures were in place nor official disinformation campaigns or media restrictions. However, there were numerous debates on where to position France on a democratic–authoritarian axis, where extraordinary top-down measures (authoritarian practice?) and strong restrictions of individual liberties (illiberal practice?) were concerned. The official presidential communication was considered too vertical and centralised, lacking explanation and transparency and infantilising the population (Le Clainche 2021). Ultimately, the combination of this dissatisfaction towards an authoritarian approach and strong expectations – leading to obedience – towards the central state and the president remains a major French enigma highlighted by the pandemic and masks, making it a political issue.

4.3 Mask as an issue: opportunities in a time of distrust

The second modality of the concept of mask is more directly political in the sense that it structured the arena of confrontations and discussions among political actors in a context in which distrust in politics is high, as seen by dissatisfaction towards pandemic management by the authorities, and where promoting masks equals public support: public opinion was frequently presented as supporting the extensions of mask-use areas throughout 2020. This situation made masks a political issue for both the opposition forces criticising the government failure and for the government smoothly appropriating masks by promoting their use.

France has become a 'society of distrust' in which citizens do not trust other individuals and the political elites (Algan et al. 2016). For instance, Cautrès and Rouban measured a higher level of distrust towards institutions in France than in Great Britain and Germany (Lazar et al. 2020, chapter 11). The erosion of public support has made it more difficult for elected leaders to govern the country and maintain relatively high popularity. This has been especially the case for the last three presidents: Nicolas Sarkozy (2007–2012, conservative), François Hollande (2012–2017, Socialist) and Emmanuel Macron (centrist) since 2017. In January 2020, before the beginning of the pandemic, Macron's approval rating was at around 30%. Contrary to other European leaders, the French president did not benefit strongly from the pandemic. His support rate rose to 44% in March but stabilised at around 38% from April to December (IPSOS 2020). In addition to political distrust, negative stereotypes of the bureaucracy contributed to spreading doubts towards public authorities (Le Clainche 2021).

The crisis management by the executive power has been evaluated more negatively in France than in other European countries (Lazar et al. 2020, chapter 12). Masks have rapidly become a symbol of the problems arising from the crisis, perceived as badly handled by Emmanuel Macron and his government. An article in *Le Figaro* from February 2021 considered, for example, the bad management of masks at the beginning of the pandemic as an 'original sin' ('*péché originel*') (Boichot 2021). Communication mistakes played a major role in feeding distrust in both the executive power and state action. Nicolas Roussellier highlighted how the initial lack of masks in France – not acknowledged by the president – revealed to the population a weakness of the technocratic dimension of state action in its capacity to organise society based on rational knowledge and expertise (*Etat planificateur*), which was an important aspect of the French economic model during the high-growth period (Roussellier 2020). This dimension materialised in *Le Figaro*, when masks came to represent, by late March, French dependency towards China before the creation of 'made in France' masks in May; it disappeared in June, when the stocks of masks were no longer an issue.

Apart from political hesitation and negative perceptions of masks as a threat – see the next part – many opinion polls revealed massive popular support for the extension of mask use. *Le Figaro* published eight surveys, from 9 April to 20 August, asking whether its readers supported making mask use 'mandatory' in their cities (9 April, 80% yes), public transportation (22 April, 93% yes), all public space (13 May, 69% yes), enclosed public spaces (13 July, 75% yes; 18 July, 89% yes), the street (1 August, 60% yes), companies (18 August, 72% yes), and everywhere outside the home (20 August, 66% yes). Although the readership of *Le Figaro* does not represent the entirety of the French people, such a strong and constant level of support reflected what the majority of the population was thinking. The anti-mask movement in France has, in fact, remained marginal, and, contrary to a common stereotype, anti-maskers have mainly belonged to the middle or upper social class and to the moderate (rather than extreme) left and right of the political spectrum (Bristielle 2020). On a larger scale, the many steps in the extension of mask use enjoyed popular legitimacy and, therefore, fostered political initiatives to promote it.

The territorial expansion of mask-wearing is concomitant with a political appropriation of masks by many political actors, both government and opposition. Starting in April 2020, heads of regions (Laurent Wauquiez and Xavier Bertrand) and mayors (François Bayrou and Anne Hidalgo), already well known in national politics, intervened to promote masks in a challenge to the executive power. For example, Laurent Wauquiez promised to provide all inhabitants of the Auvergne-Rhône-Alpes region with masks (17 April). Pau mayor François Bayrou and Paris mayor Anne Hidalgo favoured making masks mandatory in public transport (20 April). *Le Figaro* noted that 'between Macron and Bertrand, the tension rises', because of the attitude of Xavier Bertrand (head of the Hauts-de-France region), who wore a mask to protest against the instructions he claimed to have received from the Elysée (the presidential palace) that local leaders take off masks so as to obtain 'prettier' pictures (28 May). Local leaders were more present in the news in April and May, when masks were in short supply. From May 2020, national opposition figures also attacked the government on its bad mask management policy and praised the use of masks. It is noteworthy that, except for one early occurrence of the Republican senator Bruno Retailleau (9 April), all the national opponents appearing in the data belonged to the National Rally (*Rassemblement national*), a far-right opposition party, notably Marine Le Pen and Jordan Bardella. Other opposition figures who voiced their criticisms at this time did not appear in *Le Figaro*.

Emmanuel Macron and the government progressively appropriated the concept of mask by integrating it into their messages and actions. First, the new – since 16 February – health minister, Olivier Véran, declared in an interview on 20 March to *Le Figaro* that masks were 'useless for self-protection', arguing that mask-wearing was mainly intended for non-medical staff to protect others when sick. Véran explained that the risk of contamination persisted when the mask was touched with unwashed hands and concluded that masks must be reserved for health professionals. This statement constituted the official governmental position for the next few months, as this description of masks as 'useless' was replicated in newspaper articles – in order to be criticised – very frequently after 20 March (3, 6, 9, 11 and 21 April, 8 and 23 May, 14, 16, 17 and 31 July, 6, 19 and 21 August, 19 November): opponents, journalists and experts referred to this key adjective to illustrate a mistake committed by the authorities.

The official negative discourse on masks evolved on 14 April when President Macron explained that 'as of 11 May, each French person will be in capacity to acquire a ' "general public" mask' ('*à partir du 11 mai, chaque Français devrait pouvoir se procurer un masque "grand public"*'). Instead of making amends for the previous official positions, he proposed a projection over time based on a specific type of mask. Two days later, he tried to be consistent:

> I refuse today to recommend mask use for all, and the government never did it. It would be incomprehensible to recommend it. Medical staff expect to

receive more, which is normal, and it is indeed our objective and production agenda to answer this request (*Je refuse aujourd'hui de recommander le port du masque pour tous et jamais le gouvernement ne l'a fait. Si nous le recommandions, ce serait incompréhensible. Les soignants en souhaitent davantage, c'est normal et c'est bien l'objectif de notre agenda de production que de répondre à cette attente*).

However, in July, the president made a '*volte-face*' (14 July) when he explained on television that 'mask wearing will become mandatory from 1 August in enclosed public spaces' (15 July, '*Le port du masque sera obligatoire le 1ᵉʳ août dans les lieux publics fermés*'). Two days later, an article detailed the evolution of the relationship between the government and masks: it read '"Useless" for the general public in March, the mask becomes "mandatory" in July' ('"*Inutile*" *pour le grand public en mars, le masque devient "obligatoire" en juillet*').

With a new government came a new mask policy. As of summer 2020, masks were promoted by the government, starting with the new prime minister – appointed on 3 July – Jean Castex, who 'wants to extend mask wearing outside' (12 August, '*veut étendre le port du masque à l'extérieur*'). Ministers intervened within their spheres of competence to promote masks. The minister of home affairs, Gérard Darmanin, 'asks the prefects to push for mask wearing 13 August, '*réclame aux préfets de pousser au port du masque en extérieur*'); education minister Jean-Michel Blanquer explained that 'the mask will be "systematic" in class and enclosed spaces for students over 11 years old and all school staff' (21 August, '*le masque sera "systématique" en classe et dans les lieux clos pour les élèves de plus de 11 ans et tous les personnels*'). Labour minister Elisabeth Borne described the measures to be respected in companies (25 August). Ultimately, 'same as the French, the government appropriates the mask' (19 August, '*à l'image des Français, l'exécutif s'approprie le masque*'). As of the end of August, this political dimension disappeared in the data due to the general consensus on the use of masks.

4.4 Mask as a symbol: projecting the self

The third modality of the concept of mask in *Le Figaro* is symbolic: masks are vested with meanings that outweigh their nature as an object used to protect the wearer from disease. Masks became the symbol of many questions and social anxieties, especially in May, when their use became required after the first confinement period. Three dimensions are to be noted: masks related to the self, to everyday life and to altruism.

First, masks were a symbol of self-expression. As explained earlier, France had emphasised the importance of the face as a key element in citizens' presence in the public space and made it illegal to hide it in public. *Le Figaro* frequently argued that the face is the vessel of the self in the public space and that, consequently, the mask made it hard to be oneself when wearing it. Many specialists quickly expressed concern, considering masks to be a factor of collective anxiety for their negative effects on the projection of the self. Masks 'spoil the mood' in restaurants (10 June, '*plombe l'ambiance*') and 'erase expressions of effort or pleasure' (21 May, '*gomme toute expression de l'effort ou du plaisir*'). Masks were perceived as the symbol of a fearful society, or a collective fear, explained as follows by journalist Léa Salamé: 'When the sanitarily correct becomes a norm, when we stop touching others, seeing others because [they are] hidden behind a mask, it scares me' (4 June, '*L'écueil où le sanitairement correct devient la norme, où on ne se touche plus, on ne se voit plus car cachés derrière un masque me fait peur*'). The conservative author Robert Redeker opined as follows: 'The COVID-19 crisis brings a fear of others, not at the origin of society like Hobbes thought, but at its heart. The need to wear a dehumanising mask, which erases what makes us human, reinforces it' (15 October, '*La crise du Covid-19 installe la peur du prochain non plus à l'origine, comme le pensa Hobbes, mais au cœur de la société. L'obligation de porter un masque déshumanisant, qui efface l'humain, la renforce*'). Masks were described as creating psychological inhibitions (8 June), connecting self-expression and collective fear. Presenting masks as a dehumanising factor reflected some cultural characteristics inherent in French society, where mask usage has never been common, unlike Japan. Masks made explicit a hidden threat in the public space, potentially propagating anxiety and mistrust of others.

Second, masks represented everyday practical life changes, with a particular focus on how to avoid damaging one's aesthetic appearance. They were, for example, described as a threat to beards (30 March), as posing a dilemma for people wearing glasses (12 May), and as disrupting makeup habits (13 and 21 May, 9 September) and clothing habits: 'will the mask fit with a bikini?' mused political scientist Jean Viard (24 April, '*Le masque va-t-il s'accorder avec le bikini?*'). Masks were frequently described as inconvenient, especially in summer, when they could be 'suffocating' (29 May, '*suffocant*'), 'unbearable' (24 June, '*insupportable*') or just 'tedious' (21 May, 5 June, 22 and 25 September, '*pénible*'). However, many articles appearing after 12 May, highlighted how masks had become a new norm in people's lives. As Cochoy (2020) explains, masks affected self-identity without hiding it. They became a new way to express one's identity in public through different elements than the smile, such as the eyes, clothing and other aspects related to body language. Yuki et al. (2007) proposed a dual model in which the eyes and mouth were opposed as 'windows to the soul', serving as cues by which emotions could be recognised: the mouth in cultures where emotional expression was the norm (such as the United States), eyes in cultures where emotional subduction was the norm (such as Japan). On which side of the coin is French culture? Collective anxieties due to the generalisation of mask use illustrated the importance of smiling in social interactions.

Finally, masks were sometimes presented as intrinsically linked to altruism, because wearing them meant thinking of others and protecting patients (13 and 14 March). Beyond health, masks were a symbol of equality among citizens: 'Wearing a mask, we are all equal, human beings who risk dying. There are no longer social classes, almost no longer genders and ages' (25 May, '*Avec le masque, nous sommes tous pareils, des êtres humains qui risquent la mort. Il n'y a plus de classe sociale, il n'y a presque plus de genre ni d'âge*'). This last dimension was, however, of lesser importance.

4.5 Conclusion

The novelty of masks in a French context, combined with the comparative dimension inherent in a pandemic affecting various societies simultaneously, made them an interesting case for political studies. In just a few months, masks acquired great significance, taking several forms that revealed or highlighted some characteristics of the French political and social environment. This chapter distinguished between three modalities of the concept of mask within newspaper articles published in *Le Figaro* – mask as a norm, as an issue and as a symbol. For example, it revealed some cultural perceptions inherent in French society, such as the importance of showing one's face in the public space, either for political reasons related to equality or for aesthetics and self-expression. Ultimately, the rapid evolution of the meaning of masks made it difficult to clearly distinguish between their intrinsic properties as a common object for protecting one's face and the characteristics of the environment where the concept of mask appeared and made sense. In the end, it experienced an epiphany: perceived as a threat to social interactions, it became the condition for the return to social life, acquiring major symbolic value as an artefact of solidarity (Cochoy 2020, p. 27).

References

Algan, Y., Cahuc, P. & Zylberberg, A. (2016) *La Fabrique de la défiance . . . et comment s'en sortir*. Paris: Albin Michel, Le Livre de Poche.

Bedock, C. (2017) 'Une démocratie mal en point: attentes et évaluations de l'état de la démocratie en France par les citoyens'. In Gougou, F. & Tiberj, V. (eds) *La déconnexion électorale, état des lieux de la démocratie française*. Paris: Fondation Jean Jaurès.

Bergeron, H., Borraz, O., Castel, P. & Dedieu, F. (2020) *Covid-19: Une crise organisationnelle*. Paris: Presses de Sciences Po.

Boichot, L. (2021, 4 February) Covid-19: la gestion de la crise par l'exécutif ne convainc toujours pas les Français. *Le Figaro*. Available at: https://www.lefigaro.fr/politique/le-scan/covid-19-la-gestion-de-la-crise-par-emmanuel-macron-ne-convainc-toujours-pas-les-francais-20210204

Bristielle, A. (2020) '"Bas les masques!": sociologie des militants anti-masques', *Fondation Jean Jaurès*. Available at: www.jean-jaures.org/publication/bas-les-masques-sociologie-des-militants-anti-masques/ (Accessed 4 May 2021).

Cochoy, F. (2020) 'L'envers du masque'. *Esprit*, 10, pp. 24–27.

Edgell, A. B., Lachapelle, J., Lührman, A. & Maerz, S. F. (2021) 'Pandemic backsliding: Violations of democratic standards during Covid-19', *Social Science & Medicine*, 285.

Gauchet, M. (2016) *Comprendre le malheur français*. Paris: Stock.

Glaser, B. & Strauss, A. (1967) *The discovery of grounded theory: Strategies for qualitative research*. Chicago, IL: Aldine.

IPSOS (2020, 16 December) *Baromètre Politique Ipsos-Le Point: la cote de popularité d'Emmanuel Macron se stabilise, celle de Jean Castex progresse sensiblement*. Available at: www.ipsos.com/fr-fr/barometre-politique-ipsos-le-point-la-cote-de-popularite-demmanuel-macron-se-stabilise-celle-de

Latour, B. (2005) *Reassembling the social: An introduction to actor-network-theory.* Oxford: Oxford University Press.

Latour, B., Jensen, P., Venturini, T., Grauwin, S. & Boullier, D. (2012) 'The whole is always smaller than its parts – a digital test of Gabriel Tardes' monads'. *British Journal of Sociology*, 63, pp. 590–615.

Lazar, M., Plantin, G. & Ragot, X. (eds) (2020) *Le monde d'aujourd'hui : Les sciences sociales au temps de la Covid.* Paris: Presses de Sciences Po.

Le Clainche, M. (2021) 'Covid-19: Les défis de la communication de crise (mars 2020-mars 2021)'. *Revue Française d'Administration Publique*, 178, pp. 433–447.

McCombs, M. & Shaw, D. (1972) 'The agenda-setting function of mass media'. *Public Opinion Quarterly*, 36.

Ministry of Justice, Directorate of Legal and Administrative Information (2020, 3 September) *Can you hide your face in a public place?* Available at: www.service-public.fr/particuliers/vosdroits/F21613?lang=en

Rosanvallon, P. (1993) *L'État en France de 1789 à nos jours.* Paris: Seuil, Points Histoire.

Roussellier, N. (2020) 'L'Etat à l'âge de la crise sanitaire'. *Etudes*, 9, pp. 33–44.

Serres, M. (1982) *Genèse.* Paris: Grasset.

Yuki, M., Maddux, W. & Masuda, T. (2007) 'Are the windows to the soul the same in the East and West? Cultural differences in using the eyes and mouth as cues to recognize emotions in Japan and the United States'. *Journal of Experimental Social Psychology*, 43(2).

5 Between 'mouth-nose-protection' and 'muzzle'

Mask-wearing in German public debate

Joachim Scharloth

On 18 September 2021, an alleged politically motivated murder occurred at a filling station in Idar-Oberstein, Rhineland-Palatinate, Germany. According to the investigations to date, on a Saturday evening, a 49-year-old man entered the kiosk at the filling station without a mask and placed two six-packs of beer on the counter at the cash register. The 20-year-old cashier reminded him of the obligation to wear a mask. Shortly after, the man left the filling station, making threatening gestures. At around 9:45 p.m., the suspect again entered the filling station, this time wearing a mouth-to-nose mask. At the cash register, he pulled down the mask. The cashier advised the man again to comply with the requirement to wear a mask. Instead of putting the mask back on, the man drew a revolver and fired a fatal shot at the 20-year-old student from Idar-Oberstein. He then fled on foot but later handed himself into the police. He was arrested and gave as a motive that the pandemic was weighing heavily on him. He had felt cornered and 'saw no other way out' than to make a mark. He stated that the victim seemed to him to be 'responsible for the overall situation, since he enforced the rules' (SWR 2021). Furthermore, in his interview, he stated that he rejected the COVID-19 protection measures.

This event highlights how the discussion around wearing masks in the Federal Republic of Germany is far more than a question of hygiene. Rather, the mask has become a symbol that can be politically interpreted in different, sometimes radical, ways.

Germany is not a traditionally mask-wearing country, at least not in everyday life. The face is considered to be a mirror of the personality. At the same time, the mask is associated with disguise or is representative of a sophisticated game of identity. Criminals wear masks to protect themselves from identification. However, masks can also be worn in theatres or at carnivals, where reality is temporarily suspended and people can assume another identity. In years gone by, masks were used as a punishment. In the 17th and 18th centuries, delinquents – such as adulterers and slanderers – were sentenced to wear a mask of shame (known as a scold's bridle). The person was reduced to the level of their crime by the mask and made to appear as the community saw them. While the medical mask signifies hygiene, it also demonstrates the risk of infection. During the COVID-19 pandemic, it has become prevalent in everyday life, but at the same time, it has become an object of various designations.

DOI: 10.4324/9781003244127-6

This chapter will explore the debate around mask-wearing in Germany in the wake of the COVID-19 pandemic, focusing on the politicisation of the mask. As it is predominantly the radical right of the political spectrum that has framed mask-wearing as more than a hygiene measure, the analysis focuses on criticisms of masks in right-wing online discourses.

The chapter is organised as follows: Section 5.1 traces the development of the legal and institutional framework of the COVID-19 policy in Germany, with a specific focus on legal ordinances on the wearing of masks. Section 5.2 explores critical protest events to show how the anti-COVID-19 movement has become radicalised and developed into a far-right movement. Section 5.3 presents the theoretical and methodological frameworks of the study. Drawing on linguistic theory, the concept of nomination is introduced, and the power of linguistic naming as a means of structuring reality is discussed. Section 5.4 presents the data basis, and Section 5.5 presents the results of the corpus-based study: the development of interpretive frames over the course of the pandemic based on the distribution of linguistic references. The research question aims to address whether the criticism of COVID-19 policies is related to the political measures that were put in place or whether these measures were simply a pretext for a more general agenda aiming to subvert trust in Germany's political system.

5.1 The legal and institutional framework for the handling of a pandemic in Germany

The Federal Republic of Germany consists of the national state (federal government, *Bund*) and 16 partly sovereign states, the federal states (*Bundesländer*), which in turn perform their own governmental functions. In Germany, infection control is a shared responsibility of the federal and state governments. As a result, health policy measures were implemented at different times and, in some cases, in different forms in various states. Therefore, the following chronological account does not provide a detailed list of all measures but is based on the major milestones of the country's COVID-19 policy.

The general basis for government action at the federal and state levels is the Infection Protection Act (*Infektionsschutzgesetz*, IfSG). This act was ratified on 20 July 2000 and came into force on 1 January 2001. It is a federal law concerning common or communicable diseases in humans and regulates the necessary cooperation and collaboration between federal, state and local authorities, physicians, veterinarians, hospitals, scientific institutions and other stakeholders. It is intended to prevent communicable diseases, detect infections at an early stage and prevent their further spread. The law allows the authorities to sanction measures for the prevention and control of communicable diseases. While the term *prevention* refers to preventing the emergence of communicable diseases, the term *control* refers to the prevention of the spread of existing diseases. However, the IfSG restricts fundamental rights. These include physical integrity and freedom of the person, freedom of movement, freedom of assembly, mail and postal secrecy and inviolability of the home. In addition, a ban on professional activities can be imposed (IfSG 2021). The four federal Laws for the Protection of the Population in the Event of an Epidemic Situation of National Significance (*Gesetz zum Schutz der Bevölkerung bei einer epidemischen Lage von nationaler Tragweite*) enacted during the pandemic made amendments to the Infection Protection Act.

However, at the beginning of the pandemic, there was no talk of new legislative initiatives. Rather, the government assessed the risk to the German population as low and the virus, in general, as far less dangerous than SARS (Ärzteblatt 2020a). Yet uncertainty spread among the population, and as early as 29 January 2020, the day after the first confirmed case in Germany, newspapers were reporting that masks were sold out (Koopmann 2020).

The following weeks were marked by discussions about tests, tracking, possible travel restrictions and the procurement of protective material for medical professionals. On 29 February 2020, Ursula Heinen-Esser, minister of health for North Rhine-Westphalia, advised against panic buying (WDR 2020). The *Robert Koch Institute* (RKI), the German federal government agency and research institute responsible for disease control and prevention, published guidelines stating that 'there is insufficient evidence that wearing oral-nasal protection significantly reduces the risk of infection for a healthy person' (Bayerischer Hausärzteverband 2020). In early March, Germany prohibited the export of protective masks, Mediclinic gloves and hazmat suits.

The situation started to change as cases rose. On 13 March 2020, after a meeting of the Conference of Education Ministers, all states decided to close their schools. On 22 March, the federal and state governments agreed to impose comprehensive restrictions regarding social contact. Among other things, a minimum distance of at least 1.50 m between people was introduced in public spaces, and people were only permitted in public spaces either alone or with one other person from outside their household. Restaurants, cafés and numerous other service businesses were closed (Bundesregierung 2020a).

On 27 March 2020, the first Act on the Protection of the Population in the Event of an Epidemic Situation of National Significance was passed (IfSG 2020). It authorised the Federal Ministry of Health, without the consent of the Bundesrat (the legislative body that represents the 16 federated states), to take measures with regard to the supply of medicines. This meant that in addition to the administrative competence of the federal states, in the event of an epidemic emergency caused by a transboundary communicable disease spreading throughout the entire federal territory, the Federal Ministry of Health could take steps to purchase and provide narcotics, medical devices, laboratory diagnostics, medical aids, items of personal protective equipment and products for disinfection. Furthermore, it meant that they could also increase human resources in the healthcare system.

On 15 April 2020, the federal government and all states extended restrictions regarding contact and, for the first time, strongly recommended that citizens use everyday masks (*Alltagsmasken*, cloth face masks), especially on public transport and when shopping in retail stores (Bundeskanzlerin 2020). Between 22 and 29 April, all states sanctioned mandatory mask-wearing on public transport and in shops (Deutsche Welle 2020). Due to the measures showing rapid success and case numbers dropping, the first relaxations of the pandemic measures were adopted on 6 May 2020. However, contact restrictions, as well as mask mandates, remained in place. A Second Law on the Protection of the Population in the Event of an Epidemic Situation of National Significance (19 May 2020) further supplemented the regulations and measures that had already been adopted.

After a relaxed summer with very low numbers of cases, mandatory masks in schools became an important public issue with the end of the summer holidays and warnings of a seasonal increase in illness. On 20 August 2020, the Münster Higher Administrative Court approved the mandatory use of masks in school lessons. There was also controversy regarding whether masks should be mandated in outdoor public spaces. Federal Health Minister Jens Spahn spoke out against nationwide mask requirements in public spaces on national television on 24 September 2020 (NDR 2020). In October 2020, Klaus Reinhardt, president of the German Medical Association, said that if sufficient distance could be maintained, mask requirements in public spaces would be excessive (Ärzteblatt 2020b). Nevertheless, many cities and administrative districts decided that when the case numbers were high, people in outdoor public spaces had to wear mouth-to-nose coverings.

With the buildup of the second wave from October 2020, the federal government and the states agreed on a flexible reaction according to the incidence rate, the so-called *hotspot strategy* (Bundesregierung 2020b). In counties with an incidence rate above a certain threshold, restrictions on social contacts were imposed. However, when these measures did not sufficiently contain the pandemic, representatives of the federal government and the states agreed, on 28 October 2020, to enact a *lockdown light*, i.e. nationwide restrictions on public life and social contacts (Ärztezeitung 2020a). This lockdown was extended on 25 November, this time based on the third Law for the Protection of the Population in the Event of an Epidemic Situation of National Significance, which was enacted on 18 November 2020. This law allowed the government to impose the following measures, among others: ordering social distancing in public areas; an obligation to wear a mouth-to-nose covering (mask obligation); curfews or contact restrictions in private as well as public areas; prohibitions or restrictions as regards recreational, cultural and sporting events; obligation to draw up and apply hygiene measures for businesses and facilities; prohibition or restriction of overnight stays; and ordering the processing of customers' contact data, including guests or event participants.

As case numbers were still rising in December 2020, a 'hard lockdown' was agreed on 13 December (Ärztezeitung 2020b). This included the closure of most shops and service businesses. Day care centres and schools were closed or converted to distance learning. Businesses had to switch to home-based operations as much as possible. Tighter mobility restrictions were adopted for areas with high rates of infection. In addition, other infection-control measures were established, such as the obligation to wear medical masks in public transport and stores. All at-risk groups get access to free or discounted FFP2 masks, i.e. level 2 Filtering Face Pieces, comparable with N95 respirators (Bundesgesundheitsministerium

2020). From 18 January 2021, an FFP2 mandate was introduced in Germany, starting in the state of Bavaria, on public transport and in retail outlets (BR 2021).

It took until 3 March 2021 for federal and state governments to agree to gradually relax the measures but only in the case of a stable incidence rate of less than 50 new infections. Shortly after, the so-called *mask affair* became public. Politicians from the governing Christian Democrats (from the CDU and CSU parties) had made considerable profits through commissions when procuring masks during the first months of the pandemic.[1]

From 23 April to 30 June 2021, the fourth Law for the Protection of the Population in the Event of an Epidemic Situation of National Significance, colloquially known as the Federal Emergency Brake, was applied nationwide in Germany (Bundesregierung 2021). The legal regulations took effect on 24 April 2021 in all counties and independent cities where the 7-day incidence rate was exceeding 100 for 3 consecutive days. These regulations usually resulted in stricter contact restrictions. In addition, there was a curfew from 10 p.m. to 5 a.m. in the affected counties and independent cities.

5.2 Protests over COVID-19 policies

Although the anti-COVID-19 measures were judged adequate or even not extensive enough by 75% to 80% of the German population, they were opposed by about one-fifth of citizens (Infratest dimap 2021). This opposition was due to several factors, such as the restrictions on fundamental rights, the view that COVID-19 was just a mild form of influenza and finally the denial of the existence of the disease. The protest movement that had formed experienced its first peak in the summer of 2020 when the incidence rate was low. At the beginning of the movement, many different groups called for rallies, but from summer 2020, the *Querdenken* movement started to dominate the protests over COVID-19 policies. The original group from the Stuttgart area also held various demonstrations in Berlin.

On 29 August 2020, more than 43,000 people (Correctiv 2020) participated in a demonstration demanding the end of all anti-COVID-19 measures and the immediate resignation of the government. *Querdenken* founder Michael Ballweg even called for a new Constituent Assembly (Heidtmann 2020). In total, 450 to 500 people, among them many supporters of the *Reichsbürger* movement[2] and Holocaust deniers, overpowered the barriers in front of the *Reichstag* building, occupied the steps and tried to enter the building, at which point they were stopped by the police. Many of the demonstrators waved the war flags of the German Reich.

More than 10,000 people demonstrated in the immediate vicinity of the Reichstag on 18 November 2020, the day of the vote on the third Law for the Protection of the Population in the Event of an Epidemic Situation of National Significance. During the demonstration, 77 police officers were injured, and 365 demonstrators were arrested.

On 21 April 2021, around 8,000 people gathered in Berlin to demonstrate against the amendment to the fourth Law for the Protection of the Population in the Event of an Epidemic Situation of National Significance, which they compared with the Enabling Act of the National Socialists in 1933. Due to the ongoing and widespread violations of the pandemic law, the police dissolved the demonstrations. Numerous demonstrators pursued violent confrontations with the police. A total of 250 people were arrested on that day.

It is not surprising that since December 2020, regional sections of the *Querdenken* movement have been classified as extremist and monitored by the Federal Office for the Protection of the Constitution. In fact, from April 2021, the whole movement has been monitored.

The history of the COVID-19 policy protests in Germany is, as shown by these examples of critical events, one of political radicalisation regarding right-wing extremist attitudes and militancy, which aim to abolish the current liberal–democratic order.

5.3 Theoretical and methodological approach

When looking at the social meaning of an item, it is important to consider the different ways it is linguistically referred to in society. Reality is not specific. Instead, several descriptions of reality are possible. When the meaning of a cultural entity is contested in society, different competing names or labels can emerge. When certain words become established in linguistic usage, this usually signifies that a certain interpretation has become hegemonic. Whether the attack on the Capitol in Washington on 6 January 2021 is called an act of protest against state injustice, as covered by the First Amendment, or an attempted coup d'état is not simply a question of right or wrong. Both interpretations are highly plausible, at least for part of the American society in each case. Public debate will decide which term will prevail.

Language-in-politics research is concerned with strategies to designate cultural entities or politically controversial matters so that the political action of the group using them appears adequate or necessary. This approach is evident in the concept of nomination. The basis of nomination theory is that linguistic conceptualisation and object constitution go hand in hand and that it is only in acts of communication that objects or facts can be made available intersubjectively (cf. Wengeler 2017, p. 28). Linguistic object construction owes much to the principles of perspectivisation (Köller 2004) relating to hiding and highlighting (Spieß 2017, p. 99): in the use of a particular expression to refer to an object, certain aspects of meaning are emphasised, whereas others recede into the background (cf. Klein 1991).

When calling a mask a *Mund-Nasen-Schutz* (mouth–nose protection), its function of protection is at the forefront. When calling it a *Zwangsmaulkorb* (coercive muzzle), the mask is framed as a medium of coercion that, rather than protecting its wearer, provides protection for those who have imposed it. Obviously, hiding and highlighting are not simply descriptive functions of nomination. Rather, in the act of linguistic reference, an evaluation is also expressed, and with it, a deontic dimension of meaning is invoked. *Protection* is something that has a positive connotation and is, therefore, desirable. Protecting oneself and others is a socially desirable action. On the contrary, a *muzzle* is a restriction of freedom. *Muzzles* are for dangerous animals, and humans should not have to wear them.

The linguistic considerations in this section demonstrate that references to masks hold relevant specific aspects of the referenced object and hide others. They furthermore have pragmatic-evaluative and deontic dimensions. With regard to the function of the mask in public discourse, we must ask which of its aspects are often established as relevant and which, if any, are hidden. We must also consider which evaluations and attitudes are expressed by it and what calls to action are associated with the words used.

To trace the different nomination strategies in public discourse, large text corpora were examined.

To start with, as many different terms for masks as possible were identified in the text corpora. This was done by both studying central texts and specifically querying relevant lexemes used as names for masks in compounds. This group included expressions referring to parts of the body covered by masks, the excretions of respiratory organs and fabrics, garments and materials for covering or veiling. Aside from *Maske* (mask), these were the lexemes *Mund* (mouth), *Maul* (mouth), *Nase* (nose), *Rachen* (throat), *Gesicht* (face), *Knebel* (gag), *Binde* (bandage/sanitary pad), *Schal* (scarf), *Lappen* (rag), *Filter* (filter), *Atem* (breath), *Aerosol* (aerosol), *Spucke* (spit), *Rotz* (snot), *Bedeckung* (covering), *Helm* (helmet), *Burka* (burka), *Haube* (hood), *Vorrichtung* (device) and *Blocker* (blocker). This search resulted in 239 different terms for the cultural concept of 'mask'.

In the second part of the process, these lexemes were categorised into terms referring to the mask as a commercial product, terms regarding the form or function of the mask and mask-critical terms. As the focus was on mask-critical discourse, the latter category was further categorised into semantic subgroups. Subsequently, the distribution of these lexemes and lexeme categories was examined in two ways: first, the distribution in different media, and second, the frequency of their use over the course of the pandemic. The latter was correlated with critical events in public discourse and the incidence rates during the pandemic.

The final step of the analysis identified compounds in which *Maske* (mask) appeared as a modifier. This needs further explanation. In German, the most productive word formation process is compounding, creating lexemes consisting of more than one stem. Compounds are written in one word. Most compounds are endocentric compounds. They consist of a head containing the basic meaning and modifiers, which restrict this meaning. For example, a *Kinderarzt* (paediatrician) is an *Arzt* (doctor) but one taking care of *Kinder* (children). By analysing compounds with *Maske* as a modifier, one can determine which other words are modified or specified in meaning by the term 'mask'. The analysis revealed 70 lexemes of this type, e.g. *Maskenterror* (mask terror) and *Maskenlüge* (mask lie). These terms were again semantically categorised, and the frequency of occurrence of the words in each category was examined in different media corpora.

5.3.1 Corpora

The corpora were selected to represent the full spectrum of opinions in the mainstream media's discourse as represented by the daily *Die Welt*, and the discourse of critics of the COVID-19 policy, using the news platform *PI-News* as an example.

Die Welt is one of few national German daily newspapers. The paper is read by people on the bourgeois-conservative spectrum. The Internet news portal of Welt Group was launched in 1995 under the name *Welt Online*. At welt.de, users can access an electronic newspaper archive of all articles published since its digitisation in May 1995. For the present study, all articles from 1 January 2020 to 1 July 2021 were automatically downloaded and processed as part of the analysis.

The newspaper strongly criticised other media outlets for their coverage of COVID-19 and policies to curb the pandemic. For example, Andreas Rosenfelder, head of *Die Welt*'s feuilleton section, accused the media of preferring to criticise the government's detractors instead of taking a critical look at its measures. 'Or people have been critical of the critics, lumping them all into the camp of corona deniers and conspiracy theorists', he told the radio station *Deutschlandradio Kultur* in an interview in January 2021.[3]

Due to the fact that the newspaper made the effort to critically examine the effectiveness of the COVID-19 policy, allowing controversial critics to have their say and giving plenty of space to those on the fringe, it can be seen as a bridge between the *Querdenken* movement and the broad social consensus of the proponents of the measures. Therefore, it provides interesting and relevant data for the study.

The news platform *Politically Incorrect* (short form *PI-News*) was founded in 2004. The platform names its central political standpoints as 'news against the mainstream – pro-American – pro-Israeli – against the Islamisation of Europe – for the constitution and human rights'. However, media and political scientists agree that *PI-News* is a central platform for alternative news from the far right (Weisskircher 2020) and the most important online platform of the German-speaking Islamophobic scene (Schneiders 2016). Since its launch, the platform has been characterised by a monothematic and negative selection of topics and biased and distorting framing (Müller, 2008). The popularity of *PI-News* grew during the so-called refugee crisis (Weisskircher 2020). During the pandemic, the platform has been a forum for critics of measures, COVID-19 deniers and conspiracy theorists.

According to the *Reuters Institute Digital News Report* of 2019, *PI-News* ranks third in the new right's media ranking after the weekly newspaper *Junge Freiheit* and the monthly magazine *Compact* (Newman 2019). User comments play a significant role in the popularity of the platform and are often far more radical than the posts themselves (Müller 2008).

The following empirical study is concerned with both the articles and comments. All articles published from 1 January 2020 to 1 July 2021 were scraped from the online platform, together with their comments, and processed for analysis.

Table 5.1 Number of texts and number of words in each subcorpus

Source	Number of Texts	Number of Words
PI-News articles	3,800	2,059,521
PI-News comments	343,747	24,552,771
Die Welt	312,708	64,737,303

While software written by the author was used for scraping and pre-processing the data, TreeTagger (Schmid 1995) was used for lemmatisation and annotation with part of speech information. Overall, the empirical basis for the analyses in the following sections consists of three subcorpora (*Die Welt*, *PI-News* articles, *PI-News* comments), the size and composition of which are presented in Table 5.1.

5.4 Findings

5.4.1 *Mask discourse, incidence rates and critical events*

The first research question is whether public discourse regarding masks is driven by the infection rate or by political and discursive events. To answer this question, the frequency of occurrence of all 239 terms referencing a mask was counted week by week in all three corpora and correlated with the incidence rate in Germany. This assumes that an intensification of the discourse on a topic also results in an increase of thematically relevant terms. If the incidence rate increases, one could suppose that the need to wear a mask will become more obvious to the public and will, therefore, be discussed more frequently in the media.

Yet, as presented in Figure 5.1, there is no correlation between incidence rate and occurrence frequency of the terms. Only in the first phase do both incidence and the number of linguistic references increase together, which is to be expected insofar as the emergence of a new phenomenon is accompanied by a need to name it. Thus, the reason for the variation in the frequency of use of mask-related expressions must be related to events that are not directly dependent on the infection rate. Rather, the variation must be caused by political measures directly related to mask procurement and wearing as well as mask-related discursive events.

The highlighted phases in Figure 5.1 with relative maxima in the usage of mask-related terms can be attributed to the following events presented in Section 5.1:

- Phase 1, calendar weeks 14 and 15, 2020: First mask mandate in a German city. German National Academy of Sciences Leopoldina advocates for a nationwide mask mandate.
- Phase 2, calendar weeks 17 and 18, 2020: RKI, the federal government and state governments recommend wearing a mouth–nose covering. First mask

Incidence and Frequency of Mask-Related Terms

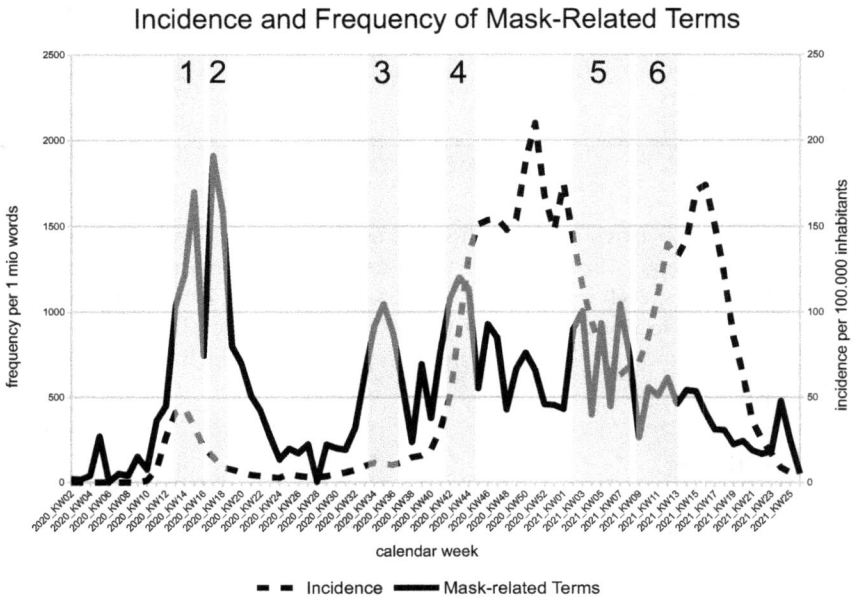

Figure 5.1 Frequency of occurrence of terms referencing masks in all subcorpora (primary y-axis) and incidence rate (secondary y-axis) per calendar week from 1 January 2020 to 1 July 2021

Source: author's own illustration

mandate in the state of Saxonia. The wearing of masks on public transport and in stores becomes mandatory across the whole of Germany.
- Phase 3, calendar weeks 35 and 36, 2020: The Münster Higher Administrative Court approves the mandatory use of masks in schools. Biggest *Querdenken* demonstration so far in Berlin with excessive violations of social distancing rules and mask mandate on August 29.
- Phase 4, calendar weeks 43 and 44, 2020: Klaus Reinhardt, president of the German Medical Association, says that the wearing of masks in public places would be excessive if sufficient distance can be maintained. A *lockdown light* is imposed.
- Phase 5, calendar week 3, 2021: FFP2 masks become mandatory on local public transport and in retail outlets.
- Phase 6, calendar week 10, 2021: News of the *mask affair* breaks. Several cases surface of members of the CDU and CSU in the German *Bundestag* and state parliaments regarding their acceptance of advantages in connection with the procurement of respiratory protection masks.

5.4.2 Nomination and framing

From a nomination-theoretical perspective, it is of interest to see which aspects of masks are defined as relevant through their specific designation in the three sub-corpora. To track down the relevant semantic dimensions, we calculated which of the 239 mask-related terms occurred significantly more often in each sub-corpus (*Die Welt*, *PI-News* articles, *PI-News* comments) when compared with the other two subcorpora. The calculation was based on a normalised frequency value (relative frequency per 1 million words). The log-likelihood ratio served as a significance measure; only words with a LLR p-value < 0.05 were considered statistically significant. The outcome of the analyses was visualised as a word cloud. The size of the words in the word cloud represents their logarithmic frequency, i.e. the more often a word occurs in the subcorpus, the bigger its size in the word cloud.

Figure 5.2 demonstrates that in *Die Welt* articles, standardised expressions and technical terms for masks were used significantly more often than in the other subcorpora.

In contrast, in articles from the far-right news platform *PI-News*, satirical expressions (*spit hood*, *pest mask*), terms that refer to the mask as a means of disguise (*taqiyya*[4] *mask, camouflage mask, character mask, balaclava*[5]), expressions that emphasise the coercive character of masks (*muzzle, corona muzzle, coercive mask, scold's bridle*) and one term using the person allegedly responsible for mask mandates as a modifier (*Merkel mask*) occur significantly more often than in the other subcorpora (Figure 5.3). It is obvious that the mask is not considered a serious method of controlling the pandemic but rather as a means of oppression

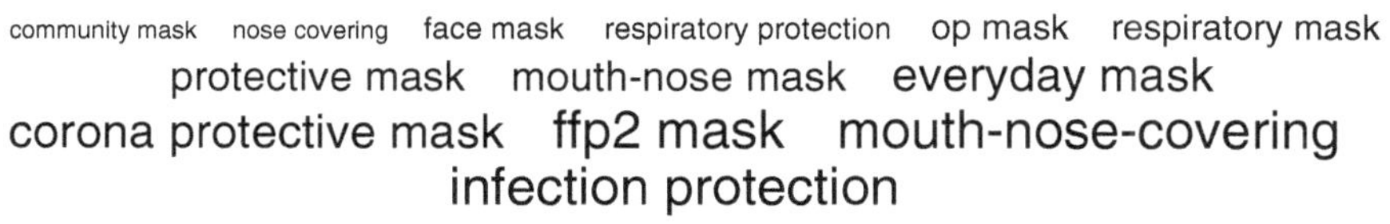

Figure 5.2 Mask-related terms occurring significantly more often in newspaper articles from *Die Welt*

Source: author's own illustration

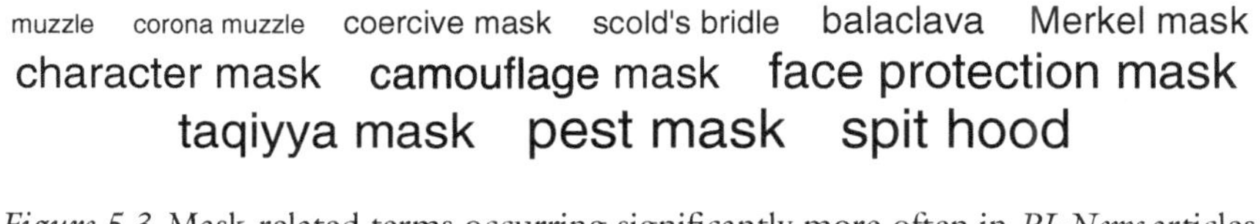

Figure 5.3 Mask-related terms occurring significantly more often in *PI-News* articles

Source: author's own illustration

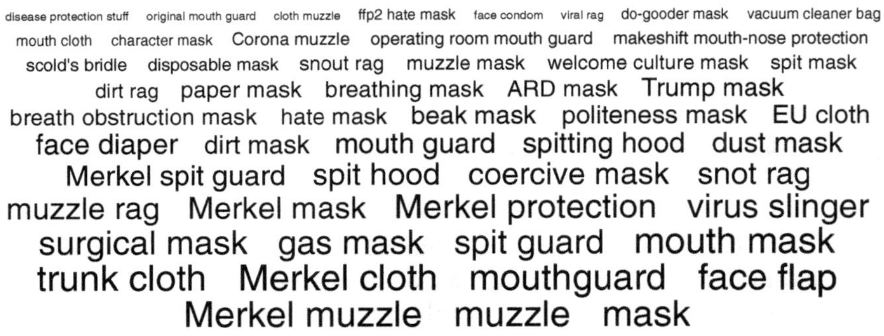

disease protection stuff   original mouth guard   cloth muzzle   ffp2 hate mask   face condom   viral rag   do-gooder mask   vacuum cleaner bag
mouth cloth   character mask   Corona muzzle   operating room mouth guard   makeshift mouth-nose protection
scold's bridle   disposable mask   snout rag   muzzle mask   welcome culture mask   spit mask
dirt rag   paper mask   breathing mask   ARD mask   Trump mask
breath obstruction mask   hate mask   beak mask   politeness mask   EU cloth
face diaper   dirt mask   mouth guard   spitting hood   dust mask
Merkel spit guard   spit hood   coercive mask   snot rag
muzzle rag   Merkel mask   Merkel protection   virus slinger
surgical mask   gas mask   spit guard   mouth mask
trunk cloth   Merkel cloth   mouthguard   face flap
Merkel muzzle   muzzle   mask

Figure 5.4 Mask-related terms occurring significantly more often in *PI-News* comments

Source: author's own illustration

and disguise. Furthermore, the mask is equated with the political leadership of the Federal Republic of Germany.

In Figure 5.4, we can see that the vocabulary used in the user comments of *PI-News* is more diversified overall. Therefore, expressions occur significantly more often than in the other subcorpora. Here, we also find satirical expressions critical of wearing masks, often questioning their effectiveness (*face condom, vacuum cleaner bag, spit mask, spitting hood, spit guard, face diaper, virus slinger, trunk cloth, breath obstruction mask*), and some that are outright derogatory (*snout rag, dirt rag, ffp2 hate mask*). Except for the term *mask*, terms that emphasise the coercive nature of the measures have the highest significance value (*muzzle, Merkel muzzle, coercive mask, muzzle mask, Corona muzzle*).

The term *muzzle* as a metaphor can be interpreted in different ways. On the one hand, a muzzle is a device that restricts the freedom of a dog, its main purpose being to protect other people or animals. In this sense, the mask can be understood as an instrument used by the government to protect itself from the population. On the other hand, the term 'muzzle' in German also figuratively refers to a ban on speech and thus to an encroachment on the freedom of expression.

Another category of expressions politicises the mask. This is done by making German chancellor Angela Merkel personally responsible for the allegedly misguided mask policies (*Merkel muzzle, Merkel mask, Merkel spit guard, Merkel protection, Merkel cloth*). Furthermore, mask and mask-wearing is also related to other policy fields, namely, migration and EU policy (*do-gooder[6] mask, welcome culture mask, EU cloth*).

Critics of the mask policy feel that wearing masks interferes with their fundamental rights. As demonstrated by the concept of the muzzle, this is in relation not only to the requirement to wear mouth–nose protection but also to the

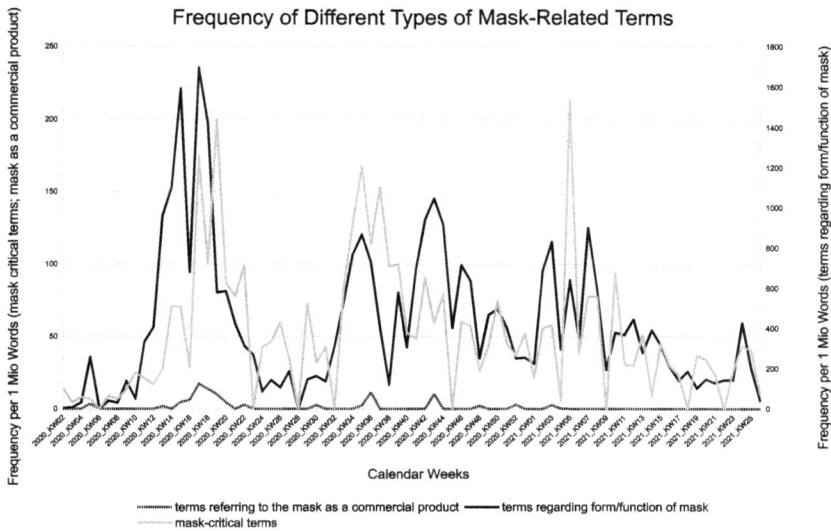

Figure 5.5 Frequency of occurrence of semantic categories of mask-related terms per calendar week from 1 January 2020 to 1 July 2021

Source: author's own illustration

democratic rights of freedom. The mask is a symbol of restrictions on freedom and a reference to a potential future dictatorship. The performative effect of the wearing of masks is that the citizen becomes a dangerous person who poses a threat to the government. Criticisms of the mask are also criticisms of the head of government as a representative of the state.

Figure 5.5 demonstrates that expressions criticising the mask and, thus, the system and its representatives did not start to take shape during the course of the pandemic but were part of the critics' repertoire from the start of the public debate. The graph shows the distribution of three categories of terms in which the 239 mask-related expressions were grouped: terms referring to the mask as a commercial product, terms regarding the form and function of masks and mask-critical terms. Even though terms regarding the form or function of masks occur about seven times more often on average, mask-critical terms appear from calendar week 13, with *muzzle* being the most popular. From calendar week 17, *Merkel muzzle* became a popular term.

The peaks in the graph representing the development of the use of mask-critical terms correspond to the big *Querdenken* demonstration in Berlin where there were excessive violations of social distancing rules and the mask mandate on August 29 (calendar week 36, 2020). They also correspond to a campaign against mandatory FFP2 masks in early February (calendar week 5, 2021). The data demonstrate that criticism of masks did not gradually develop as a result of the pandemic measures into a general criticism of the political system. Rather, the interpretation suggests that the term 'mask' was used from the start to reinforce an already widespread mood in the radical right-wing milieu, namely, that the Federal Republic of Germany is an undemocratic regime ruled by a dictatorial government.

Criticism of mask mandates is, therefore, a pretext to pursue a more general agenda aimed at subverting trust in Germany's political system. In doing so, the radical right follows a pattern that has been evident many times in the past. On virtually every political issue of national scope, the radical right and its parliamentary arm, the Alternative for Germany (AfD), occupy positions of fundamental opposition. They call for Germany to leave the euro, to leave the European Union (the so-called *Dexit*) and to suspend the basic right to asylum. Furthermore, they oppose vaccination against COVID-19 and all other measures to contain the pandemic.

Their justifications are the same: the government's policies lead to the loss of sovereignty and restrictions on citizens' freedom, allegedly pursuing the goal of abolishing Germany, replacing its population and suppressing opposition to this process. Mask mandates are inserted into this sequence as another narrative thread. Masks are stylised as a medium of dictatorial oppression that represents the restriction of fundamental rights and the gagging of the national opposition.

This interpretation is supported by the distribution of expressions in which *Maske* (mask) is used as a modifier. Expressions depicting the effectiveness of wearing masks as fake, such as *Maskentheater* (mask theatre) and *Maskenlüge* (mask lie), are comparatively rare (0.05 per 1 million words). Terms characterising the use of a mask as a collective mental disorder, such as *Masken-Wahn* (mask madness), *Maskenirrsinn* (mask insanity), *Masken-Blödsinn* (mask nonsense) and *Maskenidiotie* (mask idiocy), are also not very frequent (0.18 per 1 million words). The vast majority (3.29 per 1 million words) of terms with *Maske* as a modifier characterise mask-related regulation as coercive, e.g. *Masken-Zwang* (mask coercion), *Maskenterror* (mask terror) and *Masken-Diktatur* (mask dictatorship).

5.5 Final remarks

The mask has been transformed into a symbol representing the alleged dictatorial character of the Federal Republic of Germany and its government. This is also evident by the number of online stores of right-wing extremists where masks carrying printed political messages can be purchased. In addition to masks with the slogan *Merkel Maulkorb* (Merkel muzzle), there are also masks in which the Federal Republic is explicitly or implicitly compared with the totalitarian regimes of the 20th century. Figure 5.6 demonstrates that, on the

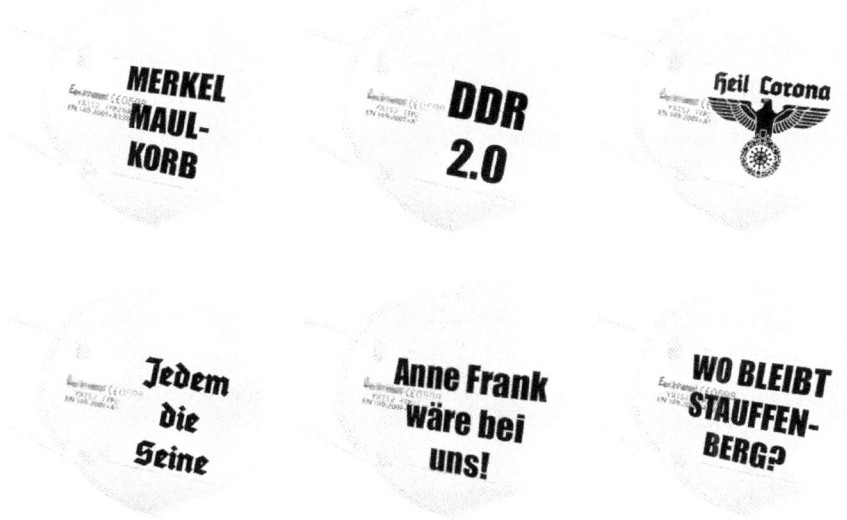

Figure 5.6 Sample masks from the radical right online shop 'politaufkleber.de'

one hand, the Federal Republic is declared to be a second German Democratic Republic (*DDR 2.0*) but that, on the other hand, the Nazi regime also serves as a benchmark.[7]

Heil Corona uses the Hitler salute, and its graphic design is reminiscent of the *Reichsadler* (Imperial Eagle) with a swastika. *Jedem die Seine* is intended to denote that everyone gets the mask they deserve. However, it is also an obvious allusion to *Jedem das Seine* (*to each what he deserves*), the motto at the entrance to the Buchenwald camp, thus comparing the mask mandate with imprisonment in a Nazi concentration camp. *Anne Frank wäre bei uns* (*Anne Frank would be one of us*) is further proof of the spiral of self-victimisation in which mask critics are caught, comparing themselves with persecuted Jews during the Nazi era. *Wo bleibt Stauffenberg?* (*Where is Stauffenberg?*) is a call to action against the German government, as Claus Schenk Graf von Stauffenberg was a key player in the assassination attempt on Adolf Hitler on 20 July 1944.

The murderer in Idar-Oberstein also operated according to this ideology. The simple obligation to wear a mask to prevent the spread of a virus had become a symbol of dictatorship. The wearing of a mask for no more than 5 minutes while buying two six-packs of beer became, in this thinking, an act of humiliation before this supposed dictatorship. As the analyses have revealed, the mask is simply a tool for right-wing radicals and extremists to further reject democracy, mobilise their activists and win new supporters.

Notes

1 Cf. *Maskenaffäre* in Wikipedia: https://de.wikipedia.org/wiki/Maskenaff%C3% A4re (in German).
2 A network of groups and people rejecting the legitimacy of the Federal Republic of Germany, claiming that the German Reich, which existed from 1871 to 1945, still exists.
3 '*Oder man hat sich kritisch mit den Kritikern befasst, indem man die alle ins Lager der Coronaleugner und Verschwörungstheoretiker eingereiht hat*' (Deutschlandfunk 2021).
4 This refers to a figurative meaning of masks as a dissimulation or denial of religious belief in Islam.
5 A warm headgear covering the neck, the whole head except for parts of the face, often made out of wool.
6 Here, the term *do-gooder* refers to people who – in the eyes of the political right – supposedly feel morally superior because they support refugees or wear masks, for example.
7 This probably requires an explanation: although the new right in Germany is author- itarian, xenophobic and anti-pluralist in orientation, it has distanced itself from the dictatorship of National Socialism and its ideology. The German New Right is ori- ented towards the völkisch groups of the Weimar period, the ideas of representa- tives of the Conservative Revolution and the early national socialists around Gregor Strasser (who was killed in 1934 during the Night of the Long Knives). Comparing something with the Nazi regime in Germany is a common way to devalue it. And even the German right wingers make excessive use of Nazi comparisons.

References

Online resources

Ärzteblatt (2020a) *Coronavirus: WHO does not declare an international emergency for the time being* (in German). Available at: www.aerzteblatt.de/nachrichten/108845/ Coronavirus-WHO-ruft-vorerst-keine-internationale-Notlage-aus (Accessed: 17 November 2021).
Ärzteblatt (2020b) *Displeasure and a lack of understanding about Reinhardt's mask statements* (in German). Available at: www.aerztezeitung.de/Politik/Unmut-und- Unverstaendnis-ueber-Reinhardts-Masken-Aussagen-413992.html (Accessed: 17 November 2021).
Ärztezeitung (2020a) *Corona 'Lockdown light' likely to begin Nov. 2* (in German). Available at: www.aerztezeitung.de/Politik/Gibt-es-ein-Corona-Lockdown-light- fuer-Deutschland-414100.html (Accessed: 17 November 2021).
Ärztezeitung (2020b) *Hard lockdown starts on December 16* (in German). Available at: www.aerztezeitung.de/Nachrichten/Harter-Lockdown-startet-am-16-Dezember- 415549.html (Accessed: 17 November 2021).
Bayerischer Hausärzteverband (2020) *Coronavirus SARS-CoV-2: Fragen und Antworten für Patienten* (as publishes by the RKI, in German). Available at: www.hausaerzte- bayern.de/images/aktuell/covid19/2020-02-28_BH%C3%84V_Presse_Statement_ Corona_Stand_28022020_002.pdf (Accessed: 17 November 2021).
BR (2021) *FFP2 mask requirement in Bavaria: What you need to know* (in German). Available at: www.br.de/nachrichten/bayern/ffp2-maskenpflicht-in-bayern-ab- heute-das-muessen-sie-wissen,SLzEfGB (Accessed: 17 November 2021).

Bundesgesundheitsministerium (2020) *Coronavirus protective masks ordinance (SchutzmV)* (in German). Available at: www.bundesgesundheitsministerium.de/service/gesetze-und-verordnungen/guv-19-lp/schutzmv.html (Accessed: 17 November 2021).

Bundeskanzlerin (2020) *Conference call between the German Chancellor and the heads of government of the federal states on April 15, 2020* (in German). Available at: www.bundeskanzlerin.de/bkin-de/aktuelles/bund-laender-beschluss-1744224 (Accessed: 17 November 2021).

Bundesregierung (2020a) *Meeting of the Federal Chancellor with the heads of government of the federal states on 22.03.2020* (in German). Available at: www.bundesregierung.de/breg-de/themen/coronavirus/besprechung-der-bundeskanzlerin-mit-den-regierungschefinnen-und-regierungschefs-der-laender-vom-22-03-2020-1733248 (Accessed: 17 November 2021).

Bundesregierung (2020b) *Telephone conference of the Head of the Federal Chancellor's Office with the Heads of the State and Senate Chancelleries of the German states on October 7, 2020* (in German). Available at: www.bundesregierung.de/breg-de/themen/buerokratieabbau/telefonschaltkonferenz-des-chefs-des-bundeskanzleramts-mit-den-chefinnen-und-chefs-der-staats-und-senatskanzleien-der-laender-am-7-oktober-2020–1796770 (Accessed: 17 November 2021).

Bundesregierung (2021) *This is what the federal emergency brake regulates* (in German). Available at: www.bundesregierung.de/breg-de/suche/bundesweite-notbremse-1888982 (Accessed: 17 November 2021).

Correctiv (2020) *No, four million people did not demonstrate in Berlin on 29 August* (in German). Available at: https://correctiv.org/faktencheck/2020/08/31/nein-in-berlin-haben-am-29-august-nicht-vier-millionen-menschen-demonstriert/ (Accessed: 17 November 2021).

Deutsche Welle (2020) *Corona live ticker from April 22: Masks mandatory throughout Germany* (in German). Available at: www.dw.com/de/corona-live-ticker-vom-22-april-maskenpflicht-in-ganz-deutschland/a-53202837–0 (Accessed: 17 November 2021).

Deutschlandfunk (2021) *Journalists too often see themselves as 'advocates of our system'.* (in German). Available at: www.deutschlandfunkkultur.de/andreas-rosenfelder-zur-corona-berichterstattung-100.html (Accessed: 17 November 2021).

Heidtmann, J. (2020) Sit-ins in the West, riots in the East (in German). In: *Süddeutsche Zeitung.* Available at: www.sueddeutsche.de/politik/demonstration-berlin-corona-massnahmen-hildmann-1.5014391 (Accessed: 17 November 2021).

IfSG (2020) Gesetz zum Schutz der Bevölkerung bei einer epidemischen Lage von nationaler Tragweite (in German). In: *Bundesgesetzblatt Jahrgang* 2020 Teil I Nr. 14. Available at: www.bgbl.de/xaver/bgbl/start.xav?startbk=Bundesanzeiger_BGBl&jumpTo=bgbl120s0587.pdf (Accessed: 17 November 2021).

IfSG (2021) Viertes Gesetz zum Schutz der Bevölkerung bei einer epidemischen Lage von nationaler Tragweite (in German). In: *Bundesgesetzblatt Jahrgang* 2021 Teil I Nr. 18. Available at: www.bundesgesundheitsministerium.de/fileadmin/Dateien/3_Downloads/Gesetze_und_Verordnungen/GuV/B/4_BevSchG_BGBL.pdf (Accessed: 17 November 2021).

Infratest dimap (2021) *Corona-COMPASS* [Recurrent Survey on Attitudes Towards Anti-COVID Measures among Germans]. Available at: www.infratest-dimap.de/umfragen-analysen/bundesweit/coronacompass/coronacompass/ (Accessed: 2 February 2022).

Koopmann, C. (2020) Masks sold out in many pharmacies (in German). In: *Süddeutsche Zeitung.* Available at: www.sueddeutsche.de/muenchen/starnberg/

coronavirus-atemschutzmasken-mundschutz-starnberg-stockdorf-1.4775079 (Accessed: 17 November 2021).

NDR (2020) *Corona blog: Spahn against nationwide mask obligation* (in German). Available at: www.ndr.de/nachrichten/info/Coronavirus-Blog-Die-Lage-am-Donnerstag-24-September,coronaliveticker540.html (Accessed: 17 November 2021).

SWR (2021) *Bloody crime in gas station: Investigations are progressing* (in German). Available at: www.swr.de/swraktuell/rheinland-pfalz/trier/toetungsdelikt-trier-tankstelle-motiv-streit-um-maske-100.html (Accessed: 17 November 2021).

WDR (2020) *Minister pleads: Hoarding purchases unnecessary* (in German). Available at: https://web.archive.org/web/20200325094136/https://www1.wdr.de/nachrichten/coronavirus-hamsterkauefe-100.html (Accessed: 17 November 2021).

Scientific literature

Klein, J. (1991) 'Kann man 'Begriffe besetzen'? Zur linguistischen Differenzierung einer plakativen politischen Metapher', ['Can one 'occupy terms'? On the linguistic differentiation of a striking political metaphor'] in Liedtke, F., Wengeler, M. und Böke, K. (eds.) *Begriffe besetzen. Strategien des Sprachgebrauchs in der Politik. [Occupying Terms. Strategies of language use in politics].* Opladen: Westdeutscher Verlag, pp. 44–69.

Köller, W. (2004) *Perspektivität und Sprache. Zur Struktur von Objektivierungsformen in Bildern, im Denken und in der Sprache. [Perspectivity and Language. On the Structure of Forms of Objectification in Images, Thought, and Language].* Berlin and New York: de Gruyter.

Müller, D. (2008) 'Lunatic Fringe Goes Mainstream? Keine Gatekeeping-Macht für Niemand, dafür Hate Speech für Alle – zum Islamhasser-Blog Politically Incorrect', ['Lunatic fringe goes mainstream? No gatekeeping power for nobody, but hate speech for everyone – on the Islam-hater blog politically incorrect.'] in *Navigationen. Zeitschrift für Medien- und Kulturwissenschaften [Navigations. Journal of Media and Cultural Studies]*, 8(2), pp. 109–126.

Newman, N. (2019) *Reuters Institute digital news report 2019.* Available at: https://reutersinstitute.politics.ox.ac.uk (Accessed: 17 November 2021).

Schmid, H. (1995) 'Improvements in part-of-speech tagging with an application to German', in *Proceedings of the EACL'95 SIGDAT Workshop.* Dublin: Association for Computational Linguistics, pp. 47–50.

Schneiders, T. G. (2016) 'Islamfeindlichkeit unter Menschen mit Migrationshintergrund', ['Islamophobia among people with an immigrant background'] in Pfeffer-Hoffmann, C. and Logvinov, M. (Hrsg.) *Muslimfeindlichkeit und Migration. Thesen und Fragen zur Muslimfeindlichkeit unter Eingewanderten. [Muslimphobia and migration. Theses and questions on Muslimphobia among immigrants].* Berlin: Mensch und Buch Verlag, pp. 85–94.

Spieß, C. (2017) 'Metaphern', ['Metaphors'.] in Roth, K. S., Wengeler, M. und Ziem, A. (eds) *Handbuch Sprache in Politik und Gesellschaft [Handbook Language in Politics and Society].* Berlin and New York: de Gruyter, pp. 94–115.

Weisskircher, M. (2020) 'Neue Wahrheiten von rechts außen? Alternative Nachrichten und der "Rechtspopulismus" in Deutschland', ['New truths from the far right? Alternative news and "right-wing populism" in Germany'] in *Zeitschrift Forschungsjournal Soziale Bewegungen [Journal of Social Movements Research]*, 33(2), pp. 474–490.

Wengeler, M. (2017) 'Wortschatz I: Schlagwörter, politische Leitvokabeln und der Streit um Worte', ['Vocabulary I: Buzzwords, leading political vocabulary and the dispute over words'] in Roth, K. S., Wengeler, M. und Ziem, A. (eds) *Handbuch Sprache in Politik und Gesellschaft [Handbook language in politics and society]*. Berlin and New York: de Gruyter, pp. 22–46.

6 The welfare state and COVID-19 countermeasures

The relationship of trust and cooperation between citizens and their governments in Sweden and Finland

Chino Yabunaga and Madoka Watanabe

6.1 Introduction

Do welfare states become more closed and authoritarian-like during a pandemic to protect their citizens from infectious diseases? In the immediate aftermath of the COVID-19 pandemic, there were some concerns that countries would move towards anti-globalisation, become more authoritarian, and bring about a resurgence of big government (e.g. Weible et al. 2020; Anttiroiko 2021). Indeed, many countries closed their borders, restricted citizens' movements, imposed lockdowns and implemented massive economic measures including monetary transfers to mitigate the impact of economic losses. However, is this an inevitable policy response in a major crisis?

Nordic countries have been known as generous welfare states with high homogeneity and large shares of public social spending. Although assessments of COVID-19 countermeasures vary greatly depending on the perspective of the assessor, journalists on featured articles in *The Wall Street Journal* (1.1.2021) and *Der Spiegel* (8.7.2021) reported high evaluations for Nordic countries because of their economic measures, degree of constraint in citizens' lives and communication with citizens, in addition to their having kept infections and mortality rates low. Moreover, these countries, as mentioned in what follows, were able to prevent their economies from fluctuating widely, far better than the Euro area average (Organisation for Economic Co-operation and Development and Statistics Finland 2021).

Among the Nordic countries, Denmark, Finland and Norway closed their borders after the World Health Organization (WHO) declared COVID-19 a pandemic and announced lockdowns under which schools were temporarily closed, restaurants were closed and unnecessary outings were restricted.[1] In contrast, Sweden did not impose a lockdown and rarely established prohibitions such as the strict movement of people and activity restrictions, for which it attracted attention as being a unique case. Separately, according to Strang (2020), Denmark and Norway emphasised the decisions of political leaders and implemented

DOI: 10.4324/9781003244127-7

decisive measures quickly, whereas Finland and Sweden chose to emphasise expert opinions and evidence. The Oxford COVID-19 Government Response Tracker also shows that Sweden and Finland both responded loosely or weakly in terms of restricting citizens' actions and in terms of policy intensity: in other words, both countries avoided authoritarian policy responses (Hale et al. 2021). In addition, Finland was able to control the impact of infectious diseases to a certain extent with a lockdown while Sweden did so to an average level without locking down. The comparative findings presented in Table 6.1 show that Finland and Sweden have stood out as different but notable cases in the COVID-19 responses in Scandinavian nations.

In this chapter, we discuss the different responses to the COVID-19 pandemic in two Nordic welfare states, Sweden and Finland. We describe both states' measures and contexts primarily during the first 6 months after the COVID-19 outbreak. First, we explain the importance of cooperation between governments and citizens. Next, we describe how actors in both states cooperatively realised their COVID-19 countermeasures with a focus on how measures constrained citizens, for instance by restricting activities or requiring masks; we also compare citizens' actions in response to these containment measures. Finally, we argue that even in a crisis such as a pandemic, welfare states attempted to minimise the restrictions on citizens' freedom, and we observed an interaction between citizens' cooperation and the minimisation of state intervention. We describe this relationship between welfare state institutions and their citizens as one of co-occurring (that is, mutual) trust.

6.2 Infectious disease control and citizens' trust in government

Studies have shown correlations between politics, institutions and trust between government and citizens and citizens' cooperative attitudes, such as their compliance with government regulations (e.g. Marien and Hooghe 2011; Lindström 2008). In situations where policy responses aim to effect behaviour change, such as with efforts to combat COVID-19, governments can promote behavioural change without restricting citizens' freedoms if citizens themselves cooperate. Reducing the impacts of infectious diseases not only saves people's health and lives but also minimises the impacts on the economy and society. Hence, it goes without saying that civic cooperation with public policies is the key to successfully combating infectious diseases. For instance, Mueller (1973) recognised that a positive rally-around-the-flag effect increased support of the government during a crisis irrespective of the appropriateness or rationality of the policy, and other researchers have confirmed this finding already in the COVID-19 crisis in European countries (e.g. Kritzinger et al. 2021; Nielsen and Lindvall 2021) as well as repeatedly in different political contexts.

However, Europe and the West showed markedly different COVID-19 responses and countermeasures than did Asian countries in the first half of 2020:

Table 6.1 COVID-19 cases and regulations in Nordic countries

		Sweden	Finland	Denmark	Norway
Population (31 Dec. 2020)		10,379,295	5,533,793	5,837,213	5,391,369
COVID-19 cases**					
31 Aug. 2020	cases	84,190	8,202	16,852	10,812
	deaths	5,827	314	624	264
31 Dec. 2020	cases	437,300	36,403	164,411	49,765
	deaths	9,658	591	1,256	429
The nature and timing of the population movement and behaviour regulations ***	Junior school closed	–	16 March	13 March	12 March
	High school/Uni changes	Distance education, 17 March	16 March	13 March	12 March
	Bans on gatherings > 500	11 March	13 March	13 March	12 March
	> 50–5	> 50 27 March	> 5 16 March	> 10 17 March	> 5 24 March
	Pubs, bars, restaurants closed	–	16 March	13 March	12 March
	Non-essential shops closed	–	4 April	18 March	12 March
	Shielding of vulnerable	16 March	17 March	13 March	12 March
	Population lockdown	–	16 March	11 March	13 March
	Border closed	–	18 March	13 March	14 March
	Travel international restrictions	11 March		13 March	12 March
	domestic	19 March	25 March	13 March	12 March
	% journeys to work in April 2020 (compared to Jan/Feb 2020)	70–80%	40–60%	50–60%	50–60%

*Sources: www.scb.se/, www.stat.fi/, www.dst.dk/en, www.ssb.no/en

** Cumulative number. Source: World Health Organization (WHO) (n.d.). There are some differences between the WHO data and the official data from the different countries' bureaus of statistics.

*** Source: Orlowski and Goldsmith (2020)

specifically, the COVID-19 strategy in Asia used the experience of SARS to prioritise economic development and promote efficient public health management; in contrast, the highest priority in Europe was civil liberties, and government measures and public acceptance of the policies determined the policies and their directions (Anttiroiko 2021). One research group examined the impacts of infectious disease on mortality and policy development during the pandemic and confirmed the importance of trust in institutions (Oksanen et al. 2020). Oksanen et al. (2020) tracked the government responses in 25 European countries along with the numbers of deaths in the early stages of the pandemic and examined factors associated with mortality and found that trust in institutions was a protective factor during the COVID-19 pandemic: countries with low citizen trust in institutions were slower to set behavioural restrictions and had to take more severe measures. In other words, the relationship between the government and citizens and their trust in each other is one of the most important perspectives in evaluating a given country's COVID-19 countermeasures.

Georgieva et al. (2021) conducted an online survey via Facebook in ten European countries and India between June and August 2020 regarding how citizens perceived COVID-19 countermeasures. They first looked at what infection-prevention actions were being constrained by the governments in each country. Next, they asked participants about the degree of compliance with infection-prevention behaviours regardless of government mandates, their levels of discomfort or feelings that their personal freedom and basic human rights were being restricted and how effective they felt the government measures were in preventing the spread of COVID-19. They found that the governments of the countries where they collected their data had instituted a number of common constraint measures: personal hygiene practises such as recommending hand-washing and wearing masks; social distancing measures to avoid physical contact such as closing schools and prohibiting gatherings and contact with vulnerable groups; containment measures such as testing, isolating and tracing infected people; and actions based on government authority such as issuing emergency declarations and enforcing penalties for violating behavioural restrictions. However, the extent to which these infection-prevention actions were mandatory varied from government to government, and the degree of compliance varied regardless of the number of mandated measures by the governments. ('Compliance' refers to the rate of adherence with the aforementioned infection-control actions and measures whether or not they are enforced by the government.)

Figure 6.1 presents the ten European countries' degrees of compliance with the different government pandemic responses.[2] In Finland and Sweden, with the high citizen compliance, high percentages felt the measures were effective, low percentages felt the measures were overly restrictive and governments imposed few of the measures. In contrast, the governments of the other countries imposed more measures, and more respondents felt their governments' measures were too restrictive. Respondents' compliance was lower in the other countries, and those respondents believed their governments' measures had not been effective.

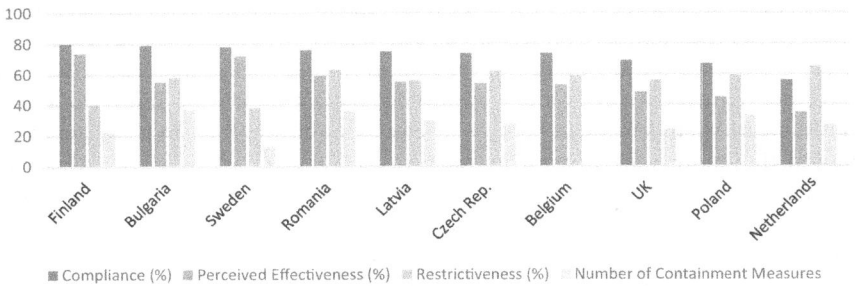

Figure 6.1 Citizens' compliance, perceived effectiveness and restrictiveness and number of containment measures by authorities

Source: data from Georgieva et al. (2021)

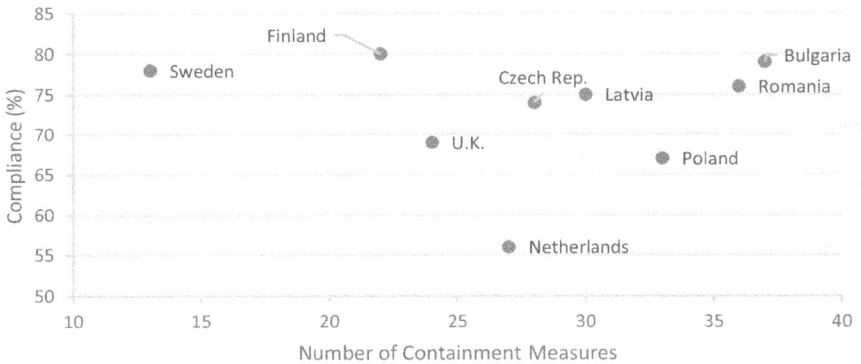

Figure 6.2 Number of containment measures and citizens' compliance

Source: data from Georgieva et al. (2021)

Figure 6.2 presents a scatter plot of the same data from Georgieva et al. (2021), and it still indicates that compliance with infection-control measures was higher in Sweden and Finland despite their fewer containment measures than the other countries.[3] In terms of the relationships between variables, their analysis made it clear that citizens' sense of the effectiveness and the restrictiveness of containment measures affected their compliance with those measures. For instance, the data show negative correlations between compliance with measures and the perception of the restrictiveness of such measures, which included mask-wearing as well as social distancing, cancellation of events, hand washing recommendations and lockdowns. The data reveal positive correlations of compliance with the sense of effectiveness of containment measures, trust in hospitals and governments and credibility of government announcements.

Based on these discussions, we can assume that citizens properly followed infection-control actions during the pandemic in Sweden and Finland and that they did so because they had high trust in the institutions that directed the infection-control actions regardless of constraint; they considered that the authorities' announcements had high credibility; and they felt that the government measures had imposed few constraints. So next, we more carefully scrutinise the situations in Sweden and Finland to see how their respective governments actually implemented their infectious disease-control measures and how citizens reacted. In an Annex table, we present a timeline of the COVID-19 countermeasures in Sweden and Finland.

6.3 Sweden

6.3.1 Behavioural restrictions (excluding masks) and public reaction to COVID-19 policy

Sweden's COVID-19 policy attracted global attention. However, according to a speech to the WHO by Lena Hallengren, Minister for Health and Social Affairs (23 April 2020), there was no 'unique' Swedish policy for COVID-19; the country's policies were similar to those in other countries but simply more relaxed. The objectives of the policies were the same as those in many countries with lockdown policies: to delay infection and save lives. However, as the minister stated, the specifics of Sweden's policy were as follows:

- Although the Swedish government had overall responsibility, public health measures relied heavily on advice from experts, and policy decisions were knowledge and evidence based.
- The top priority was protecting the elderly and at-risk groups. Accordingly, the government issued a strong request that people refrain from going out, discouraged visits to institutions for the elderly and encouraged people aged 70 and older to avoid physical contact with other people.
- Social distancing and 'stay at home' were key policies.
- Sick leave was originally easy to obtain in Sweden; notably, the government encouraged people to take leave even for very slight symptoms. However, originally, 'the period allowed for sick leave without a doctor's diagnosis' was unpaid on the first day, although later legislation changed this.
- Sweden's public health response built in flexibility to add measures whenever needed.

On observation, these measures (Government Offices of Sweden 2020) were similar to those of other countries except for the lockdowns; furthermore, despite what international media commonly reported, Sweden was not following a policy of herd immunity.

Other measures enforced by law included a ban on gatherings of more than 50 people and restrictions on the distance between customers at restaurants. The government recommended that high schools and universities offer online classes, that businesses offer remote work, and that all citizens refrain from unnecessary travel.

Sweden also chose not to close nurseries and primary and junior high schools simultaneously; the government aim was to keep essential workers such as medical staff from having to take time off for child care given that children were unlikely to spread the infection. Furthermore, there were concerns about increased abuse in the home as a side effect of closing public spaces.

Sweden enacted less restrictive measures than did other countries for three constitutional reasons: (1) guarantee of freedom of movement, (2) guarantee of independence of public authorities and (3) guarantee of autonomy of local authorities. (Jonung 2020).

In terms of the public's response to the measures, in the early days of pandemic in the spring of 2020, approximately 80% of respondents to a survey said that they had changed their behaviours to slow down the transmission of coronavirus, even though the Swedish government was not enforcing COVID-19 policies, as policy was not enforced by law (Folkhälsomyndigheten 2020a). Moreover, in a survey of the public's trust in ministries, agencies and institutions as of August 2020, 79% of respondents said they trusted hospitals the most, but a majority (52%,) also trusted the government (Kantar Sifo 2020).

Foreign-born citizens (former refugees and immigrants) account for approximately 20% of the Swedish population (Statistiska centralbyrån 2021b). Here, we discuss the damage they suffered and the support they received related to COVID-19. Since the spring of 2020, there have been many cases of infections, serious injury, injury and deaths among foreign-born people who work as part-time caregivers, and language factors have been cited as a cause. In response, several ministries and agencies cooperated to conduct investigations in several languages and to disseminate information beginning in spring 2020 (Myndigheten för samhällsskydd och beredskap 2021). However, the high proportion of foreign-born citizens among COVID-19 deaths did not change. In autumn 2020, the proportion of foreign-born citizens among all deaths in Sweden was still much higher than in previous years, although not as high as in spring 2020 (Statistiska centralbyrån 2021a).

In an analysis of the relevant factors, the Public Health Agency of Sweden reported that

> Socioeconomic factors and housing conditions account for a large part of the reason for the high number of foreign-born deaths. Income and education are also clear factors and raising people's awareness of socioeconomic needs is necessary for equal health. Inequalities risk spreading COVID-19 to foreign-born populations.
>
> (Folkhälsomyndigheten 2021c)

The report established 'equitable health' in 2018 as the country's new public health policy framework and goal (*God och jämlik hälsa – en utvecklad folkhälsopolitik* – Good Equitable Health – Developmental Public Health Policy). Its target areas are broad and include, for example, education, income and housing. Currently, foreign-born citizens in Sweden are 'the most affected among self-employed people' (Sverigeradio 25.2.2021), and the path ahead does not seem straightforward. However, the Public Health Agency, in cooperation with other ministries, aims to work on better social and economic policies towards the aim of good and equitable health.

6.3.2 Mask policy and public reaction

In Sweden, masks for daily use outside of medical and institutional settings have been far from obligatory. Masks were not even recommended since the beginning of the pandemic because 'the evidence that they are beneficial in fighting COVID-19 is weak' and 'wearing a mask could be used as an excuse not to stay indoors, which could be counterproductive'. In an August 2020 survey of 1,000 people commissioned by a private TV station, only 13% of respondents said yes to the statement 'Masks are necessary in all environments', while 60% said no. However, two out of five respondents affirmed the necessity of wearing masks on crowded public transportation (Omni 2020).

Here, we offer a timeline of the social developments regarding masks that took place at the end of 2020, when Sweden decided to recommend masks on public transport, and at the beginning of 2021. Why was Sweden reluctant to recommend masks during 2020, and why did it finally decide to partially recommend them at the end of 2020?

During the winter of 2020, the second wave of infections in Sweden led to more deaths. On 29 October 2020, the government raised the regulations to recommend not entering stores and other buildings unless necessary for living but did not include a mask recommendation (Folkhälsomyndigheten 2020b).

In response, on 16 November, Mike Ryan, WHO's head of crisis preparedness, said, 'It is understandable that Sweden has tightened its restrictions in response to the infection situation, but in such a widespread area, mask recommendations are also necessary for coronavirus control. Masks work well'. Mr. Ryan was responding to a question from a Swedish reporter (Svenska Dagbladet 16.11.2020).

On 17 November, Ebba Bush, leader of the country's Christian Democrats, sent a letter to Prime Minister Stefan Löfven's secretary, asking questions such as, 'Why do you not recommend masks?' (Svenska Dagbladet 20.11.2020).

Around that time, European countries strengthened regulations, and demonstrations and protests against them increased. On 18 November, there was a demonstration of 5,000 people in Germany against the government's coronavirus policy. When the demonstrators refused to comply with the police's call to wear masks, the police sprayed water on them (Sydsvenskan 19.11.2020). However, constitutionally speaking, it was difficult for Sweden to enforce such policies on its citizens; the only option for the Swedish government was to rely on its citizens' autonomy without forcing them to comply with COVID-19 containment measures, including masks; therefore, gaining citizens' trust without a confrontation was essential for Sweden's COVID-19 policy. For the Public Health Agency, the confrontation between the government and citizens in Germany was a bad situation that should have been avoided. Nevertheless, the rest of the world condemned Sweden's avoidance of masks in 2020.

Meanwhile, in response to the Swedish government's avoidance of enacting a policy on masks, the expert group on COVID-19 of the Royal Swedish Academy of Sciences issued a statement on 19 November saying it was 'very important for the Public Health Agency to come up with measures for wearing masks indoors and in public transport' (Kungl. Vetenskapsakademien 2020); the government was under pressure from both domestic and international sources to recommend masks. On the same day, Karin Tegmark Wisell, the head of the Public Health Agency at the time, said at a press conference that 'Both the WHO and the European Infection Agency recommend masks as a supplementary measure when it is not possible to maintain a distance between people. That is the same as the Swedish measure'. Earlier, in August 2020, the Public Health Agency had already stated that 'In Sweden, too, masks can be used as a supplementary measure at a certain stage. There is not much difference', and 'When it comes to mask policy, equality must also be considered because it is a personal purchase' (Expressen 19.11.2020). There was much criticism of this statement later. For example, Tove Lifvendahl, political editor-in-chief of *SvD*, one of the nation's newspapers, criticised the comment as follows: 'Equality in policy can only be achieved if the policy saves many lives in a pandemic' (Svenska Dagbladet 22.11.2020).

However, the next day, 20 November, a Danish study on masks and COVID-19 infection made headlines in the media. Although the results were favourable to the Public Health Agency's claim that 'there was no clear evidence that masks reduce coronavirus infections' (Svt Nyheter 7.12.2020), the study led to more discussions in newspapers about the agency and its mask policy (Svenska Dagbladet 20.11.2020). Researchers not only of the Danish study but also of many other studies on the effects of masks through spring 2021 concluded that masks were not particularly effective in reducing COVID-19 infection. In response, Anders Tegnell, a state epidemiologist for the Public Health Agency, said, 'There is no scientific basis for masks' (Dagens Nyheter 8.11.2020). Meanwhile, Mr. Wisell had said in August, 'If the problem of infection grows again, we will consider measures such as masks' (The Local 2020).

On 22 November 2020, Prime Minister Löfven held a press conference to call for public action, saying, 'Sweden is now being tested, and if everyone does not accept the regulations and recommendations, more people will die' (Expressen 22.11.2020). At this point, the government was not recommending masks to the public; consequently, the regulations and recommendations the Prime Minister mentioned mainly included social distancing, handwashing, self-isolation at home if one was even slightly unwell and limiting the number of people at events. However, most newspapers argued that 'the Prime Minister's call to the people is like water sprinkled on a desert, and the effect of the call is limited. We need more effective policies, such as mask recommendations' (Svenska Dagbladet 24.11.2020).

On 26 November 2020, an article appeared in the online TV edition of the popular newspaper *Aftonbladet* (11.26.2020) explaining how to wear a mask. Then, on 30 November, Andreas Fischer, the president of the professional association of medical doctors, Sjukhusläkarna, in Stockholm, said, 'We need to wear masks in shopping centres, for example. Personal responsibility is important, but in the event of a pandemic the authorities must not be inadequate' (Svenska Dagbladet, 11.30.2020). At this time, the Public Health Agency had not yet recommended masks, but many ministries and government offices were already supplying them, and wearing masks had become somewhat mandatory. In December, the WHO tightened its guidelines on the use of masks in areas where COVID-19 had spread (WHO 2020).

On 16 December, as the country headed into Christmas, the Swedish royal family's annual words to the nation were broadcast on television. In the program, each member of the royal family reflected on the year 2020, with the king saying, 'We failed. A lot of people died, and it was terrible. We are all hurting. The people of Sweden have suffered very much in difficult circumstances. Some of you may think of people who have died in situations where they could not even say goodbye to their families. Such a situation, without a warm goodbye, is a really heavy and deeply traumatic experience'. He continued with words of compassion for the people (Svt Nyheter 17.12.2021).

Newspaper articles appeared in Sweden in large space, since the message from the king in December was a Christmas custom in Sweden, but people were comparatively calm. Moreover, the article titles Swedish people saw daily changed gradually from shocking statements such as, 'King on Pandemic: "I Think We Have Failed"' (Svt Nyheter 17.12.2020) to calmer expressions such as, 'King said to people: "The light comes back"' (Aftonbladet 25.12.2020).

However, it is well known that the news that focused only on the initial words was broadcast widely and sensationally on television in the United Kingdom from 17 December onwards and travelled around the world (BBC News 17.12.2020). In Sweden, the media reported with surprise that the news was being sensationalised in other countries, with reports including one expert's statement that the king's words were not a criticism of the government but an expression of compassion for the people (Aftonbladet 17.25.2020). Because Sweden's is a symbolic monarchy, there are no restrictions on the government, whether the king's comments were intended as criticism or not.

On the same day (17 December), at a daily COVID-19 press conference, state epidemiologist Tegnell responded as follows to a reporter's question: 'I have no opinion on what the King thinks'. The pandemic was reaching its peak in the second wave, with an increasing number of infections and deaths. Data from the Public Health Agency showed that on 17 December alone, the number of people infected was 9,640 and the number of deaths was 116; this was the very peak of illness in the country (Folkhälsomyndigheten 2021b).

Finally, on 18 December, Prime Minister Löfven announced that 'from 7 January 2021, it will be recommended to wear masks on public transport only during certain hours'. This remained not a legal mandate but a recommendation (Krisinformation 2021).

On the surface, one could easily argue that the government had shifted to recommending masks in response to the king's statement just before the announcement of the recommendation. However, as already mentioned, scientific evidence on the effectiveness of masks was somewhat limited during 2020. Further, there was much more resistance to wearing masks in Europe than in Asia, as reflected in demonstrations against mandatory masks in other European countries. Thus, in Sweden, where the government could not make masks compulsory because it was essential to gain the public's trust for constitutional reasons, it was difficult even to make the recommendation. However, as the second wave of infections and deaths reached its peak, there were requests from experts, doctors, and the WHO to recommend masks in Sweden, and finally, there was pressure from inside and outside the country over the King's comments. All these factors are thought to have led to the initial mask recommendation.

As of December 2020, and for the first time in Sweden during the pandemic, the government was recommending that the general public apart from medical personnel wear masks on public transport, although only during certain hours. We investigated the public's actual reactions and found mixed results. In parts of the country with low population density and little commute traffic, the percentage of people wearing masks did not increase, but near the central train station in Stockholm, approximately 60% of people wore masks. On 7 January, three weeks after the announcement recommending masks, sales of masks almost doubled (Dagens Nyheter 7.1.2021). Moreover, in interviews around town, people said, 'I think masks are effective in crowded places such as during commuting hours. I was surprised that so many people were following it, but I think it's a good trend'. Thus, many people had a positive view of the policy (Sverigeradio 8.11.2021).

Meanwhile, Tegnell said, 'If used incorrectly, masks can be harmful' and 'Masks are not a panacea, especially in schools' (Olsson 2021).

The recommendation as of February 2021 was that people wear masks all day long, not just during commute rush hours. However, three months later, in May, the incidence of mask-wearing on public transport had declined, perhaps because the second wave of infection, which had peaked in December, had settled (Svt Nyheter 23.5.2021). Following several months of decline in infections and deaths, the national recommendation to wear masks was lifted on 1 July 2021 (Folkhälsomyndigheten 2021a). Some municipalities still recommended masks, for example, 'in the event of the emergence of an infected person in the workplace' (Borgholms Kommun 2021). In addition, many companies require their employees to wear masks almost compulsorily, and train announcements still include mask recommendations.

We separately investigated whether there had been any pressure on foreign-born citizens to wear masks and found that as of July 2021, there were no major conflicts or research studies that would have led to newspaper articles on the issue, possibly because the mask recommendation in Sweden was fairly limited in general. Rather, we received via e-mail interview a comment from one immigrant in Stockholm that it appeared to have been foreign-born individuals who were wearing their masks. This could have been because, as we mentioned earlier, there were many COVID-19 victims among former refugees and immigrants in Sweden.

6.3.3 Public trust in and support for the government's COVID-19 policy

In Sweden, trust is seen as an integral part of society. In fact, since 1997, the government has regularly conducted a multifaceted survey called the Trust Barometer (Förtroendebarometern). The March 2021 trust survey stated, 'Trust binds people in society together like glue. And when society is in a state of disquiet, trust is tested' (Kantar Sifo 2021a). In Subsection 6.3.1, we explained 'more relaxed', which is similar to those of other countries except for the lockdowns, than those in other countries for constitutional reasons which derive in part from trust:

> Since the constitution provides for coronavirus measures in Sweden, the government has to rely on information and recommendations in order to influence the behaviour of the public, and the impact of this type of policy instrument is closely related to the level of trust in society.
>
> (Jonung 2020)

In the most recent survey in July 2021, in response to the question of whether the Public Health Agency 'had done a good job on coronavirus policy', 68% of the public responded that the Public Health Agency's efforts had been good, very good, or extremely good; 81% of the public reported trusting the agency on health care in the most recent survey (Kantar Sifo, Medieakademin 2021b).

One reason for the high level of public trust in the agencies that direct Sweden's COVID-19 policy, and in the medical care that plays such an important role in combating COVID-19, could have been the daily press conferences held at 2:00 p.m. by Anders Tegnell and others who directed the policy. Every day, they talked directly to the public about the ever-changing situation and countermeasures, showing graphs and other images. Afterwards, they asked and answered live questions with the news media, who came from all over Sweden and sometimes even from abroad, in front of the public, with unlimited time for Q&A based on scientific evidence. If there were any mistakes in data Tegnell provided previously, he admitted they had been wrong and informed the public. Consequently, the public felt gradual relief from the anxiety they had felt in the early days of the pandemic.

Sweden has a long history of systems for building trust, with the first being its information disclosure policy. On 2 December 1766, Sweden enacted His Royal

Majesty's Gracious Ordinance Relating to Freedom of Writing and of the Press, a freedom-of-the-press act (Kongl 1766; Nordin 2015). This is considered the world's oldest information disclosure law, and it is reflected in the high information transparency in Sweden. In a recent example, emails Mr. Tegnell exchanged were released at journalists request and are now available online to everyone (Karlsten 2020).

In addition, the constitution and the administrative code in Sweden clearly stipulate that whenever a new bill is submitted to the Parliament, remiss, a system of listening to opinions, is mandatory, and the exchange of opinions, including which groups submitted what opinions, how the government responded to them and whether the government amended the bill as a result, is all open to the public (Watanabe 2006).

We believe that the national trust in Sweden's government that had derived from its combination of efforts to keep the public informed underpinned Sweden's measures against the COVID-19 pandemic.

6.4 Finland

In Finland, the first infected person (a foreign tourist) was confirmed at the end of January 2020 in a tourist area in the north of the country; by the time the pandemic was declared on 11 March, there were approximately 60 infected people in Finland. The country applied the Emergency Powers Act (1552/2011) on the Monday following the declaration and placed the whole nation under a state of emergency on the 17th. A state of emergency can only be imposed for a limited time, but the government can exercise special powers to protect people without waiting for parliamentary approval.

6.4.1 Behavioural restrictions (excluding issues except wearing masks) and public response to the coronavirus policy in Finland

Whereas Sweden expected citizens to act responsibly and voluntarily to prevent infection and prioritised individual freedom of movement and the independence of public authorities, Finland emphasised citizen responsibility while simultaneously imposing practical restrictions. Under the state of emergency, the Finnish government took measures to prevent infection in educational settings (closure of educational facilities except child day cares and shifting to remote classes, closure of cultural and sports facilities, etc.); prevent infection among high-risk groups (restricting gatherings, discouraging interpersonal contact among people over 70, restricting visits to facilities for elderly persons, prohibiting gathering in public places, etc.); secure and allocate medical resources (redistributing medical functions, restricting the sales of medicines, reducing urgent health and medical services, issuing exemptions from the Working Hours Act (872/2019) and the Annual Holidays Act (162/2005), requiring welfare, medical and security professionals to work, etc.); and contain COVID-19 (making preparations for border closures, partially suspending transportation, adjusting employment during quarantine periods, requesting that citizens return home, etc.). Simultaneously, the Ministry of the Interior listed 98 essential worker jobs, both public and private, that were exempt from the restrictions (Valtioneuvosto 2020a). Most of these measures were recommendations and restrictions based on the Communicable Diseases Act (1227/2016). The only exceptions using special powers under the Emergency Powers Act were closing the schools, suspending restaurant services, restricting movement in the Uusimaa region including the capital, Helsinki, and suspending non-urgent treatment to expand ICU beds (Tiirinki et al. 2020).

During the lockdown (March-May 2020), parents who took time off work to care for their children at home received a temporary infectious-disease subsidy (€723.5 per month, with parents themselves determining their need); additionally, the unemployment insurance system was temporarily relaxed to cover self-employed persons whose income fell below a certain level. However, other than these two measures, matters of income and unemployment were managed within the framework of the ordinary welfare system. The number of applications for unemployment benefits doubled, and the number of applications for housing benefits increased by 36%, but there was little increase in the number of applicants for the infectious-disease allowance. This allowance provided full compensation for loss of income during the quarantine period, and there were few applicants because there were few infected persons in Finland. The government announced a package of economic measures totalling €15 billion, including a provisional €5 billion when the state of emergency was declared, and additional economic measures to help businesses were enacted four days later, on 20 March (Valtioneuvosto 2020b). Subsequently, approximately 60% of workers switched to teleworking, and 30% saw their working hours reduced, compared with 37% and 50%, respectively, in the 27 EU countries (Kangas 2020), and this indicates that the smooth transition to telework was less damaging to jobs than in other European countries.

Amid reports of the spread of COVID-19 infections around the world, Finnish experts, the government and politicians did not provide clear guidelines for prevention until applying the Emergency Powers Act (e.g. Väliverronen et al. 2020; Jallinoja and Väliverronen 2021); during this period, they were subjected to intense criticism in the media and on social networking. After the government declared the state of emergency and the overall picture of the measures to be taken against the coronavirus became clear in the following week, a united front formed which included citizens (e. g. HS 19.3.2020; 12.4.2020). No entity submitted to the parliament a resolution of censure against the government or a no-confidence vote in any ministers until autumn (Yle 2.10.2020).

In terms of the public response to the COVID-19 countermeasures, surveys conducted by in April and June 2020 revealed ratings of good and very good combined for the results achieved by the key actors in these countermeasures in April as follows: 56% for the Finnish Institute for Health and Welfare (THL), 49.5% for the Ministry of Social Affairs and Health (STM), 66.6% for the cabinet, 74% for the president and 45.3% for the WHO. In addition, 92.6% of the respondents said that they 'acted according to the government's instructions', and these figures remained almost unchanged in June, when the state of emergency was lifted. In addition, only 12.1% (April) and 18.7% (June) of respondents reported that their personal freedom was excessively restricted (Jallinoja and Väliverronen 2021). These figures reflect that most Finnish citizens trusted the government and followed its instructions. The Citizens' Pulse survey, which the government has been conducting since April 2020, shows similar results (Valtioneuvosto n.d.; Tilastokeskus n.d.).

Still, cultural minorities such as foreign-born citizens tended to be left behind in such countermeasures against the infectious disease. In mid-April, about one month after the WHO declared COVID-19 a pandemic, the City of Helsinki announced that the infection rate among Somali-speaking citizens (1.8%) was much higher than that for all its citizens in general (0.2%) (City of Helsinki 2020b). In addition, the infection rate by district, shown on a map every other week on the city's website, illustrated that areas in which immigrants congregated were the first to show high infection rates (City of Helsinki 2020a). In response, the Somali community protested, pointing out that the map as presented fostered discrimination and that they were frequently essential workers, which increased their virus exposure (Yle 14.4.2020). However, True Finns, a nationalist party, criticised the lifestyle of immigrants, including their usage of certain shopping centres, and objected to public subsidies for immigrant services (Suomen Uutiset 2020). According to Statistics Finland, foreign-born people accounted for 5% of COVID-19 deaths in 2020, more than double the overall COVID-19 mortality rate of 2%. Other data indicated more clearly that COVID-19 deaths were concentrated among foreign-born citizens. Although their share of all deaths in 2020 was 4%, the foreign-born share of COVID-19 deaths was 20% (Tilastokeskus 2021).

6.4.2 Policy on wearing masks and public reaction

Immediately after the pandemic declaration, there were problems with masks in Finland, including low stockpiles and a procurement scandal; in addition, experts had different views on the effectiveness of masks (e.g. HS 14.4.2020). Eventually, the STM issued a verification report stating that there was no clear effect of wearing masks, which became the official government position (STM 2020). Consequently, little progress was made on wearing masks (IL 2.8.2020). Then, on 3 June 2020, the government issued guidelines on individual infection-prevention measures to take once the COVID-19 state of emergency special measures were lifted (Valtioneuvosto 2020d), and masks were de-emphasised. Rather, priority was given to preventing infection by maintaining physical distance, washing hands thoroughly and following coughing and sneezing etiquette. Not only were masks not recommended as a way to prevent infection, they had the potential to increase the risk of infection if they were not put on and taken off correctly. However, masks could be used to protect others in crowded places. To improve their effectiveness, the THL publicised their correct use (THL 2020, 2021b).

It was a 13 August THL recommendation to the general public that prompted the wearing of masks in Finland, which began to be discussed domestically in parallel with the increasing numbers of cases across Europe around the beginning of August (THL 2020). Newspapers reported that the public was divided, with some questioning the necessity and timing of the project and others questioning the cost burden, while still others called for stronger regulations (HS 13.8.2020; IS 3.8.2020). In its recommendation, the THL stressed that masks do not protect the wearer but are effective in preventing the spread of infectious disease via airborne droplets. The agency also noted that private organisation requests that employees and others wear masks should consider the Non-Discrimination Act (1325/2014) and that organisations should take reasonable care for those who are unable to wear them and make available alternative means and services (THL 2021a). However, it was left up to the individual to decide whether to wear a mask.

Meanwhile, there was also concern that there would be peer pressure on those who did not wear masks. Helsinki Region Transport, for example, expressed the view through the media that 'citizens cannot require others to wear masks' (HS 17.8.2020). In September, the government formulated an action plan of long-term measures to address the disease and its spread from autumn onwards (Voipio-Pulkki 2020). In accordance with this plan, the specific guidelines for wearing masks varied depending on domestic infection levels. For instance, in October, when the infection was again spreading domestically, disputes about masks decreased, and mask instructions differed by region.

The evening newspaper *Ilta-Sanomat* conducted a poll in November 2020 that asked about mask-wearing habits. In it, 68% of respondents said they regularly wore masks and approximately 79% said they wore masks on public transportation (IS 25.11.2020). Many of those who said they did not wear masks explained that they did not use public transportation or they used alternative transportation methods that did not require them to wear masks. Only a small number of respondents explained that they did not wear masks because 'they are uncomfortable' (6.2%) or because they 'do not think they are effective' (5.0%). Although there has been no significant debate about or opposition against the wearing of masks, such as protests, there have been concerns in the media regarding individuals' possible physical reactions to masks (Yle 30.11.2020) and the peer pressure to wear them (Yle 30.11.2020). An online survey by the Finnish national broadcaster Yleisradio (Yle) in December 2020 found that physical ill health, mental ill health and discrimination against not wearing a mask were problems associated with mask-wearing (Yle 16.12.2020).

6.4.3 Trust in government, experts and science

Although the COVID-19 outbreak arrived later in the Nordic countries than in the rest of European countries, Finland's policy decisions before and after the WHO declared the pandemic were even more delayed than those of Denmark, Norway and Sweden (see Table 6.1). While other Scandinavian and European countries closed schools and cancelled flights, there was criticism of the Finnish government's slow response, mainly from opposition parties (Yle 21.3.2020). Before the Emergency Powers Act was applied, local governments had already started to respond by closing schools of their own accord. Finland's counter-measures tended to be opportunistic, as the prime minister and the cabinet struggled to coordinate with the president under the semi-presidential system and made decisions based on other countries' statuses and citizens' reactions while being aware of Sweden's choices.

There was a clear difference of opinion between the STM, the ministry in charge, and the THL, a specialised national research institute, on the effectiveness of masks and recommendations for their use, which caused confusion among the public (Yle 14.4.2020; 28.7.2020). For example, at a press conference in April, Markku Tervahauta, director-general of the THL, argued for the benefits of wearing masks, saying that masks could prevent others from becoming infected despite studies showing that many people worldwide are asymptomatically infected. However, in agreement with the STM, the THL took the official position that it would not issue recommendations or guidelines to the general public on mask-wearing. While the field experts and the THL mainly supported their effectiveness, the STM continued to oppose them (IS 29.7.2020). The STM still had to prioritise securing masks and other personal protective equipment for medical personnel (Valtioneuvosto 2020c), primarily because of mask procurement challenges (Yle 5.5.2020). Reportedly, the STM ignored the THL's position on masking, and the THL was under the STM's supervision during the state of emergency; indeed, there was media criticism of the STM's control, grounded in the argument that the THL should have been independent (IL 12.10.2020; IS 12.10.2020). The professional body should have been able to make scientific judgements based on evidence, and instead, its independence had been undermined.

Nevertheless, communication with the public in Finland was relatively smooth overall, and trust remained mutual between citizens and the government, including specialised institutions. Jallinoja and Väliverronen (2021) conducted surveys asking about the reliability of COVID-19-related information from experts and the government, and more than 80% of the respondents understood that there were multiple positions on scientific opinions; approximately 70% considered university researchers and professional organisations to be the most reliable, more than 80% thought that the government's instructions for action on infection-prevention were well reasoned, and less than 20% thought that the government's COVID-19 measures were based on a false outlook.

One of the reasons organisations involved in infection control were able to maintain smooth communication and mutual trust with citizens is the well-developed information and communication technology (ICT) public health care infrastructure. The Omaolo application, which has been in development since 2016, allows users to assess their symptoms, obtain instructions for self-care, and receive feedback from health care providers and other professionals over the Internet. The Kanta service, whose development began in 2010, operated by the Social Insurance Institution, Kela, registers users' health information, including medical records, immunisation status, prescriptions and consent to medical treatment (Yle 3.1.2020). With a user's consent, data can also be transferred and shared among health- and welfare-related institutions, and the individual user can also check their own information. As of November 2019, about one-third of people aged 65 and over were using the Kanta system. Separately, a free emergency-assessment medical helpline, 116117, that was introduced in 2018 assesses the need for an emergency call; if the call is not urgent, experts are consulted on the spot who provide the necessary instructions and advice. At the time of the COVID-19 outbreak, this helpline was in the process of being introduced, although it did cover 74.5% of the population. Finally, the Communicable Diseases Act was amended to develop a contact-tracking application, Koronavilkku (THL n.d.; HS 13.10.2021), which collected information on infections and provided contact tracing and tracking of persons who had possibly been exposed to infected persons. The application was made available for download as of 31 August for first use beginning 1 September. On the very first day, one million people downloaded the application, about one-fifth of the population, and at its peak, about half the population was using it. The widespread use of ICT, which had been developed to improve the quality and efficiency of welfare provision in a sparsely populated country, contributed to building trust by enabling mutual contact between citizens, especially in situations in which physical contact is restricted, such as during infectious disease outbreaks.

6.5 Discussion

As we have discussed, the Swedish and Finnish measures against COVID-19 were implemented on the principle of minimising restrictions on citizens' freedom. In Sweden, the constitutional guarantee of freedom of movement and the principle of the independence of public authorities and local autonomy made it difficult for the Swedish to mandate restrictions on movement; instead, the government's policy was to rely on expert advice, basing policy decisions on knowledge and evidence and relying on citizens' autonomous compliance with public health measures. Out of consideration of these constitutional freedoms, Sweden did not adopt a containment policy, and the country's infection and mortality rates were extremely high compared with those of other Nordic countries. However, despite this open strategy, Sweden's infection and mortality rates one year since the pandemic have been at the same level or even lower than those of other (non-Nordic) European countries that implemented lockdowns.

Finland has maintained very low infection and mortality rates compared with the rest of Europe, but in contrast with Sweden, Finland had a temporary lockdown. Finland's response measures were decided through the state's separated power structure (between the cabinet and the president) by observing the situations in other countries, the reactions of Finnish citizens and available data from Sweden. The government measures took optimal advantage of the existing system, and the special authority provided in the Emergency Powers Act was very limited. Finland's choice was not as definitive as Sweden's, with various agencies involved and ambiguous directions. However, the government's cautious approach, the adherence to infection-prevention behaviours by citizens who trusted the government and a well-developed ICT environment helped to reduce infections. In addition, Finland's success in controlling the spread of infection may have been partly due to its good fortune in being able to implement regulations and recommendations at an early stage because of the relatively late onset of the pandemic in the country.

Both countries chose policies that, at first glance, appear to be contrasting. Nevertheless, policies restricting citizens' freedom were kept to a minimum, and citizens did not find them overly restrictive at least during the early stage of the pandemic, the first six months. In addition, citizens in both countries had high trust in the experts and their political leaders; citizens faithfully followed the recommended infection-control measures with few notable conflicts between citizens and the state. This relationship of trust between citizens and the government can be attributed to the results of the COVID-19 measures in both countries. A survey of ten European countries revealed that in both Sweden and Finland, citizens felt the need to take COVID-19 countermeasures voluntarily and adhered to their governments' recommended measures; they perceived the contexts of the relatively loose behavioural restrictions as described earlier. Citizens in both countries also considered that their governments' COVID-19 measures had been highly effective. In both countries, the relatively moderate restrictions on citizens and citizens' accompanying compliance with infectious disease countermeasures were based on mutual trust between the government and citizens. This raises the question of how such a combination emerged.

Rothstein (Rothstein and Stolle 2002, 2003; Rothstein 2005) discussed that general trust depends not on politics itself but on how institutions implement policies. In the context of this study, universal welfare systems with no room for discretion generate people's general trust. Further, people's general trust is known to be positively correlated with economic equality and high-quality institutions (e.g. Stiglitz et al. 2018). In other words, the relationship of trust between government and citizens in the welfare state is rooted in the general trust that the universal welfare state has fostered over the years.

Citizens' trust in the government and autonomous compliance with government recommendations are grounded in high policy transparency, high citizen literacy in policy and natural science (i.e. human capital) and, in Finland, well-developed ICTs that allowed for smooth transitions to telework, which allowed for more effective social distancing. Strong systems such as Finland's rely on high ICT literacy among populations rather than knowledge concentrated among a few elites. As Greve et al. (2021) argued, high incomes, economic stability and high social equality enabled the Nordic countries to cope with the challenges posed by the pandemic and to sustain themselves better than other countries, although as we discussed, ethnic inequalities remain a challenge.

While trust from citizens is important, it is also necessary to consider the government's trust in its citizens; governments that do not trust citizens to comply voluntarily enforce stronger constraints. Anttiroiko (2021) evaluated the approaches of Denmark, Finland and Sweden as 'well-developed and successful Nordic countries' and identified that those nations' success was accompanied by an emphasis on civic responsibility. Orlowski and Goldsmith (2020) explained that Sweden's strategy of choosing more explicit collaboration between the government response and citizens' individual responsibility was grounded in the national *folkvett*, the common sense of the people as a collective. In Finland, meanwhile, although the government did issue some temporary restrictions, individuals were left to make their own decisions on whether to comply with the restrictions such as staying at home or not wearing masks. In other words, in both countries, the government trusted their citizens and gave them discretionary power. What emerged from these circumstances was that citizens trusted their governments' infectious-disease-control measures, and governments respected their citizens' rights and trusted them to follow recommendations responsibly.

Finally, it is important to point out the dangers posed by emotional traits in this cooperative relationship between government and citizens. In a Finnish survey by Jallinoja and Väliverronen (2021), 85.2% and 84% of the respondents, respectively, agreed with the notions that 'protection against infectious diseases takes precedence over personal freedom' and 'individuals who ignore government instructions pose a major threat to Finland'. Regarding instructions to wear masks, some respondents said they were uncomfortable doing things differently from others or being treated differently if they did not wear masks. Even when there was initial resistance to wearing masks, when it was positioned as a prosocial act, national sympathy was encouraged, and there was peer pressure to wear them (Pfattheicher et al. 2020), particularly if authority figures explained that masks effectively and directly protected others. Meanwhile, Orlowski and Goldsmith (2020) noted that Sweden is a nation of individualists with deeply personal behaviour within a framework of a strong state and governance. They explained that the guiding principle for decisions regarding COVID-19 was to measure the impacts of comprehensive stay-at-home measures on the alliance between the Swedish state and its people. Thus, the line that separated Sweden from Finland in domestic pandemic response was the degree of individualism among each respective nation's citizens.

6.6 Conclusion

During the COVID-19 pandemic, to be an economically and socially sustainable society, it is necessary to minimise the impacts of infectious-disease-control measures on economic activities and people's daily lives. In Asia, authoritarianism permitted efficient, effective countermeasures against COVID-19 with learning from earlier infectious-disease experiences. However, we observed here that countermeasures can be effective without authoritarian moves to restrict citizens' freedoms. In Finland and Sweden, the two states discussed in this chapter, relatively modest behavioural restrictions were combined with citizens' autonomous compliance with disease-control measures based on mutual trust between the government and citizens. Additionally, science, expertise, and trust in the government did encourage citizens to voluntarily protect themselves as Finnish case indicated.

The two countries' different choices regarding lockdown reflected the national degrees of individualism. In Sweden, there was no constitutional authority to restrict individual movement, and state intervention had to be minimised, whereas Finland proceeded with minimal restrictions on freedom and balanced policy decisions while evaluating the situations in other countries.

Both cases display that the affluence and equality of the welfare state increase the capacity of individuals and societies to respond to crises and minimise state intervention in individual lives during national emergencies. Although there were disparities between native citizens and immigrants and cultural minorities, these were less pronounced. Meanwhile, in both countries, autonomous citizen cooperation was greater than it was in other countries grounded in mutual trust between the citizens and their governments. We described this situation as enabling a relationship of co-occurring trust and cooperation between government and citizens, and this was grounded in the stability of a universal welfare state that fostered general trust.

In this chapter, we discussed COVID-19 controls in Sweden and Finland with our observations and interpretations of the latest findings as well as previous studies. At the time of writing, the pandemic has not yet ended, and it is likely too early to draw any clear conclusions. We leave further investigations to future research.

Annex Table Timeline for COVID-19 controls in Sweden and Finland

Sweden	Finland
10 March 2020	4 March 2020
Advice to the public: avoid unnecessary visits to medical and elderly-care facilities.	Reminder to public authorities to prepare for applicating Emergency Powers Act.
Interview with the Public Health Agency (Fälkhelsomyndigheten, FHM): Those with symptoms should take time off work.	Each medical area prepared for Emergency Plans.
	9 March
	Announcement of the timetable for the application of the Emergency Powers Act.
9 March	12 March
Test recommendations for symptomatic travelers from foreign countries identified as high risk.	The cabinet meeting decides on recommendations and responses.
11 March	Recommendation to stop gatherings of more than 500 people in accordance with the Infectious Diseases Act.
Ban on gatherings of more than 500 people.	13 March
12 March	Joint meeting of the cabinet and the president. Decision to apply the Emergency Powers Act.
Education minister announces at a press conference that there will be no simultaneous closure of schools for the time being.	Local administrative authorities ban gatherings of more than 500 people.

Sweden	Finland
13 March	16 March
Advice: If you are unwell, stay at home.	Declaration of the application of the 'state of emergency' under the Emergency Powers Act. The government may exercise special powers to restrict the rights and lives of citizens. Announcement of the details of the special measures to be taken during the state of emergency. €5 billion economic stimulus package.
Provisional rules set for when school closures are necessary.	
16 March	
Avoid contact with older people over 70.	
Stay at home and work from home as much as possible.	
The government orders the Social Affairs Agency to distribute protective equipment (including masks) as required.	
	17 March,
	'State of Emergency' applied (16 June)
17 March	18 March
Remote education in secondary and higher education recommended.	Implementation of special measures.
Travel ban outside the EU.	20 March
19 March	Decision to increase funding by €ten billion, mainly for employers. Strengthening the guarantee of equal rights for pupils receiving distance education. Obligation to provide face-to-face tuition for children in the lower grades (up to third year at comprehensive school) (entered into force 23 March).
Parliament approves the government's decision to close all schools when necessary.	
Unnecessary travel to be avoided.	
23 March	
Cancellation of national school examinations.	
24 March	27 March
Restaurants and other places of eating and drinking: social distancing of customers.	Travel restrictions across the Uusimaa region.
	4 April
Customers should sit down and eat their meals.	Closure of restaurants, cafes and nightclubs.
27 March	9 April
Prohibition of gatherings of more than 50 people.	Decision to extend special measures (until 13 May).
30 March	15 April
No visits to elderly-care institutions.	Travel restrictions across the Uusimaa region lifted.
Increased testing for corona infection.	22 April
Advice: social distancing.	Revision of the coronavirus strategy (temporarily called the hybrid strategy).
7 April	
Comprehensive corona policy issued by the government.	3–4 May
16 April	Consideration of lifting various restrictions.
The Infectious Diseases Act increases the powers of the government.	6 May
23 April	Adoption of the hybrid strategy.
Poster on COVID-19 and care of the elderly (later translated into ten languages).	13 May
	End of application of emergency response legislation.

(*Continued*)

Annex Table (Continued)

Sweden	Finland
NBHW asks all municipalities (kommun) to distribute anti-infectives. * A number of other companies lock down their own facilities from April. **5 June** WHO recommends wearing masks on public transport and in crowded places such as shopping. However, the Swedish authorities did not recommend wearing masks except in medical and elderly-related situations. **13 June** Travel restrictions in Sweden relaxed. **1 July** Further relaxation of travel restrictions in Sweden. **12 August** Karolinska Hospital in Stockholm recommends wearing a mask when social distancing is not possible. **18 August** The Public Health Agency announces that it is conducting a national study on face masks and that it may recommend wearing them locally in the future. Then, on 18 December 2020 It is announced that masks will be recommended from 7 January to be worn on public transport at specific times of the day. **7 January 2021** Recommendation to wear masks on public transport. **1 July** Recommendation to wear masks on public transport lifted.	**14 May** Resumption of normal school hours. Lifting of restrictions on movement within the Schengen area. Conditional reopening of outdoor sports facilities. **29 May** Announcement of policy allowing domestic travel. **1 June** Easing of restrictions on gatherings. The maximum number of people allowed to gather is reduced to 50. **3 June** Guidelines on the use of masks issued. Priority given to safe distances, hand washing and cough hygiene to prevent infection. **16 June** State of emergency lifted. **23 June** Lifting of restrictions on travel to and from countries with a similar incidence of infected people. **1 July** Ban on outdoor gatherings of more than 500 people lifted. **13 August** Masks are recommended. **31 August** The Koronavilkku contact tracing application is released. It was downloaded more than one million times on the first day. **6 September** Hybrid strategy revised, with three levels of infection to be applied as guidelines for each health area. **23 October** Guidelines for the second wave applied in some areas.

Source: Authors

Notes

1 Sweden had many more infections and deaths and higher proportions of both than did the other three countries. However, the number of deaths as of March 2021 (126.7 per 100,000 people) was close to the average among the 30 European Union/European Economic Area member states (121.1 per 100,000; European Centre for Disease Prevention and Control n.d.).

2 We excluded India from consideration here because of the significant sample bias: 82.3% of respondents in India had completed higher education (compared with rates of 15.5% to 79.7% in other countries), and 26.8% of Indian respondents worked in health care (compared with 4.3% to 31.4% in other countries).
3 In Sweden and Finland, fewer government-imposed measures and higher compliance rates indicate that citizens autonomously took measures to prevent infection.

References

Anttiroiko, A.-V. (2021) 'Successful Government Responses to the Pandemic: Contextualizing National and Urban Responses to the COVID-19 Outbreak in East and West', *International Journal of E-Planning Research* (IJEPR), vol. 10, no. 2. doi: 10.4018/IJEPR.20210401.oa1.

Borgholms Kommun (2021). 'De flesta regionala rekommendationer upphör – munskydd vid smitta på arbetsplats ska användas'. Available at: www.borgholm.se/de-flesta-regionala-rekommendationer-upphor-munskydd-vid-smitta-pa-arbetsplats-ska-anvandas/ (Accessed: 16 August 2021).

City of Helsinki (2020a) 'Helsingin koronavirustilannekatsaus'. Available at: www.hel.fi/helsinki/korona-fi/sote-palvelut/korona-tilanne/ (Accessed: 20 August 2021).

City of Helsinki (2020b) 'Somalinkielisten koronavirustartunnat ovat lisääntyneet Helsingissä – Luuqadda soomaliga dadka ku hadlo cudurka korona wuu ku soo siyaadey magaalada Helsinki', 14 April. Available at: www.hel.fi/uutiset/fi/kaupunginkanslia/somalinkielisten-koronavirustartunnat (Accessed: 20 August 2021).

European Centre for Disease Prevention and Control (n.d.) 'Download COVID-19 datasets, COVID-19'. Available at: www.ecdc.europa.eu/en (Accessed: 15 September 2021).

Folkhälsomyndigheten (2020a) *Beteende, oro och informationsbehov Genomförda och pågående undersökningar under covid-19.* Stockholm: Fälkhelsomyndigheten. Available at: www.folkhalsomyndigheten.se/contentassets/9fd20c6bde8e4fd188 6bb589fa09e202/beteende-oro-informationsbehov.pdf (Accessed: 29 July 2021).

Folkhälsomyndigheten (2020b) *Beslut om skärpta allmänna råd i Stockholms län, Västra Götalands län och Östergötlands län.* Stockholm: Fälkhelsomyndigheten. Available at: www.folkhalsomyndigheten.se/nyheter-och-press/nyhetsarkiv/2020/oktober/beslut-om-skarpta-allmanna-rad-i-stockholms-lan-vastra-gotalands-lan-och-ostergotlands-lan/ (Accessed: 2 December 2021).

Folkhälsomyndigheten (2021a) *Anpassning av åtgärder mot spridning av covid-19 Antal fall av covid-19 i Sverige – data till och med föregående dag publiceras varje tisdag-fredag.* Stockholm: Fälkhelsomyndigheten. Available at: www.folkhalsomyndigheten.se/smittskydd-beredskap/utbrott/aktuella-utbrott/covid-19/skydda-dig-och-andra/anpassning-av-atgarder-mot-spridning-av-covid-19/ (Accessed: 6 August 2021).

Folkhälsomyndigheten (2021b) *Antal fall av covid-19 i Sverige – data till och med föregående dag publiceras varje tisdag-fredag.* Stockholm: Fälkhelsomyndigheten. Available at: https://experience.arcgis.com/experience/09f821667ce64bf7be6f9 f87457ed9aa/page/page_0/ (Accessed: 23 July 2021).

Folkhälsomyndigheten (2021c) *Utrikesfödda och covid-19 Konstaterade fall, IVA-vård och avlidna bland utrikesfödda i Sverige.* Stockholm: Fälkhelsomyndigheten. Available at: www.folkhalsomyndigheten.se/contentassets/2dddee08a4ec4c25a0a59aa c7aca14f0/utrikesfodda-och-covid-19.pdf (Accessed: 16 August 2021).

Georgieva, I., Lantta, T., Lickiewicz, J., Pekara, J., Wikman, S., Loseviča, M., Raveesh, B. N., Mihai, A. and Lepping, P. (2021) 'Perceived Effectiveness, Restrictiveness, and Compliance with Containment Measures against the COVID-19

Pandemic: An International Comparative Study in 11 Countries', *International Journal of Environmental Research and Public Health*, vol. 18, no. 7. doi:10.3390/ijerph18073806.

Government Offices of Sweden (2020) *Speech by Minister for Health and Social Affairs Lena Hallengren at WHO Briefing 23 April, 2020*. Stockholm: Government Offices of Sweden. Available at: www.government.se/speeches/2020/04/speech-by-minister-for-health-and-social-affairs-lena-hallengren-at-who-briefing-23-april/

Greve, B., Blomquist, P., Hvinden, B. and van Gerven, M. (2021) 'Nordic Welfare States – Still Standing or Changed by the COVID-19 Crisis?', *Social Policy Administration*, vol. 55, pp. 295–311. doi:10.1111/spol.12675

Hale, T., Angrist, N., Goldszmidt, R., Kira, B., Petherick, A., Phillips, T., Webster, S., Cameron-Blake, E., Hallas, L., Majumdar, S. and Tatlow, H. (2021) 'A Global Panel Database of Pandemic Policies (Oxford COVID-19 Government Response Tracker)', *Nature Human Behaviour*, vol. 5, pp. 529–538. doi:10.1038/s41562-021-01079-8.

Jallinoja, P. and Väliverronen, E. (2021) 'Suomalaisten Luottamus Instituutioihin ja Asiantuntijoihin COVID19-Pandemiassa', *Media & Viestintä*, vol. 44, no. 1, pp. 1–24. doi:10.23983/mv.107298

Jonung L. (2020) 'Sweden's Constitution Decides Its COVID-19 Exceptionalism', in *Lund University Department of Economics School of Economics and Management Working Paper 2020:11*. Lund: Lund University. Available at: https://project.nek.lu.se/publications/workpap/papers/wp20_11.pdf (Accessed: 28 July 2021).

Kangas, O. (2020) 'Finland: Policy Measures in Response to the COVID-19 Pandemic', ESPN Flash Report 2020/59, European Social Policy Network (ESPN). Brussels: European Commission. Available at: https://ec.europa.eu/social/BlobServlet?docId=23058&langId=enKangas (Accessed: 20 August 2021).

Kantar Sifo (2020) *Katar Rapport om förtroende, oro och beteende under coronakrisen 21 mars-3 augusti Rapport till MSB*. Stockholm: Kantar Sifo. Available at: www.msb.se/siteassets/dokument/aktuellt/pagaende-handelser-och-insats/coronaviruset – covid-19/resultat-fran-kantar-sifos-undersokningar/augusti-2020/200803-kantar-sifo-resutat-coronaundersokning.pdf (Accessed: 29 July 2021).

Kantar Sifo (2021a) *Kantar Allmänhetens tillit, tankar och beteende under coronapandemin Publicerade och egna undersökningar från Kantar Sifo 11–24 mars 2021*. Stockholm: Kantar Sifo. Available at: www.kantarsifo.se/sites/default/files/reports/documents/kantar_sifo_allmanhetens_tillit_tankar_och_beteende_under_coronakrisen_26_mars.pdf (Accessed: 10 August 2021).

Kantar Sifo (2021b) *Kantar Public Allmänheten om anseendet för svenska myndigheter*. Stockholm: Kantar Sifo. Available at: www.kantarsifo.se/sites/default/files/reports/documents/sifo_anseendeindex_myndigheter_2021_kantar_public.pdf (Accessed: 10 August 2021).

Karlsten, E. (2020) 'Här är kontext till de publicerade Tegnell-mejlen'. Available at: https://emanuelkarlsten.se/har-ar-kontext-till-de-lackta-tegnell-mejlen/ (Accessed: 10 August 2021).

Kongl, M. (1766) *Nådige Förordning, angående Skrif-och Tryck-friheten; Gifwen Stockholm i Råd Cammaren 2*. December.

Krisinformation (2021) 'Kantar Munskydd i kollektivtrafiken, Krisinformation. se'. Available at: www.krisinformation.se/detta-kan-handa/handelser-och-storningar/20192/myndigheterna-om-det-nya-coronaviruset/andra-sprakother-languages/lattlast1/nyhetsarkiv-lattlast (Accessed: 6 August 2021).

Kritzinger, S., Foucault, M., Lachat, R., Partheymüller, J., Plescia, C. and Brouard, R. (2021) ' "Rally round the flag": The COVID-19 Crisis and Trust in the National Government', *West European Politics*, vol. 44, no. 5–6, pp. 1205–1231. doi:10.10 80/01402382.2021.1925017.

Kungl. Vetenskapsakademien (2020) 'Ny rapport om munskydd och ventilation från Vetenskapsakademiens expertgrupp om COVID-19'. Available at: www.kva.se/sv/pressrum/pressmeddelanden/ny-rapport-om-munskydd-och-ventilation-fran-vetenskapsakademiens-expertgrupp-om-covid-19 (Accessed: 4 December 2021).

Lindström, M. (2008) 'Social Capital, Political Trust and Purchase of Illegal Liquor: A Population-Based Study in SOUTHERN SWEDEN', *Health Policy*, vol. 86, no. 2–3, pp. 266–275. doi:10.1016/j.healthpol.2007.11.001.

Marien, S. and Hooghe, M. (2011) 'Does Political Trust Matter? An Empirical Investigation into the Relation between Political Trust and Support for Law Compliance', *European Journal of Political Research*, vol. 50, pp. 267–291. doi:10.1111/j.1475-6765.2010.01930.x

Mueller, J. E. (1973) *War, Presidents, and Public Opinion*. New York: John Wiley & Sons.

Myndigheten för samhällsskydd och beredskap (MSB) (2021) *Information om coronaviruset på andra spark*. Sweden. Stockholm: MSB. Available at: www.msb.se/sv/aktuellt/pagaende-handelser-och-insatser/msbs-arbete-med-anledning-av-coronaviruset/information-pa-andra-sprak – other-languages/ (Accessed: 29 July 2021).

Nielsen, J.H. and Lindvall, J. (2021) 'Trust in Government in Sweden and Denmark during the COVID-19 Epidemic', *West European Politics*, vol. 44, no. 5–6, pp. 1180–1204. doi:10.1080/01402382.2021.1909964.

Nordin, J. (2015) *1766 års tryckfrihetsförordning Bakgrund och betydelse*. Stockholm: Kungl Biblioteket. Available at: www.kb.se/Dokument/Aktuellt/publikationer/TF%201766,%20Nordin,%20liten.pdf (Accessed: 10 August 2021).

OECD (Organisation for Economic Co-operation and Development) and Statistics Finland (2021) *Finland: Road to Recovery after COVID-19*. Paris: OECD Publishing. Available at: www.oecd.org/sdd/its/Finland-COVID-Report-May-2021.pdf (Accessed: 10 August 2021).

Oksanen, A., Kaakinen, M., Latikka, R., Savolainen, I., Savela, N. and Koivula A. (2020) 'Regulation and Trust: 3-Month Follow-up Study on COVID-19 Mortality in 25 European Countries', *JMIR Public Health and Surveillance*, vol. 6, no.2. doi:10.2196/19218.

Olsson, E. (2021) 'Tegnell: "Då är munskydd smittorisk" ', *Läraren.se*, 26 January. Available at: www.lararen.se/nyheter/coronaviruset/tegnell-da-ar-munskydd-smittorisk (Accessed: 3 August 2021).

Omni (2020) 'Två av fem vill se krav på munskydd på buss och tåg', *Omni*. Available at: https://omni.se/tva-av-fem-vill-se-krav-pa-munskydd-pa-buss-och-tag/a/zGWAGq (Accessed: 4 August 2021).

Orlowski, E.J.W. and Goldsmith, D.J.A. (2020) 'Four Months into the COVID-19 Pandemic, Sweden's Prized Herd Immunity Is Nowhere in Sight', *Journal of the Royal Society of Medicine*, vol. 113, no. 8, pp. 292–298. doi:10.1177/0141076820945282.

Pfattheicher, S., Nockur, L., Böhm, R., Sassenrath, C., and Petersen, M. B. (2020) 'The Emotional Path to Action: Empathy Promotes Physical Distancing and Wearing of Face Masks During the COVID-19 Pandemic'. *Psychological Science*, vol 31, no. 11, pp. 1363–1373. doi:10.1177/0956797620964422.

Rothstein, B. (2005) *Social Traps and the Problem of Trust.* Cambridge: Cambridge University Press.

Rothstein, B. and Stolle, D. (2002) 'How Political Institutions Create and Destroy Social Capital: An Institutional Theory of Generalized Trust', Paper prepared for the 98th Meeting of the American Political Science Association in Boston, MA, August 29–2 September 2002.

Rothstein, B. and Stolle, D. (2003) 'Social Capital, Impartiality and the Welfare State: An Institutional Approach', in Hooghe and Stolle (eds), *Generating Social Capital.* New York: Palgrave Macmillan, pp. 191–230.

Statistiska centralbyrån (2021a) *Tabell 9a, Antal rapporterade dödsfall till SCB för inrikes och utrikes födda per vecka åren 2015–2021.* Stockholm: Statistiska centralbyrån.

Statistiska centralbyrån (2021b) Utrikes födda i Sverige. Available at: www.scb.se/hitta-statistik/sverige-i-siffror/manniskorna-i-sverige/utrikes-fodda/ (Accessed: 16 August 2021).

Stiglitz, J., Fitoussi, J. and Durand, M. (eds) (2018) *For Good Measure: Advancing Research on Well-being Metrics Beyond GDP.* Paris: OECD Publishing. doi:10.1787/9789264307278-en.

STM (Sosiaali- ja Terveys Ministeriö) (2020) Selvitys väestön kasvosuojusten käytöstä COVID-19-epidemian leviämisen ehkäisyssä, Sosiaali- ja terveysministeriön raportteja ja muistioita. Available at: http://urn.fi/URN:ISBN:978-952-00-5421-2 (Accessed: 20 August 2021).

Strang, J. (2020) 'Why do the Nordic countries react differently to the covid-19 crisis?', *Nordics info*, 6 April. Available at: https://nordics.info/show/artikel/the-nordic-countries-react-differently-to-the-covid-19-crisis (Accessed: 20 August 2021).

Suomen Uutiset (2020) 'Ronkainen ja Rantanen maahanmuuttajien korkeammista koronatartuntaluvuista: "Ei ole syrjintää tai rasismia vaatia samoja varotoimenpiteitä"', *Suomen Uutiset*, 24 October. Available at: www.suomenuutiset.fi/ronkainen-ja-rantanen-maahanmuuttajien-korkeammista-koronatartuntaluvuista-ei-ole-syrjintaa-tai-rasismia-vaatia-samoja-varotoimenpiteita/ (Accessed: 20 August 2021).

THL (Terveiden ja Hyvinvointi Laitos) (2020) 'THL suosittaa kasvomaskin käyttöä toisten suojaamiseksi – käsienpesu ja turvavälit ovat tärkeimmät keinot ehkäistä koronatartuntoja', *Tiedote*, 13 August. Available at: https://thl.fi/fi/-/-thl-suosittaa-kasvomaskin-kayttoa-toisten-suojaamiseksi-kasienpesu-ja-turvavalit-ovat-tarkeimmat-keinot-ehkaista-koronatartuntoja (Accessed: 20 August 2021).

THL (Terveiden ja Hyvinvointi Laitos) (2021a) 'Can a private service provider or event organiser require mask use? How should service providers that require mask use act if a person cannot wear a mask due to a disability or for health reasons?', in Questions and answers about face masks. Updated 31 March 2021. Available at: https://thl.fi/en/web/infectious-diseases-and-vaccinations/what-s-new/coronavirus-covid-19-latest-updates/transmission-and-protection-coronavirus/recommendation-on-the-use-of-face-masks-for-citizens/questions-and-answers-about-face-masks (Accessed: 20 August 2021).

THL (Terveiden ja Hyvinvointi Laitos) (2021b) 'Recommendation on the use of face masks for citizens'. Updated 4 August 2021. Available at: https://thl.fi/en/web/infectious-diseases-and-vaccinations/what-s-new/coronavirus-covid-19-latest-updates/transmission-and-protection-coronavirus/recommendation-on-the-use-of-face-masks-for-citizens (Accessed: 20 August 2021).

THL (Terveiden ja Hyvinvointi Laitos) (n.d.) 'Tartuntaketjujen katkaisua tehostava sovellus, Koronavilkku'. Available at: https://thl.fi/fi/web/infektiotaudit-ja-rokotukset/ajankohtaista/ajankohtaista-koronaviruksesta-covid-19/

tarttuminen-ja-suojautuminen-koronavirus/tartuntaketjujen-katkaisua-tehostava-sovellus (Accessed: 20 August 2021).

Tiirinki, H., Tynkkynen, L.K., Sovala, M., Atkins, S., Koivusalo, M., Rautiainen, P., Jormanainen, V. and Keskimäki, I. (2020) 'COVID-19 Pandemic in Finland – Preliminary Analysis on Health System Response and Economic Consequences', *Health Policy Technology*, vol. 9, no. 4, pp. 649–662. doi:10.1016/j.hlpt.2020.08.005.

Tilastokeskus (2021) 'Koronavirustauti kuolemansyynä vuonna 2020', *Tilastokeskus*, 21 May. Available at: www.tilastokeskus.fi/ajk/koronavirus/koronavirus-ajankohtaista-tilastotietoa/miten-vaikutukset-nakyvat-tilastoissa/koronavirus_kuolemansyyna (Accessed: 20 August 2021).

Tilastokeskus (n.d.) 'Kansalaispulssi'. Available at: www.stat.fi/tup/htpalvelut/tutkimukset/kansalaispulssi.html (Accessed: 20 August 2021).

Väliverronen, E., Laaksonen, S-M., Jauho, M. and Jallinoja, P. (2020) 'Liberalists and Data-Solutionists: Redefining Expertise in Twitter Debates on Coronavirus in Finland', *Journal of Science Communication*, vol. 19, no. 5. doi:10.22323/2.19050210.

Valtioneuvosto (2020a) 'Yhteiskunnan toiminnan kannalta kriittisten alojen henkilöstö', Governmental press release, *Tiedote 145/2020*, 17 March. Available at: https://valtioneuvosto.fi/-/10616/yhteiskunnan-toiminnan-kannalta-kriittisten-alojen-henkilosto (Accessed: 20 August 2021).

Valtioneuvosto (2020b) 'Hallitus esittää laajoja taloustoimia koronavirusepidemian haittojen minimoimiseksi', Valtioneuvoston viestintäosasto, *Tiedote 158/2020*, 20 March. Available at: https://valtioneuvosto.fi/-/10616/hallitus-esittaa-laajoja-taloustoimia-koronavirusepidemian-haittojen-minimoimiseksi (Accessed: 20 August 2021).

Valtioneuvosto (2020c) 'Sosiaali- ja terveydenhuollon suojavarusteiden tilannekuva päivitetty', Sosiaali- ja terveysministeriö, Työ- ja elinkeinoministeriö, *Tiedote 138/2020*, 3 June. Available at: https://valtioneuvosto.fi/-/1271139/sosiaali-ja-terveydenhuollon-suojavarusteiden-tilannekuva-paivitetty (Accessed: 20 August 2021).

Valtioneuvosto (2020d) 'Hallitus linjasi neuvottelussaan kasvosuojuksista ja keskusteli rajaliikenteestä', Valtioneuvoston viestintäosasto, *Tiedote 387/2020*. 3 June. Available at: https://valtioneuvosto.fi/-/10616/korjaus-hallitus-linjasi-neuvottelussaan-kasvosuojuksista-ja-keskusteli-rajaliikenteesta (Accessed: 20 August 2021).

Valtioneuvosto (n.d.) 'Kansalaispulssi'. Available at: https://valtioneuvosto.fi/tietoa-koronaviruksesta/kansalaispulssi (Accessed: 20 August 2021).

Voipio-Pulkki, L.M. (2020) 'Toimintasuunnitelma hybridistrategian mukaisten suositusten ja rajoitusten toteuttamiseen covid-19-epidemian ensimmäisen vaiheen jälkeen', *Sosiaali- ja terveysministeriö*, 7 September. Sosiaali- ja terveysministeriön julkaisuja 2020:26. Available at: http://urn.fi/URN:ISBN:978-952-00-7176-9 (Accessed: 20 August 2021).

Watanabe, M. (2006) 'The roll of remiss system in decision-making procedure in Sweden- in the case study of Ädel reform (medical and welfare reform of elderly care)', in *Northern Europe Study. Second vol. 2005*. Tokyo: Northern Europe Association.

Weible, C. M., Nohrstedt, D., Cairney, P., Carter, D. P., Crow, D. A., Durnová, A. P., Heikkila, T., Ingold, K., McConnell, A. and Stone, D. (2020) 'COVID-19 and the Policy Sciences: Initial Reactions and Perspectives', *Policy Sciences*, 1–17. doi:10.1007/s11077-020-09381-4.

WHO (World Health Organization) (2020) 'Coronavirus disease (COVID-19): Masks', 1 December. Available at: www.who.int/news-room/questions-and-answers/item/coronavirus-disease-covid-19-masks (Accessed: 14 December 2021).

WHO (World Health Organization) (n.d.) 'COVID-19 Dashboard'. Available at: https://covid19.who.int/ (Accessed: 20 August 2021).

News media (excluding those published by political parties)

Aftonbladet	www.aftonbladet.se/
BBC News	www.bbc.com/news
Dagens Nyheter	www.dn.se/
Der Spiegel	www.spiegel.de/
Expressen	www.expressen.se/
HS (Helsingin Sanomat)	www.hs.fi/
IL (Iltalehti)	www.iltalehti.fi/
IS (Ilta-Sanomat)	www.is.fi/
Svenska Dagbladet	www.svd.se/
Sverigeradio	https://sverigesradio.se/
Svt Nyheter	www.svt.se/
Sydsvenskan	www.sydsvenskan.se/
The Local	www.thelocal.se/
The Wall Street Journal	www.wsj.com/
Yle (Yleisradio)	https://yle.fi/uutiset

7 The unlawful and unequal wearing of masks

The case of Poland during COVID-19

Łukasz Czarnecki and Monika Skowrońska

7.1 Introduction

Coronavirus disease 2019 (COVID-19) was not the first virus that deeply transformed both legal and social relations worldwide.[1] During this pandemic, however, masks were imposed globally, with some differences in each country (PDA 2020). During 2020 and 2021, new legal provisions were established in Poland, and the country's legal framework regarding mask-wearing went through many different stages of legal transformation. The objective of this chapter is to shed light on the legal and social consequences in Poland of mask mandates.

The Polish legislature passed measures in the form of limitations, orders, and prohibitions that significantly limit the exercise of freedoms constituting human rights subject to legal protection under the Polish constitution and international law. The measures imposed affect such rights and freedoms as personal freedom,[2] especially when it comes to the obligation to cover the mouth and nose, and the right to privacy.[3] The Polish Constitutional Tribunal defines personal freedom as 'the possibility for an individual to make decisions according to his own will, to freely choose how to proceed in public and private life, unrestricted by other persons'.

The pandemic is an 'unprecedented and massive scale sanitary crisis', the management of which requires extraordinary measures (Council of Europe 2020, p. 2). Some of these measures, however, interfere with human rights, as indicated by the Secretary General of the Council of Europe, Marija Pejčinović Burić: 'The virus is destroying many lives and much else of what is very dear to us. We should not let it destroy our core values and free societies' (Council of Europe 2020, p. 2).

In this situation, 'actions by authorities that impose restrictions on human rights and freedoms should be justified, necessary, limited in time and proportionate to the threat posed by the spread of the COVID-19 virus' (Granowska 2020, p. 4). Governments can use people's fear of the disease to introduce unjustified restrictions on human rights or cover up human rights violations, so it is imperative – especially at present – to analyze the various actions of governments (Amnesty International 2020).[4]

To address the questions of how Poland's legal framework transformed regarding wearing masks and how and to what extent mask-wearing shed light on inequalities reproduced during COVID-19, the authors will first analyze the

DOI: 10.4324/9781003244127-8

country's legal framework (Section 7.2) and then its reproduction of power (Section 7.3).

7.2 Legal framework

The Polish legislature introduced measures to combat and contain an infectious disease that poses a threat to human life. The reaction of Polish authorities to the COVID-19 pandemic raised serious concerns, however. Polish courts also raised these concerns, asserting in many cases the government's inability to apply these provisions as a basis for legal sanctions against entities that disregarded them.

The principles and procedures for preventing and combating human infectious diseases in Poland are defined in the Act of 5 December 2008, which does not mention COVID-19.[5] The Act does, however, provide for the competence of the Minister of Health to include a disease other than those listed if there is a risk of its spreading.

On this basis, on 27 February 2020, before the disclosure of the first case of coronavirus in Poland, the Minister of Health announced that 'SARS-CoV-2 coronavirus infection was covered by the provisions of the Act on preventing and combating infections and infectious diseases in humans'.[6] The Act of 5 December 2008 originally did not contain provisions related to the obligation to cover the mouth and nose but rather provided for a general obligation to 'comply with the orders and bans of the State Sanitary Inspection aimed at preventing and combating infections and infectious diseases' (Article 5.1.3).

The COVID-19 pandemic forced the legislature to amend the act many times. First, on 8 March 2020, the competence of the Council of Ministers was established to issue a regulation specifying restrictions, orders and bans in the event of an epidemic or epidemic threat of a nature and size exceeding the capacity of the bodies that already had such powers, the Minister of Health and voivodes.[7] The authorisation initially included the possibility of establishing the requirement of 'the use of other preventive measures and treatments by sick and suspected sick persons', and on 29 November 2020, expanded to 'the obligation to use other preventive measures and treatments' and 'the order to cover the mouth and nose, in certain circumstances, places and facilities and in specific areas, together with how to implement this order'.[8]

The reaction of Polish legislators to the pandemic was to introduce regulations that required covering the mouth and nose and included other obligations aimed at preventing the spread of the disease. Although regulations are one of the sources of universally binding law, they have an executive nature in relation to acts. Regulations are not issued by the Parliament but by bodies of executive power (e.g. the Council of Ministers and ministers). Meanwhile, taking into account that the measures selected by the legislature interfere with human rights, regulations should be implemented in the form of acts in accordance with existing legal provisions.[9]

It is also important that, according to Poland's constitution, regulations may be issued by specific organs of executive power on the basis of a detailed authorisation contained in an act or law for the purpose of its implementation.[10] Such statutory delegation should not only define the authority competent to issue the regulation but also set the scope of matters to be regulated as well as the guidelines regarding the content of the act. The anti-COVID-19 regulations do not meet this criterion.

The general obligation to cover the mouth and nose in public places was issued by regulation on 15 April 2020. According to this regulation: 'The person is required to uncover the mouth and nose at the request of: (1) authorised bodies in the case of identifying the person to establish his identity; (2) another person in connection with delivering services or the performance of professional or official activities, including in the case of the need to identify or verify the identity of a given person'.[11]

In other words, until 29 November 2020, when the Act of 2008 was amended to provide for the obligation to 'take preventive measures and treatment' of covering the mouth and nose, it only applied to people who were sick or suspected to be sick. In a case regarding the failure of others to fulfill their duty to cover their mouths and noses during the period from 16 April to 28 November 2020, the court refused to hold them liable.

In the justification to the amendment, which entered into force on 29 November 2020 and introduced the power of the Council of Ministers to establish in the regulation 'an order to cover the mouth and nose, in certain circumstances, places and objects and in specific areas, together with the manner of implementing this order', it was indicated that its purpose was 'clarification of the existing provisions to avoid interpretation doubts as to the possibility of establishing the obligation to apply specific preventive measures and treatments'.[12] This is, of course, an incorrect definition of the nature of the amended provisions. Because the possibility of introducing the obligation to apply certain preventive measures was previously explicitly reserved, this is not only a change for clarification but also a substantive change in legal status.

For Polish society to understand the purpose of this new legal framework, it was not desirable that regulations on these measures were introduced in various laws, sometimes of a similar nature, because these laws were frequently changed, and the legislative period was very short.

By exercising only one of the many statutory delegations contained in the Act of 5 December 2008, the Council of Ministers, based on projects prepared by the Ministry of Health, adopted as many as 78 regulations that introduced or changed restrictions, orders and prohibitions regarding the pandemic.[13] The regulations entered into force within 2 to 4 days of their adoption by the Council of Ministers and were published in the Official Journal on the day they were adopted or the day after.

As noted, the basic principles for the prevention of infectious diseases were set out in the Act of 5 December 2008, which was enacted more than 11 years before the advent of COVID-19. The Minister of Health co-opted its use during the pandemic, and on 2 March 2020, the act on special solutions related to the prevention and combating of COVID-19, other infectious diseases and the crisis situations caused thereby (the so-called special anti-COVID-19 law) was passed. This law is more detailed and not only is intended to counteract COVID-19 but also refers to certain financial consequences of applying measures to counteract it. It is unclear, however, why both laws contain regulations aimed at achieving the same goal. For example, to secure certain scarce goods (in particular for medical personnel), the Act of 5 December 2008 empowered public administration bodies to establish restrictions or prohibitions on trade or use (on the basis of which they are obliged to notify the intention to export or sell certain types of masks outside Poland). In contrast, the Special Act of 2 March 2020 empowers another authority to set the maximum or upper limits on wholesale and retail margins used for the sale of goods 'essential for the protection of health'. This legislative chaos was exacerbated by transferring pandemic-related regulations from one legal act to another. For example, the restrictions on the export or sale of certain types of masks, which were initially governed by the provisions of the regulation of the Minister of Health on the declaration of an epidemic threat and later on the state of an epidemic, were repealed and introduced into the regulation of the Council of Ministers on the establishment of certain restrictions, orders, and bans due to the epidemic.

According to the Council of Ministers' regulation, the new amendment published at the end of September extended wearing masks in public places until 31 October 2021.[14]

7.3 Reproduction of power during the pandemic

The emergence of the pandemic is not the result of biomedical procedures such as human interaction with the environment. On the contrary, it can be viewed as a reproduction of such power structures that Jaime Breilh (1986) observed in his book titled *Epidemiology: Economics, Medicine and Politics*. In addition, Ivan Illich considered that international pharmaceutical corporations produce and reproduce the idea of medicalisation of human beings, of someone who should be constantly under medical vigilance (Illich 1982).

In the 1990s, Amartya Sen, a Nobel Prize laureate in economic sciences, emphasised the need to understand health issues in much broader terms. According to Sen, 'the health aspects relate to the social environment, to the provision of medical care, to the pattern of family life, and to a variety of other factors, and a purely income-based analysis of poverty cannot but leave that story half told' (Sen 1992, p. 114). Based on the capitalist logic of commodifying access to all goods, a hegemonic model of healthcare has been imposed during those times, during which access to healthcare varies with respect to social status (Menéndez 1990). The relationship between society and disease is a relationship based on the context of class relations (Almeida-Filho 2000).

Neoliberal policies have developed the 'scientific area' of medicine aimed at the individual without developing the premises of collective (environmental) health that deals with practices, policies, technologies and instruments of a collective approach, hence the complete disappearance of 'social medicine' as a science. This paradigm deals not only with health but also with the violence that shapes it (Tetelboin-Henrion et al. 2018). For example, Ana Cristina Laurell (2015) developed a critical stance against the conventional, biomedical and epidemio-logical visions that hide social processes, naturalise social relations and shift the focus to the individual.

The pandemic has revealed all these issues regarding the reproduction of power and the hegemonic model of power itself.[15] Moreover, the pandemic has demonstrated how separate the health sector has become from social and public policies, often with the acceptance of pharmaceutical companies, for which ensur-ing health by providing appropriate medications is not entirely certain.

7.3.1 Social reproduction

Social reproduction refers to social forces conducted mostly by women in soci-ety, 'those available for birthing and raising children, caring for friends and fam-ily members, maintaining households and broader communities, and sustaining connections more generally' (Fraser 2016, p. 99). Thus, women play significant roles in society, and the pandemic has negatively affected social reproduction forces. Social reproduction recognises gender differences among women and men (Gordon-Bouvier 2021) and refers to our everyday life split into categories with respect to gender, age and education differences.

In Poland, women account for 55.2% of infection cases and men account for 44.8% of the cases (GIS 2020). COVID-19 imposed social distancing, in which wearing masks plays a particular role (Jarynowski et al. 2020).

The Foundation Center for Public Opinion Research (CBOS in Polish) launched a study on masks and the pandemic and masks.[16] When asked whether wearing respiratory masks primarily protects against infection, persons with basic vocational education were most often convinced that masks equally protect both persons wearing masks and those around them (Table 7.1). Interestingly, the percentage of respondents who claim that masks do not protect anyone increases with the level of education and is the highest among people with higher educa-tion, approximately 20% (CBOS 2020).

Persons with only primary education tend to believe that the masks primarily protect those who wear them, whereas respondents with higher education know that they primarily protect those around them (CBOS 2020).

In the CBOS study, people over 45 most often believed that wearing a mask protects both themselves and those around them. At the same time, persons over 65 years old tended to believe that masks protect against infecting primarily themselves (13%). Young people from 18 to 24 years old (29%) primarily believe that the mask mainly protects surrounding individuals. At the same time, younger Poles most often contest the effectiveness of this preventive measure and believe that the masks are not protecting anyone. This is the opinion of almost every third person aged 25 to 34 and almost every fourth aged 18 to 24 and 35 to 44.

More than half of adult Poles agree with the statement that wearing a mask and inhaling air through it for a considerable amount of time is harmful and can lead to serious lung diseases. Women (57%) are more convinced of the harmfulness of masks than men (52%).

Table 7.1 Does wearing respiratory masks primarily protect against infection? (in percentages)

Education	It protects persons wearing masks	It protects others, with whom a person in a mask has contact	It protects in a similar degree the ones wearing them and others	It protects nobody from infection	Hard to tell
Elementary/ lower secondary	13	15	52	14	7
Basic vocational	5	14	60	16	4
High school	6	26	43	18	6
Higher	4	29	45	19	4
Age					
18–24	6	29	38	23	4
25–34	3	23	37	32	6
35–44	3	23	45	23	6
45–54	8	25	51	14	2
55–64	5	21	57	11	6
≥65	13	17	59	5	6

Source: Own based on CBOS (2020: 8)

The COVID-19 pandemic revealed deep inequalities with respect to class position and the hierarchy of the labour structure. The highest socioeconomic sector of Polish society demonstrated high mobility in February and March 2020; businessmen and corporate bosses, often returning from winter holidays from resorts in Austria, Switzerland or Colorado, were at the top of the list. The pandemic reinforced the happening of the accumulation of capital at one end of the spectrum and the pauperisation of the workforce at the other. The second category includes the health care and security services, which protect health and safety, and the third category includes lost professions: hairdressers, restaurant workers, etc. that suffered during the pandemic. The fourth includes workers who are not affected by social distancing, including employees of transnational plants, such as Amazon, and state-owned companies, such as coal and energy, among others.

7.3.2 Reproduction of economic power: the case of the Polish Sewing Works program

At the beginning of the pandemic, masks became a scarce commodity, and the attention of state authorities focused on securing them for certain professional groups, in particular medical personnel. This focus was also reflected in the provisions of early pandemic regulations. The Act of 28 October 2020 stipulated the possibility for the competent minister in matters of the economy to determine the maximum prices or margins for the sale of goods 'of significant importance for the protection of human health or safety'. Masks as a commodity effectively became a source of economic power.

The activities of entrepreneurs in the field of setting prices of certain products, including hygiene measures to protect against coronavirus infection, were at the center of interest for the Polish authority for competition and protection – the president of the Office of Competition and Consumer Protection (UOKiK 2020).

In an effort to provide masks produced by national companies, one of the government's anti-COVID-19 activities was the establishment of the Polish Sewing Works program (*Polskie Szwalnie*).[17] The effort ended up with massive fraud, however.[18] This program implemented by the state controlled the Industrial Development Agency (*Agencja Rozwoju Przemysłu*, hereafter ARP) aimed to ensure the production of safe and effective face masks in Poland during the COVID-19 pandemic. Despite this goal, useless products were produced, and secret and lucrative contracts appeared in the background. While many unanswered questions remain about the scale of irregularities in the government program, the ARP prevents access to information that should be public. The ARP conducted the program under the patronage of the president of Poland, Andrzej Duda, and after just a few months announced that 178 million Polish protective masks were produced for a total sum of 258 million PLN (almost 63 million USD).[19] It turns out, however, that it was a lucrative and accumulative example of economic power in which ministers, governmental agencies and politicians were participating and profiting. The Supreme Audit Office took over control of the program after it was discovered that the factory in the city of Stalowa Wola never produced any masks and that the Industrial Development Agency purchased 22 million masks from China.[20]

7.4 Conclusions

State authorities on different administrative levels have regulated wearing masks in Poland during the pandemic. It was the central government that imposed mask regulations on Polish citizens, however. Since then, contradictions and confusion in applications of legal frameworks have occurred.

Pertinent legal discourse stressed that covering the mouth and nose by everyone in generally accessible places was possible in an emergency state; however, in the 'ordinary' state, this obligation may apply only to persons suspected of being infected or sick. Due to the state of the epidemic, bans, orders and restrictions were introduced by subsequent Council of Ministers regulations starting on 31 March 2020. While one of these was the obligation to cover the mouth and nose with masks in generally accessible places, the regulation was implemented without a legally binding framework.

Moreover, the Polish Ombudsman (RPO 2020) emphasised that the order to cover the mouth and nose in generally accessible places was issued in violation of the rules of lawmaking. According to the constitution, this should be provided for by acts of law and not by government regulations.

In the Act of 28 October 2020, which made amendments in connection with counteracting the crises related to the occurrence of the COVID-19 pandemic, a provision was added that imposed obligations on healthy people, including the obligation to wear a mask.[21] From the date of entry into force of the amendment

(29 November 2020), non-compliance with this provision was an offense punishable by a fine. According to Art. 54 of the Code of Offenses,[22] persons who do not comply with the regulations on behavior in public places may be fined up to PLN 500 (almost 121 USD). In addition, the lack of a mask in stores has become a justified basis for refusing to sell. It is worth remembering, however, that the problem of legal basis is still not solved comprehensively because the order to cover the nose and mouth itself should be included in the act.

Masks are associated with different and heterogeneous medical factors,[23] but there are also social impacts such as social reproduction that must be considered. With respect to economic power relations, money laundering occurred in the Polish Sewing program, one of the principal activities touted by the government as part of the fight against the spread of the coronavirus. In sum, these two forces – unlawful legal binding and social inequalities – are irrefutably interrelated to the usage of masks.

Abbreviation

Dz. U. (*Dziennik Ustaw*): Journal of Laws

Notes

1 For example, in 1351 Pope Clement VI reported that 23,840,000 people died of the Black Death, when the population of Europe decreased from 94 million to 68 million between 1400 and 1300. According to Scheidler, the plagues somehow compensated for the changing ratio of land to work, reducing the value of the former and increasing the value of the latter (Scheidler 2017, p. 292).
2 Art. 41 Constitution of Poland (Dz. U. 1997, nr 78, 483, with amendments), Art. 6 Charter of Fundamental Rights of the European Union (CFREU, http://data.europa.eu/eli/treaty/char_2016/oj), and Art. 5.1 European Convention on Human Rights (ECHR, www.echr.coe.int/documents/convention_eng.pdf).
3 Art. 47 Constitution of Poland, Art. 7 CFREU, and Art. 8 ECHR.
4 A particular problem in Poland was the introduction of restrictions on the freedom of assembly in a situation where Poles wanted to jointly and directly express their protest against the ruling issued in autumn 2020 by the Constitutional Tribunal (accused of politicising) stating the unconstitutionality of some provisions that prohibited abortion in Poland.
5 Act of 5 December 2008 on preventing and combating infections and infectious diseases in humans [Ustawa z dnia 5 grudnia 2008 r. o zapobieganiu oraz zwalczaniu zakażeń i chorób zakaźnych u ludzi], Dz. U. 2020, 1845.
6 § 1 of the Regulation of Minister of Health 27 February 2020 r. on coronavirus SARS-CoV-2 infections [Rozporządzenie Ministra Zdrowia z dnia 27 lutego 2020 r. w sprawie zakażenia koronawirusem SARS-CoV-2], Dz. U. 325, with amendments.
7 Voivode is a head of administrative provinces in Poland and represents government there. Poland is divided into 17 administrative provinces.
8 The amendment was introduced by Art. 15.2c of the Act of 28 October 2020 amending certain acts in connection with counteracting crises related to the occurrence of COVID-19. Dz. U. 2112, with amendments.
9 The form of the act (*ustawa*) is required by the general limitation clause regarding all constitutional rights and freedoms according to Art. 31 sec. 3 of the

Constitution of the Republic of Poland and strictly with regard to personal freedom, also Art. 41 sec. 1 *in fine* of the Constitution. This form is also required by Art. 52 sec. 1 of the EU Charter.

10 For the purpose of our chapter, we used 'act' and 'law' equally to mean *ustawa* in Poland.

11 Regulation of the Council of Ministers of 15 April 2020 amending the regulation on the establishment of certain restrictions, orders, and bans in connection with the occurrence of an epidemic [Rozporządzenie Rady Ministrów z dnia 15 kwietnia 2020 r. zmieniające rozporządzenie w sprawie ustanowienia określonych ograniczeń, nakazów i zakazów w związku z wystąpieniem stanu epidemii], Dz. U. 2020, 673.

12 Dz. U. 2020, poz. 2112.

13 Fifteen regulations introduced such measures for a limited period, others (more than 60) amended these regulations.

14 § 25 Regulation of the Council of Ministers of 6 May 2021 on the establishment of certain restrictions, orders, and bans in connection with an epidemic (*Rozporządzenie Rady Ministrów z dnia 6 maja 2021 r. w sprawie ustanowienia określonych ograniczeń, nakazów i zakazów w związku z wystąpieniem stanu epidemii*), Dz. U. 2021.861.

15 In a way, how Antoni Gramsci analysed the hegemony paradigm.

16 The study was conducted in a mixed mode on a representative sample of adult Polish residents.

Each respondent chose one of the methods on his own: direct interview with the interviewer (CAPI method), telephone interview after contacting a CBOS (CATI) interviewer or self-completion of an online questionnaire. In all three cases, the survey had the same set of questions and structure. The study was carried out from 18 to 27 August 2020 on a sample of 1,149 people (including: 72.7% using the CAPI method, 17.0% – CATI and 10.4% – CAWI).

17 See: Polish Sewing Companies program, 2021 www.gov.pl/web/rozwoj-technologia/100-mln-maseczek-z-polskich-szwalni (18.10.2021).

18 Masks and Polish Sewing Companies. 2021 https://wiadomosci.radiozet.pl/Polska/Maseczki-ochronne-i-kontrowersje-w-programie-Polskie-Szwalnie.-Posel-KO-Wniesiemy-o-kontrole-NIK (10.18.2021).

19 See: Fiasko rządowego programu 'Polskie szwalnie', www.politykazdrowotna.com/74839,fiasko-rzadowego-programu-polskie-szwalnie (18.10.2021).

20 See: RP 2020, *Jak rząd kupował maseczki w Chinach*, www.rp.pl/swiat/art765311-jak-rzad-kupowal-maseczki-w-chinach (12.14.2021).

21 Act of 28 October 2020 on amending certain acts in connection with counteracting crises related to the occurrence of COVID-19 (*Ustawa z dnia 28 października 2020 r. o zmianie niektórych ustaw w związku z przeciwdziałaniem sytuacjom kryzysowym związanym z wystąpieniem COVID-19*) Dz. U. 2020.2112.

22 Art. 54, Code of Offenses (*Kodeks wykroczeń*), Dz. U.2021.281.

23 Matusiak Ł, Szepietowska M, Krajewski PK, Białynicki-Birula R, Szepietowski JC (2020). The use of face masks during the COVID-19 pandemic in Poland: A survey study of 2315 young adults. *Dermatol Ther.* 33(6).

References

Almeida-Filho, N. (2000) *La ciencia tímida. Ensayos de deconstrucción de la epidemiología*. Buenos Aires: Lugar. [*Shy science. Essays on Epidemiology's Deconstruction*].

Amnesty International (2020) *COVID-19 i prawa człowieka. Jak chronić nasze prawa i wolności w czasach pandemii?* https://amnesty.org.pl/covid-19-i-prawa-czlowieka/. [*COVID-19 and human rights. How to protect our rights and freedoms in times of a pandemic?*]

Breilh, J. (1986) *Epidemiologia: economía, medicina y política: hacia una investigación médica en la transformación de la investigación en salud*. Barcelona: Fontamara. [*Epidemiology: economics, medicine and politics: towards medical research in the transformation of health research*]

CBOS (2020) *Polak w maseczce lub bez maseczki* (Nr 110/2020). Warsaw: Fundacja Centrum Badania Opinii Społecznej. [*Pole with or without a mask*]

Council of Europe (2020) *Respecting democracy, rule of law and human rights in the framework of the COVID-19 sanitary crisis. A toolkit for member states*, Information Documents SG/Inf(2020)11, 7 April 2020. https://rm.coe.int/sg-inf-2020-11-respecting-democracy-rule-of-law-and-human-rights-in-th/16809e1f40

Fraser, N. (2016) 'Contradictions of capital and care', *New Left Review*, vol. 100, pp. 99–120.

Gordon-Bouvier, E. (2021) 'Vulnerable bodies and invisible work: The Covid-19 pandemic and social reproduction', *International Journal of Discrimination and the Law*, vol. 21, no. 3, pp. 212–229.

Granowska, J. (2020) *Przestrzeganie praw człowieka w dobie pandemii COVID-19. Stanowisko Rady Europy, Opracowania tematyczne OT – 684*. Warsaw: Senate Republic of Poland. www.senat.gov.pl/gfx/senat/pl/senatopracowania/193/plik/ot_684.pdf. [Respect for human rights during the COVID-19 pandemic. Position of the Council of Europe, Thematic studies OT – 684].

Illich, I. (1982) *Medical Nemesis: The Expropriation of Health*. New York: Pantheon.

Jarynowski, A., Wójta-Kempa, M. & Belik, V. (2020) 'Percepcja koronawirusa w polskim Internecie do czasu potwierdzenia pierwszego przypadku zakażenia SARS-CoV-2 w Polsce', *Pielęgniarstwo i Zdrowie Publiczne (Nursing and Public Health)*, vol. 10, no. 2. [*Perception of the 'coronavirus' on the Polish Internet until the first case of SARS-CoV-2 infection in Poland*].

Laurell, A. C. (2015) 'Three decades of neoliberalism in Mexico: The destruction of society', *International Journal of Health Services*, vol. 45, no. 2, pp. 246–264.

Matusiak, Ł., Szepietowska, M., Krajewski, P. K., Białynicki-Birula, R. & Szepietowski, J. C. (2020). 'The use of face masks during the COVID-19 pandemic in Poland: A survey study of 2315 young adults', *Dermatology and Therapy*, vol. 33, no. 6.

Menéndez, E. (1990) Antropología médica en México. Hacia la construcción de una epidemiología sociocultural. In: *Antropología médica. Orientaciones, desigualdades y transacciones*. Mexico: Centro de Investigaciones y Estudios Superiores en Antropologia Social, pp. 24–49. [*Medical anthropology in Mexico. Towards the construction of a sociocultural epidemiology*].

PDA (2020) Wearing face masks in Public: Approach of different countries across the world. *Pharmacists' Defence Association*. www.the-pda.org/wp-content/uploads/002-Face-masks-Global-Iman-V2.pdf (accessed 19 October 2021).

RPO (2020) *Koronawirus. Noszenie maseczek zasadne, ale taki nakaz powinien wynikać z ustawy – nie z rozporządzenia*. Warsaw: RPO Office. https://bip.brpo.gov.pl/pl/content/koronawirus-rpo-nakaz-zakrywania-ust-nosa-niezgodny-z-zasadami-tworzenia-prawa (accessed 18 October 2021). [*Coronavirus. Wearing masks is justified, but such an order should result from the act – not from the regulation*]

Sen, A. (1992) *Inequality Reexamined*. Oxford: Oxford University Press.

Scheidler, W. (2017) *The Great Leveler*. Princeton: Princeton University Press.

Tetelboin-Henrion, C., Czarnecki, L. & Vargas Chanes, D. (2018) 'Depression and diabetes in Mexico. A relation to explore from the social sciences', *Salud Problema*, vol. 24, pp. 54–71.

Legal acts

Act amending certain acts in connection with counteracting crises related to the out-break of COVID-19. [*Poselski projekt ustawy o zmianie niektórych ustaw w związku z przeciwdziałaniem sytuacjom kryzysowym związanym z wystąpieniem COVID-19.*] Dz. U. 2020 poz. 2112

Act of 5 December (2008) On preventing and combating infections and infectious diseases in humans [*Ustawa z dnia 5 grudnia 2008 r. o zapobieganiu oraz zwalczaniu zakażeń i chorób zakaźnych u ludzi*], Dz. U. 2020, 1845.

Act of 28 October (2020) On amending certain acts in connection with counteracting crises related to the occurrence of COVID-19 (*Ustawa z dnia 28 października 2020 r. o zmianie niektórych ustaw w związku z przeciwdziałaniem sytuacjom kryzysowym związanym z wystąpieniem COVID-19*), Dz. U. 2020.2112.

Charter of Fundamental Rights of the European Union (CFREU, http://data.europa.eu/eli/treaty/char_2016/oj)

Code of Offenses (*Kodeks wykroczeń*), Dz. U. 2021.281.

Constitution of Poland (Dz. U. 1997, nr 78, 483, with amendments).

European Convention on Human Rights (ECHR, www.echr.coe.int/documents/convention_eng.pdf)

Regulation of the Council of Ministers of May 06, 2021, on the establishment of certain restrictions, orders and bans in connection with an epidemic (*Rozporządzenie Rady Ministrów z dnia 6 maja 2021 r. w sprawie ustanowienia określonych ograniczeń, nakazów i zakazów w związku z wystąpieniem stanu epidemii*), Dz. U. 2021.861.

Regulation of Minister of Health 27 February 2020 r. on coronavirus SARS-CoV-2 infections (Dz. U. 325, with amendments).

Regulation of the Council of Ministers of 15 April 2020 amending the regulation on the establishment of certain restrictions, orders and bans in connection with the occurrence of an epidemic [*Rozporządzenie Rady Ministrów z dnia 15 kwietnia 2020 r. zmieniające rozporządzenie w sprawie ustanowienia określonych ograniczeń, nakazów i zakazów w związku z wystąpieniem stanu epidemii*], Dz. U. 2020, 673.

Other multimedia sources

Fiasko rządowego programu 'Polskie szwalnie,' 2021, www.politykazdrowotna.com/74839,fiasko-rzadowego-programu-polskie-szwalnie (accessed 18 October 2021).

GIS 2020, *Główny Inspektorat Sanitarny*, www.gov.pl/web/gis/struktura-zachorowanna-covid-19-w-podziale-ze-wzgledu-na-plec-w-polsce

Masks and Polish Sewing Companies, 2021, https://wiadomosci.radiozet.pl/Polska/Maseczki-ochronne-i-kontrowersje-w-programie-Polskie-Szwalnie.-Posel-KO-Wniesiemy-o-kontrole-NIK (accessed 18 October 2021).

Polish Sewing Companies program: 100 mln maseczek z polskich szwalni, 2021, www.gov.pl/web/rozwoj-technologia/100-mln-maseczek-z-polskich-szwalni (accessed 18 October 2021).

RP 2020, Jak rząd kupował maseczki w Chinach, www.rp.pl/swiat/art765311-jak-rzad-kupowal-maseczki-w-chinach (accessed 14 December 2021).

UOKiK 2020, Wysokie ceny – działania UOKiK, www.uokik.gov.pl/aktualnosci.php?news_id=16322&news_page=9.

8 Attitudes towards mask-wearing in Greece

Athanasia Chalari

8.1 Mask mandates

Social protection measures, including mask mandates, have been implemented on a global scale to help protect individuals and communities from the impacts of the COVID-19 pandemic (Rontos et al. 2021). Independently of the COVID-19 pandemic, mask-wearing has been a common practice in many countries (particularly in Asia). According to Burgess and Horii (2012), face coverings have been used in Asian societies long before the COVID-19 pandemic and can be culturally interpreted as a boundary between the clean self and the contaminated outside. On a more practical level, Kim and Kim (2021) explain that the common practice of mask-wearing in Korea resulted from air pollution problems. From a social-psychological perspective, wearing face masks in public can be regarded as a specific behaviour ultimately resulting from one's cognitive decision-making processes (Zhao and Knobel 2021). In terms of mask-wearing as a measure to prevent the spread of COVID-19, relevant literature indicates notable differences in the extent to which mask-wearing guidelines have been successfully implemented in different countries (Mahalik et al. 2021; Kim and Kim 2021; Zhao and Knobel 2021), although a limited number of studies have been conducted in that respect.

For example, studies conducted in the United States (US) seem to agree that Americans' adaptation to mask-wearing measures varied significantly at both individual and community levels (Mahalik et al. 2021). Interestingly, 18 US states have adopted an anti-masking law, and in some states, such laws have transitioned from protecting against the Ku Klux Klan (this is the origin of the purpose of anti-masking regulations) to protecting those who put communities in danger by refusing to wear a face covering during the COVID-19 pandemic (Shiram et al. 2021). Nevertheless, the refusal of part of the population to wear masks was still notable in the US, and a similar attitude has been observed (and reported to a certain extent) in European countries. According to Zhao and Knobel (2021), unlike China, European countries have followed different guidelines regarding mask-wearing along with different levels of enforcement. The same study explains that the personal preference for not wearing masks has influenced the decision of this study's participants in Europe. Although few studies have examined why a part of the population has refused to wear masks during the

DOI: 10.4324/9781003244127-9

COVID-19 pandemic, it might be relevant to discuss some of the reasons behind such attitudes. Kim and Kim (2021), for example, state that although breathing can be uncomfortable with a mask on, people's physical discomfort may be based on preconceptions to some extent. Using the health belief model developed in the 1950s, they explain that individuals value disease avoidance and expect that their specific health behaviours will prevent diseases. However, specific barriers may prevent such health behaviours, including physical, psychological and financial barriers (Lin et al. 2005). In that respect, according to He et al.'s (2021) study on relevant tweet responses, common reasons for opposition to mask-wearing included physical discomfort and side effects. It was also claimed that masks were ineffective and unnecessary or inappropriate for certain people or under certain circumstances. For example, the mask-wearing requirement for children became a controversial topic of discussion in various countries (e.g. the United Kingdom did not impose this measure in primary schools, whereas Greece did). Spitzer (2020) explains that parents of school-aged children have concerns about the potential harms of mask-wearing for the health and socio-emotional development of children (e.g. masks potentially prevent adequate communication in the classroom, blocking emotional signalling between teachers and children).

According to Rontos et al. (2021), socioe-conomic deprivation seems to be inextricably linked with the COVID-19 pandemic, because the way disease spread has been controlled by authorities depends upon the specific local infrastructure and socio-economic inequalities in each context. Thus, socio-economic factors should be taken into consideration when implementing public health interventions, including mask-wearing measures. An additional social factor is that of gender; research results indicate that men, in particular, seem to be less willing to wear masks than women. Men are likely to feel stigma from wearing a mask, as it might be viewed as a sign of weakness (Capraro and Barcelo 2020). Women report greater social distancing, handwashing and mask-wearing (Okten et al. 2020). Courtenay (2000) explains that masculinity is understood as a social construct that incorporates health risk behaviours as an integral part of what it means to be a man. Kim and Kim's (2021) study also showed that gender (along with education, income and information on harmful effects) can affect health beliefs and mask-wearing behaviours.

From a social psychological perspective, individual obedience to health advice has also been associated with trust in the government and health systems (Larson et al. 2018). As Zhao and Knobel (2021) explain, mask-wearing in China is less a function of whether one likes face masks or experiences difficulties wearing face masks and of with a function of obedience to advice from local health authorities. By contrast, European participants indicated that their personal preferences about wearing face masks influenced their actions. Additionally, people's trust and confidence in scientific experts and the perceived value of science-informed health policy also reportedly relate to whether persons follow scientific recommendations concerning the pandemic (Plohl and Musil 2020). High levels of mask defiance may be related to the lack of confidence in those scientific experts making people less receptive to following public health recommendations. This discourse has been more popular in some countries (e.g. Greece and Cyprus) than in others (e.g. Japan and China). Carpenter (2010) explains that people are more likely to adopt recommended health practices if they believe that those practices will produce benefits (e.g. keep their loved ones healthy, end the pandemic) that outweigh their perceived barriers/costs (e.g. inconvenience, wearing masks makes one look weak or afraid).

An additional and rather crucial explanation for mask-wearing is that people might feel empathy (or not) towards persons who are vulnerable to COVID-19. Pfattheicher et al. (2020) explain that feelings of empathy for vulnerable persons are significantly related to the motivation to self-quarantine, remain in isolation if infected, maintain social distance and follow rules imposed by the government. Mahalik et al. (2021) argue that empathy for persons who are vulnerable to COVID-19 should relate to people's attitudes towards mask-wearing; refusal to wear masks may be associated with lower levels of empathy for vulnerable persons, making people less likely to have positive attitudes toward public health recommendations.

In conclusion, this review discussed possible reasons (or barriers) that have prevented the universal implementation of mask-wearing as a measure to prevent the spread of the COVID-19 pandemic. Those reasons can be summarised as follows: socio-historic reasons; personal preferences; physical discomfort; physical, psychological and financial barriers; inappropriateness for certain people or under certain circumstances (e.g. children); socio-economic and gender factors; education; trust towards the government and towards the scientific community; and potential lack of empathy towards vulnerable people. The following section introduces the Greek social context to fully comprehend the specific mask-wearing measures implemented by the Greek government.

8.2 Greek society and dominant Greek mentalities

Greece is a geographically unique country consisting of a mainland and a large number of islands, located in the southeast edge of Europe, whose shared borders with Europe and Asia allow continued cultural, economic, political and social interactions. Greece's long history (among the longest in the region) has allowed a rather complex socio-political mosaic to be formed within its territory.

Modern Greek society and the modern Greek state have suffered ongoing discontinuities over a prolonged period, which has significantly delayed social, political and economic development. Greek society has always suffered from certain dysfunctions especially concerning economic and political orientation. Modern Greek society (the beginning of the so-called Greek crisis) has undergone additional complexities, especially since 2008, due to the global economic recession, which resulted in 10 years of deep recession, the implementation of repeated austerity measures and a complex mixture of unprecedented political, economic and social consequences. Greece's difficulty in surviving the global economic recession is explained by its extremely poor politico-economic fundamentals, which led Greek society to become exposed and particularly vulnerable to such crises (Chalari 2014).

In that context, the COVID-19 pandemic hit Greece only two years after the official completion of a 10-year-long recession involving substantial social alterations and psycho-social dislocation (Chalari and Serifi 2018). To better comprehend the attitudes of Greeks towards mask-wearing practices during the COVID-19 pandemic, it would be beneficial to review how dominant Greek mindsets have been depicted by relevant literature, notably in relation to how Greeks interact among themselves and towards established authorities. Greek mindsets have been identified by Greek scholars as forming distinct ways of collective thinking and acting within the Greek socio-historic context and culture.

Mouzelis (2012) focuses on the socio-historic origins of the Greek mindset, tracing elements of that mindset to the more than 400-year-long Ottoman occupation, arguing that certain customs and patterns of behaviour have therefore become inherent in the operation of Greek society and the Greek state. Alexakis (2008) and Voulgaris (2006) add that one of the main characteristics of the Greek mentality is a tendency to act in an individualistic manner, acting in one's personal interest, rather than in the collective interest; they maintain that such tendencies may relate to the struggle of the Greeks to protect themselves and their families during the 'dark' years of Ottoman occupation.

Panagiotopoulou (2008) echoes this view and further argues that it was extremely difficult for Greek society to follow the development and fully absorb the values, principles and ways of thinking of Western Europe, since Greek society had been influenced by the Eastern (Ottoman) way of life while Western Europe was evolving mentally, scientifically, politically and socially[1]. Furthermore, the entire 20th century was of extreme political, social and economic turbulence for Greece,[2] which did not allow Greek society to take form and be freely and fully organised. Sotiropoulos (2004) explains that, especially after the fall of the military junta (1967–74), democracy in Greece was restored rapidly but not systematically and thoroughly.

Elder (1974) explained that human agency is limited by social, historic and economic change, meaning that the Greeks had to find a way to adjust to a constantly recreated social reality – one which had been repeatedly disrupted. Therefore, to understand how the Greeks are experiencing the current pandemic situation, it is vital to understand that Greek society has been constantly reinventing itself over the last few centuries. Silbereisen et al. (2007) argue that how individuals handle changes depends on their resources and opportunities, but they are also constrained by these and by social transformations; this means that the Greek cultural and historic heritage represents a major parameter to the Greek handling of the so-called Greek crisis (austerity measures implemented during a decade: 2008–2010) as well as the COVID-19 pandemic crisis.

Now that we have briefly reviewed some of the parameters that have contributed to the formation of modern Greek society, it may be easier to portray the complexity of dominant Greek mindsets. A core characteristic of modern Greek society relates to the lack of rational organisation of the Greek state, which ultimately leads to the dysfunction of Greek society (Tsoukalas 2008; Alexakis 2008). This context encourages Greeks to act in an individualistic manner, acting in their own personal interest, rather than in the collective interest (Voulgaris 2006). The Greek mentality of 'tzampatzis' ('free rider': those who are only concerned about their own personal benefit) largely explains why Greek society remains dysfunctional and incapable of forming and maintaining a comprehensive and efficient state and effective political system (Tsoukalas 2008). In this vein, several studies have revealed the prolonged, ongoing and profound distrust among Greek people and between the Greeks and their government (Chalari and Koutantou 2020, Koniordos 2014; Mouzelis 2012, Panagiotopoulou 2008), which may be related to collective attitudes of suspicion and mistrust formed during the military junta (1967–74) or even earlier, during the Greek civil war (1946–49) and especially during the German occupation (1940–44). Thus, distrust can be seen as an inherited characteristic of Greek society, which has served its purpose during several unstable and rather critical periods of recent Greek history. More recently, additional characteristics of the mosaic of dominant Greek mindsets have been identified in the form of Greek nepotism, corruption, fraud, cartelisation, patronage, familial and cliental links, lack of reforms and political instability (Chalari and Koutantou 2020) within a social context of 'persistent stagnating conditions' (Tsekeris et al. 2015), including profoundly individualistic forms of Greek interactions characterised by 'anarchic individualism' and 'amoral familism' (Marangoudakis 2018).

Furthermore, we should not exclude the intervening relationship between the Greek state and the church, occasionally resulting in polarisation within Greek society, especially when nationalistic and conservative values have been threatened (Chrysoloras 2008; Sakellariou 2019). Kordas (2021) maintains that especially during the COVID-19 pandemic, the Greek Church adopted an active role as a protector of the nation and religion, whereas anti-systemic rhetoric overshadowed the power of political parties. Such rhetoric is also linked to conspiracy theories arguing that both Greek society and the Greek nation are threatened by the pandemic, masks and vaccines. This depiction of the current pandemic situation strengthens further the relationship of suspicion and distrust that some Greeks have with the state and even the church by revealing the openness of Greeks to primarily extreme-right conspiracy theories (Kordas 2021).

Having portrayed some of the dominant components of Greek society and mentalities, we may now focus on how Greek authorities have implemented mask-wearing measures in Greece during the COVID-19 pandemic and, more importantly, try to review the practices Greeks followed in relation to this specific measure.

8.3 Methods and research objectives

The aim of this study is to identify possible attitudes of the Greek people towards mask-wearing measures. To explore how mask-wearing measures have been received by the Greek people, a large-scale survey or dataset would have been relevant. However, an initial pilot online research study revealed the limited governmental sources and statistical data that are made available by the Greek government. The main source of data related to governmental documents regarding the implemented policies on mask-wearing measures. Document/textual analysis (Rapley 2018) on those documents can assist in depicting the policy context of this particular measure. However, such analysis would not be sufficient to reveal civilian attitudes towards this particular measure. The lack of reliable or official data on Greek popular attitudes pointed towards digital media research, as according to Mahata and Agarwal (2015), online forms of media can provide a platform to instantly tap into a huge audience. More specifically, the major news media play a central role in popular culture, given their relationship to social institutions that, in turn, have adopted much of the logic and format of these media (Altheide 1996). Consequently, digital news media were selected as an additional suitable source for this project.

In this vein, the objective of this study was to collect two kinds of targeted digital data in the Greek language, covering the period between March 2020 and October 2021: (a) official documents/announcements published online by the Greek government in 2021 and (b) online publications derived from online Greek newspapers and news-related websites.

Given the exploratory nature of this study, a simple, targeted sampling strategy was used. Sampling was accommodated by a Google search in the Greek language, which included a limited variety of search words directly related to mask-wearing policies, practices and attitudes. The search words were derived from the research question and ultimately formed the protocol for data collection (Altheide 1996). The selected documents and publications (units of analysis) were chosen based on their relevance to the protocol and the legitimacy of their content. Only official governmental announcements were used, published through the official Greek government websites, and popular (to Greek audiences) online newspapers and news-related websites were included. As the researcher is Greek, familiarity with Greek culture enabled the efficiency of this selection. Qualitative thematic analysis (Boyatzis 1998; Guest et al. 2011) of governmental documents and newspapers/news-related websites has been conducted based on the relevance of their content to mask-wearing policies, practices and attitudes in Greece.

The purpose of this targeted online data collection was to depict how the Greek people have reacted to mask-wearing measures. The objective was to create a digital database consisting of the following:

Nine official governmental documents derived from five official governmental institutions

Table 8.1 Official governmental documents

No. of Documents	Source of Document
1	Greek National Health Organisation
2	Ministry of Health
3	Greek Government/Home Office
1	Greek Parliament
2	Greek Statistical Authority

Table 8.2 Greek newspaper

No. of Publications	Newspaper	Political Position
2	*The Step*	Centre-Right
3	*The News*	Centre-Right
2	*First Issue*	Centre-Right
2	*Marine/Commercial*	Conservative
1	*The Nation*	Centre-Left
1	*The Newspaper*	Centre-Left
1	*Avgi*	Left

Table 8.3 News-related websites

No. of Publications	Website	Content
1	Skai News	News
1	News 24/7	News
1	Greek Church	Religious
1	Cnn.gr	News
1	CityPortal	News-Related
4	Lifo	News-related/magazine
1	Protagon	News-related
1	TechieChen	Independent
2	Deutsche Welle.gr	News
2	European Commission	Governmental
1	Labour Resistance	Independent website
1	FortuneGreece	magazine
1	UK Pharmacist Defence Association	Independent

Twelve publications derived from six Greek newspapers

Eighteen publications deriving from 13 news-related websites (seven news websites, one magazine, one church website, three independent websites and the European Commission)

While the data could have been examined using a quantitative media content analysis approach, thematic analysis prevailed. The amorphous nature of the subject makes formal coding very disparate and thus unsuitable for exploratory research of the kind being done here. In contrast, thematic analysis is a powerful tool for theory building from empirical data (Boyatzis 1998; Guest et al. 2011). Thematic analysis in this study was based on the protocol followed and concentrated exclusively on identifying the relevance of the analysed documents/publications in relation to the mask-wearing policies, practices and attitudes. The following themes emerged: (a) policy context, (b) compliance with and necessity of the measure, (c) resistance towards mask-wearing measures and (d) resistance towards vaccination measures.

8.4 Policy context: mask-wearing measures by Greek authorities

In accordance with an official policy first announced by the Greek Home Office in March 2020, the following mask-wearing measures remain in force in Greece: mask-wearing is compulsory in all public closed spaces (including schools) and in public transportation (Greek National Public Health Organisation 2021). Regarding the exact ways that masks should be used, the Greek Ministry of Health published a relevant official document online stating that the mask should fully cover the nose and mouth, should adjust completely to the face and should only be touched with clean hands (Ministry of Health 2021a).

The Greek government has encouraged the usage of masks for children over 2 years old (Greek government 2020a). The measures the Greek government has taken during the COVID-19 pandemic have varied significantly. A general lock-down was initially implemented in March 2020 along with compulsory mask-wearing. Additional measures included the prohibition of free movement through fines for unnecessary movement and the prohibition on non-Greeks entering the country. During spring 2020, the Greek government (Greek Government 2020b) announced a series of related policies to implement mask mandates: a fine of 150 euros to the civilians who fail to wear masks in public places and 300 euros in case they are in hospitals. Organisers of gatherings could be fined 3,000 euros, and in cases of repeat offenders, the fine increased to 5,000 euros. Owners of restaurants, cafes, etc., could be fined 5,000 euros if they admitted more customers than allowed (depending on the capacity of the premise), and an employer could be fined 1,000 euros if an employee failed to wear a mask.

In the summer of 2020, most of the measures were lifted except mask mandates within closed spaces (Ministry of Health 2021b). During the winter lock-down, such measures as limitation of movement after late-evening hours, closing of all public services/organisations and shops, introduction of home schooling and compulsory mask-wearing under all circumstances were reintroduced. During the disrupted school year (September 2020–June 2021), students of all ages (including preschool) had to wear masks during the school day (Greek Parliament 2021). In May 2021, most of the measures were again lifted, although mask-wearing remained compulsory only in indoor spaces (Greek Government 2021). The latest lifting of measures is also related to the percentage of vaccinated Greek residents, which in November 2021 was 58% (18th out of the 27 EU countries) (Greek Statistical Authority 2021a). The measures taken in Greece are among the strictest in the EU, including compulsory mask-wearing even outside closed spaces during critical periods of the spread of COVID-19. Relevant data reveal the different approaches European countries have adopted with regard to mask-wearing in public (UK Pharmacists Defence Association 2020), showing that mask mandates in open spaces has not been adopted universally. Failure to comply with mask mandates in Greece results in a fine (as discussed), and daily controls in public places by the police have resulted in more fines (The Newspaper 2021).

8.5 Compliance with and necessity of the mask-wearing measures

According to a survey conducted in September 2020 by a popular Greek TV channel, 78% of respondents were convinced of the need to wear masks by emphasising the even higher percentages among older respondents (Skai News, survey published 24/9/2020). A similar survey conducted by a popular online newspaper revealed comparable results, indicating that 66.5% of respondents wore face masks all or most of the time (News 24/7, survey published 21/5/2020). According to a third survey conducted by the Greek Association of Traders, 61% of the participants were willing to continue wearing masks while shopping within closed shopping areas, whereas 12% of the participants declared that they had already stopped wearing masks regardless of the relevant mandatory measures; 27% of the participants intended to stop wearing masks 'shortly' (Greek Church 2021). Unfortunately, no official statistics are available regarding the success of mask-wearing measures in Greece, and therefore any analysis followed should be treated as indicative rather than generalisable.

Despite the lack of official data on the obedience of Greeks to mask mandates, it seems safe to argue that most Greeks have been using face mask protection. Greek infectious-disease specialists argue that this particular measure should remain mandatory because if it became optional, Greeks would refuse to continue wearing masks (The Step 2021a). This possibility should be avoided due to the relatively large proportion of Greeks (one-third) who have not been vaccinated (Greek Statistical Authority 2021b) regardless of the relevant and repeated calls by the government and the additional measures to reinforce the necessity of vaccination (Marine/Commercial 2021a). The same group of experts often use social media to advocate the necessity of mask-wearing and encourage parents in particular to provide their schoolchildren with masks (The News 2020a; cnn.gr 2021).

8.6 Resisting mask-wearing measures

Based on such indicative data, it is understood that mask-wearing has not been universally adopted in Greece; in this vein, the refusal of some Greeks to use face masks has been covered by Greek digital media. On several occasions, digital media have depicted cases of provocative ideological groups advertising and encouraging mask defiance as a way to express resistance and disobedience to authority, or simply because they do not like to do what they are told because they distrust authority (government or the scientific community). Characteristic examples are as follows:

Despite the lack of systematic published data collection or analysis of how several groups have expressed their disobedience to mask mandates, news-related media and particularly newspapers have repeatedly published calls from experts towards the Greek public, asking them to continue wearing masks even if they have been vaccinated (The Nation 2021). Digital media have targeted specific individuals in institutional roles, while they exercise their choice of not wearing

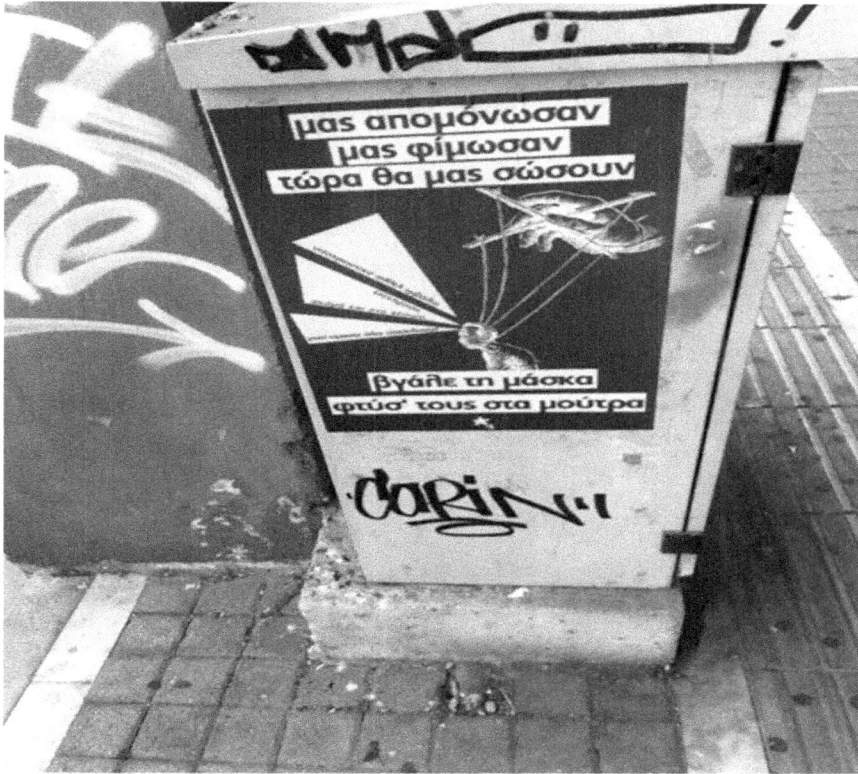

Figure 8.1 Street poster displayed in public places in Athens. Translation: 'They have isolated us, they have silenced us, and now they will save us? – take off the mask, spit in their face'

Source: Lifo (2020a)

masks. Most such cases have involved religious leaders and politicians in governmental posts. The following pictures illustrate such occasions:

Furthermore, specific leaders of Greek political parties (typically, representing extremist political ideologies) have publicly declared their opposition to mask mandates. The public opposition to masks influenced by certain religious leaders can be associated with the church's attempt to protect both religion and nation by demonstrating the superior power of its members against the threat of infection and against governmental restrictions. The tendency of the church to act independently from the Greek state (even in conflicting ways) has been evident in the past, whereas mostly right-wing/conservative politicians have traditionally supported the acts of the church, primarily for populist reasons (Kordas 2021).

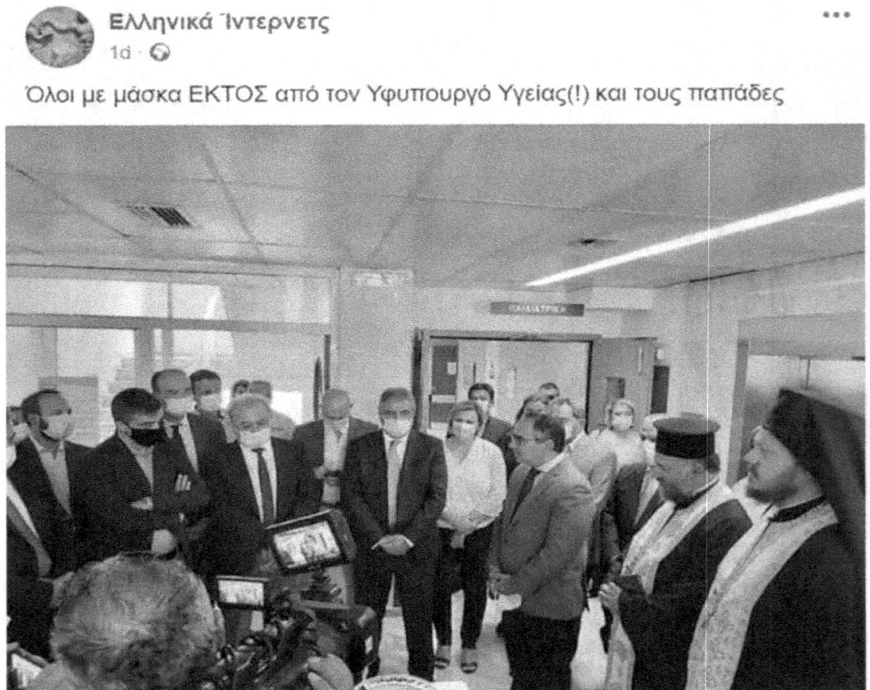

Ελληνικά Ίντερνετς
1d · ☺

Όλοι με μάσκα ΕΚΤΟΣ από τον Υφυπουργό Υγείας(!) και τους παπάδες

Figure 8.2 State and church

The Greek vice-minister of health visited a Greek hospital with representatives of the Greek Orthodox church. The vice-minister himself and the priests do not wear masks. The medical staff are masked.

Source: Lifo (2020b)

Thus, the contradiction in the picture between politicians representing the government, which issues regulations, while refusing to wear masks illustrates the rather common stance of several Greek politicians who try to show respect or obedience to the church, even as they also serve the priorities and policies of the current government. It might also be relevant to note that the popularity of the Greek government has been gradually decreasing, especially since October 2020, although it faces a lack of threatening opposition (Avgi 2022).

Additionally, some famous individuals – Greek 'celebrities' – have also used their public voice to oppose mask mandates (usually followed by a refusal to get vaccinated) (Protagon 2021). Digital media have also published cases of parents who refuse vaccination for themselves and prohibit their children from having COVID tests (PCR or rapid tests) or wear masks. They are motivated by their distrust towards experts and restrictive governmental policies (FirstIssue 2021a), expressing their opposition towards what they see as the elimination of human rights and freedom of choice. For example, a Greek father has been recently convicted for violently insisting on his child's admission to school while refusing to allow his child to follow the mask mandate or take the required COVID test before the start of the school day (Cityportal 2021).

Greek digital media has been preoccupied by a prolonged debate related to conspiracy theories and people's need to believe in controversial and very often unjustified concepts (Lifo 2020c). The Greek government has even made available an official guideline on how to recognise conspiracy theories (European Commission 2021a). Media have often presented various extreme ideas that describe COVID-19 as being part of a conspiracy against humanity (DeutscheWelle.gr 2021a). On many occasions, conspiracy theories are presented critically, portrayed as a controversial set of beliefs that some people choose to follow (FortuneGreece 2020; The News 2020b). Nevertheless, believers in conspiracy theories (even if they are not termed as such) use various electronic sources to reinforce their beliefs and ultimately influence their attitudes towards COVID-19 measures (for example: LabourResistance 2021). Notably, though, such beliefs are not only seen within the Greek context. Relevant demonstrations have taken place in other countries, revealing that part of the wider population is indeed convinced by such approaches (Marine/Commercial 2020b, Kordas 2021).

8.7 Resistance towards vaccination

Such controversial approaches are also relevant to Greek attitudes towards vaccination; according to a survey conducted by a digital magazine (Lifo 2021, published 21/7/2021), one third of Greeks have not been vaccinated. Some respondents refuse to be vaccinated because they do not 'believe in vaccination' or are afraid of the side effects. A similar article published in another popular newspaper claims that one quarter of Greeks refuse vaccination because of distrust towards the government and/or because of fear of side effects (FirstIssue 2021b). A similar publication based on a related survey also finds that one third of the respondents refused vaccination for the same reasons: mistrust towards the government, fear of side effects and belief that the vaccine had not been adequately tested yet (The News 2021c).

Furthermore, Greeks prefer specific brands of vaccines to others due to public fear of being vaccinated by the 'damaging' one (The Step 2021b). While the Greek government is informing the public about the safety and necessity of vaccines through official and credited sources (European Commission 2021b), Greek digital media occasionally share stories of certain individuals who advocate against the necessity and safety of vaccination (TechieChan 2020). Even medical professionals have refused vaccination, reinforcing the refusal of those who deny having received it (DeutscheWelle.gr 2021b). Although the data used to review Greek attitudes towards the vaccine are not derived from official sources but from surveys and publications found on digital media, it becomes apparent that a significant portion of the Greek population refuses to be vaccinated for very specific reasons (mistrust towards the government and the scientific community). Due to lack of official data, it is currently impossible to quantify the exact share of the population that intentionally refuse vaccination, as it is impossible to do the same for those who intentionally refuse to wear masks. However, it may be argued that according to the indicative data presented here, one-third of Greeks tend to refuse vaccination, and approximately the same share of the population refuse to wear masks. We cannot argue that this one-third (if accurate) consists of the same individuals, although the reasoning behind the refusal to follow those two measures is common.

8.8 Factors leading to opposition to mask-wearing in Greece

Although this chapter was unable to use concrete data that would have allowed adequate generalisations, the present study has managed to depict indicative attitudes among Greek citizens towards mask mandates. It is safe to conclude that mask mandates have not been fully or universally adopted by the Greeks. It may be relevant to compare those who refuse vaccination with those who refuse or avoid wearing masks; ultimately, both attitudes involve a refusal to follow the guidance of experts and resistance to the implementation of COVID-19 measures. Therefore, given that mask mandates have not been unanimously adopted and followed in Greece, there is scope for identifying possible reasons for such attitudes, which may also be related to the attitudes towards vaccine mandates.

The findings of the present analysis are based on official announcements related to Greek government measures and how the reaction towards these measures was depicted in the Greek digital media. Due to lack of concrete data, this study concludes by avoiding quantitative assumptions about the proportion of the Greek population who are not following the relevant measures. The review of the data used in this study has indicated the following: (a) that the Greek government has implemented strict measures (compared to other EU countries) including mask mandates; (b) that experts have repeatedly used social media to reinforce the necessity of this measure; (c) that this particular measure was initially accepted by most Greeks, whereas, currently, this attitude has been dropped; and (d) that digital media have identified the following cases of those who have publicly refused to follow this measure: (i) parents prohibiting their children from attending school without wearing masks, (ii) anti-authority movements advertising and encouraging refusal to wear masks, (iii) individuals in institutional roles (politicians and religious leaders), (iv) conspiracy theorists (even if they do not self-identify as such) refusing to follow this measure and (v) those who refuse vaccination. Notably, some individuals may display multiple characteristics.

Furthermore, according to the media depictions used in this chapter, the reasoning behind the refusal to wear masks is related to very specific attitudes: (a) mistrust towards the government (including a rather provocative anti-authoritarian ideology), (b) mistrust towards the scientific community (including the effectiveness, safety and necessity of mask-wearing) and (c) public disobedience towards

measures by individuals representing political, governmental and religious institutions. This particular attitude depicts a contradictory attitude associated with
power relations between the Greek Orthodox church and the state (Kordas 2021)
as well as a populist form of political behaviour followed by certain governmental
representatives and right-wing politicians. It might also be relevant to note that
the popularity of the Greek government has gradually decreased, especially since
October 2020, although it lacks a threatening opposition.

8.9 Conclusion

This study has identified dominant negative attitude(s) and reason(s) (or barriers)
that have prevented the universal implementation of mask-wearing as a measure
to avert the spread of the COVID-19 pandemic in Greece: the dominant negative attitude(s) ultimately relate(s) to distrust towards authority (represented by
government and/or scientific expertise). Such a finding should not come as a surprise, as relevant research (already discussed) has already identified a lack of trust
towards the government and towards the scientific community as a distinct barrier (Zhao and Knobel 2021; Plohl and Musil 2020; Larson et al. 2018). As part
of this wider negative attitude, relevant and more specific barriers could be summarised as follows: (a) the reluctance of parents to accept COVID-19 measures
that affected their children, which has already been identified as a barrier (Spitzer
2020; He et al. 2021); such an attitude from Greek parents should perhaps have
been expected; (b) the barrier related to the discourse around conspiracy theories
in Greece has also been noted by relevant literature related to preconceptions
and psychological barriers towards mask mandates (Kim and Kim 2021). Perhaps
such discourse could also be perceived as a distinct psychological barrier, as those
who refuse to follow mask mandates because of specific beliefs around such discourse do so due to consequential strong feelings preventing their obedience to
specific measures. Barriers related to socio-economic (i.e. class), educational and
gender factors have not been identified due to lack of concrete and systematic
data. Finally, the data used in this study have not touched upon the relevance of
empathy, although lack of empathy has been identified by literature as a distinct
barrier (Pfattheicher et al. 2020; Mahalik et al. 2021). Although the review of
the present data has not identified lack of empathy as a separate barrier, it might
be regarded as a consequential finding; the refusal of some Greeks to follow the
COVID-19 mask and vaccination mandates ultimately allows a gap in the protection of the wider public that inevitably has a greater impact on vulnerable individuals. Thus, potential lack of empathy towards vulnerable people (Mahalik et al.
2021) can be included as a consequential effect of the generic attitude of mistrust
towards the government and the scientific community. The findings of this study
also reinforce the more generic findings of relevant literature identifying personal preferences as a barrier towards the universal implementation of COVID-
19 measures (Zhao and Knobel 2021) including mask-wearing and vaccination.

  Notably, the negative attitude of some Greeks, related to mistrust towards
dominant forms of authority (government and scientific authority), is indeed a

very familiar one within the Greek context. As already discussed, lack of trust among Greeks and between Greeks and their government has been repeatedly identified by relevant literature (Chalari 2021; Koniordos 2014; Mouzelis 2012; Panagiotopoulou 2008) and can be described as an inherent component of dominant Greek mindsets related to profound socio-historic developments in modern Greek history, particularly during the last century. An additional way to depict this individualistic rather than collectively driven attitude is related to Marangoudakis's (2018) concept of 'anarchic individualism' as well as Tsoukalas's (2008) concept of 'tzampatzis'. The resistance or avoidance to mask mandates (or vaccination) has an ultimately negative effect on others, and particularly on vulnerable individuals. Thus, people who make such choices are primarily driven by individualistic rather than collective motives. The study of Shiram et al. (2021) on American society has also identified the socio-historic origins to the negative attitudes of some Americans towards mask mandates.

Therefore, the negative attitude of some Greeks towards the adaptation of or even defiance towards mask mandates should not come as a surprise. To the contrary, it may be perceived as an active and rather persistent component of Greek society, as it derives from socio-historical factors that have taken shape independently of the COVID-19 pandemic, albeit embedded within Greek culture and dominant Greek mindsets. The inevitable question that arises is whether this particular attitude has already served its purpose during the critical periods of Greek history or whether such attitudes may serve an actual and topical objective. If this is the case, perhaps concrete data followed by systematic analysis is needed in order to understand, explain and ultimately evaluate such a purpose.

Notes

1 The first independent Greek state was formed in 1827. This means that compared with most Northern European states, Greece is a relatively young state.
2 The main historical episodes in Greece during the 20th century are as follows: 1914–1918: 1st World War; 1940–1944: 2nd World War (German occupation); 1946–1949: civil war; 1950s and 1960s: massive migration waves; 1967–1964: military junta; 1974: restoration of Greek democracy.

References

Alexakis, M. (2008) 'Each one for oneself and everyone against anyone: Political space, political culture and social conflict in Greece' – "Καθένας για τον εαυτό του και όλοι εναντίον όλων: Θέσμιση του δημοσίου χώρου, πολιτική κουλτούρα και κοινωνικές συγκρούσεις στην Ελλάδα", στο Κονιόρδος, Σωκράτης (επιμ), Ανθολόγιο. Όψεις της Σύγχρονης Ελληνικής και Ευρωπαϊκής Κοινωνίας, ΕΑΠ, Πάτρα 2008, σ. pp. 91–129.
Altheide, D.L. (1996) *Qualitative media analysis.* London: SAGE.
Boyatzis, R.E. (1998) *Transforming qualitative information: Thematic analysis and code development.* London and Thousand Oaks, CA: SAGE.
Burgess, A. and Horii, M. (2012) 'Risk, ritual and health responsibilisation: Japan's 'safety blanket' of surgical face mask-wearing', *Sociology of Health & Illness* 34(8): 1184–1198.

Capraro, V. and Barcelo, H. (2020) 'The effect of messaging and gender on intentions to wear a face covering to slow down COVID-19 transmission', *Annual Review of Genomics and Human Genetics* 21: 231–261. http://doi.org/10.31234/osf.io/tg7vz

Carpenter, C.J. (2010) 'A meta-analysis of the effectiveness of health belief model variables in predicting behavior', *Health Communication* 25: 661–669. http://doi.org/10.1080/10410236.2010.521906.

Chalari, A. (2014) 'The subjective experiences of three generations during the Greek economic crisis', *World Journal of Social Science Research* 1(1): 89–109.

Chalari, A. and Koutantou, E. (2020) 'Narratives of leaving and returning to homeland: The example of Greek Brain Drainers living in the UK', *Sociological Research Online* 26(3): 544–561.

Chalari, A. and Serifi, P. (2018) 'The crisis generation: The effect of the Greek Crisis on youth identity formation', GreeSE: Hellenic Observatory Papers on Greece and Southeast Europe. London School of Economics. Paper No 123: 1–23.

Chrysoloras, N. (2008) 'Why orthodoxy? Religion and nationalism in Greek political culture', *Studies in Ethnicity and Nationalism* 4(1): 40–61.

Courtenay, W.H. (2000) 'Constructions of masculinity and their influence on men's well-being: A theory of gender and health', *Social Science & Medicine* 50: 1385–1401. http://doi.org/10.1016/s0277–9536(99)00390–1

Elder, G.H. (1974) *Children of the great depression*. Chicago, IL: University of Chicago Press.

Guest, G., MacQueen, K.M. and Namey, E.E. (2011) *Applied thematic analysis*. London and Thousand Oaks, CA: SAGE.

He, L., He, C., Reynolds, T.L., Bai, Q., Huang, Y., Li, C., Zheng, K. and Chen, Y. (2021) 'Why do people oppose mask wearing? A comprehensive analysis of U.S. tweets during the COVID-19 pandemic', *Journal of the American Medical Informatics Association* 28(7): 1564–1573. http://doi.org/10.1093/jamia/ocab047

Kim, J. and Kim, Y. (2021) 'What predicts Korean citizens' mask-wearing behaviors? Health beliefs and protective behaviors against particulate matter', *International Journal of Environmental Research and Public Health* 18(6). https://doi.org/10.3390/ijerph18062791

Koniordos, S. (2014) 'Economic Crisis and Social Crisis of Trust' "Κοινωνικό Κεφάλαιο και Εμπιστοσύνη (και Κοινωνία Πολιτών) – Ταύτιση ή Απόκλιση;" στο Κονιόρδος Σ. (επιμ.), *Κοινωνικό Κεφάλαιο, Εμπιστοσύνη και Κοινωνία των Πολιτών*. Αθήνα: Παπαζήσης, σελ. 99–129.

Kordas, G. (2021) 'Covid-19 in Greece: From the Government's clash with the Greek Church to the diffusion of anti-mask supporters', *The Open Journal of the Sociopolitical Studies* 14(1): 241–260.

Larson, H.J., Clarke, R.M., Jarrett, C., Eckersberger, E.Z., Schulz, W.S. and Paterson, P. (2018) 'Measuring trust in vaccination: A systematic review', *Human Vaccines & Immunotherapeutics* 14(7): 1599–1609.

Lin, P., Simoni, J.M. and Zemon, V. (2005) 'The health belief model, sexual behaviors, and HIV risk among Taiwanese immigrants', *Aids Education and Prevention* 17: 469–483. https://doi.org/10.1521/aeap

Mahalik, J.R., Di Bianca, M. and Harris, M.P. (2021) 'Men's attitudes towards mask-wearing during COVID-19: Understanding the complexities of mask-ulinity', *Journal of Health Psychology* 1–18. https://doi.org/10.1177%2F1359105321990793

Mahata, D. and Agarwal, N. (2015) 'Identifying event-specific sources from social media', in Kawash, J. (ed.) *Online social media analysis and visualization*. Canada: Springer International.

Marangoudakis, M. (2018) *The Greek crisis and its cultural origins: A study in the theory of multiple maternities*. London: Palgrave Macmillan.

Mouzelis, N. (2012). Developments leading to the Greek crisis. Presented at the Workshop on Social Change: Theory and Applications (the case of Greek Society). 9 March. Hellenic Observatory, London School of Economics.

Okten, I.O., Gollwitzer, A. and Oettingen, G. (2020) 'Gender differences in preventing the spread of coronavirus', *Behavioral Science & Policy*. Available at: https://behavioralpolicy.org/journal_ issue/COVID-19/ (accessed 18 September 2020).

Panagiotopoulou, R. (2008) 'Rational practices of an irrational political system' -Ορθολογικές πρακτικές στα πλαίσια ενός "ανορθολογικού" πολιτικού συστήματος", το οποίο δημοσιεύτηκε στον τόμο που επιμελήθηκαν οι Χ. Λυριτζής, Η. Νικολακόπουλος και Δ. Σωτηρόπουλος, Κοινωνία και Πολιτική: Όψεις της Γ΄ Ελληνικής Δημοκρατίας 1974–1994, εκδόσεις Θεμέλιο, Αθήνα 1996, pp. 139–160, στο Κονιόρδος, Σωκράτης (επιμ), Ανθολόγιο. Όψεις της Σύγχρονης Ελληνικής και Ευρωπαϊκής Κοινωνίας, ΕΑΠ, Πάτρα.

Pfattheicher, S., Nockur, L., Böhm, R., Sassenrath, C. and Petersen, M. (2020) 'The emotional path to action: Empathy promotes physical distancing during the COVID-19 pandemic', *Psychological Science* 31(11): 1363–1373.

Plohl, N. and Musil, B. (2020) 'Modeling compliance with COVID-19 prevention guidelines: The critical role of trust in science', *Psychology, Health & Medicine* 26: 1–12. https://doi.org/10.1080/13548506.2020.

Rapley, T. (2018) *Doing conversation, discourse and document analysis*. London: SAGE.

Rontos, K., Syrmali, M.E. and Salvati, L. (2021) 'Unravelling the role of socioeconomic forces in the early stage of COVID-19 pandemic: A global analysis', *International Journal of Environmental Research and Public Health* 18: 1–14.

Sakellariou, A. (2019) 'Authoritarianism and the Greek Orthodox Church: Historical and contemporary aspects', *Risa Luxemburg Stiftunk*. Available at: https://www.rosalux.de/en/publication/id/40942/#_ftn18

Shiram, S.K., Gigerich, W., Patel, M. and Miller, K. (2021) 'State mask mandates to address COVID-19 have been complicated by anti-mask measures often dating back to the 19th century', *American Politics and Policy*. Available at: https://blogs.lse.ac.uk/usappblog/

Silbereisen, R.K., Best, H. and Haase, C. (2007) 'Editorial: Agency and human development in times of social change', *International Journal of Psychology* 42(2): 73–76.

Sotiropoulos, D. (2004) 'The civil society in Greece: Inadequate or invisible?' "Η κοινωνία πολιτών στην Ελλάδα: Ατροφική ή Αφανής;", στο Σωτηρόπουλος, Δημήτρης (επιμ) (2004), Η Άγνωστη Κοινωνία των Πολιτών, Αθήνα, Εκδόσεις Ποταμιανός, pp. 117–157.

Spitzer, M. (2020) 'Masked education? The benefits and burdens of wearing face masks in schools during the current corona pandemic', *Trends Neuroscience Education* 20: 100138–100238. https://doi.org/10.1016/j.tine.2020.100138.

Tsekeris, C., Pingule, M. and Georga, E. (2015) 'Young people's perception of economic Crisis in contemporary Greece: A social psychological pilot study', *Crisis Observatory, ELIAMEP* 19: 1–26.

Tsoukalas, K. (2008) 'Τζαμπατζήδες' στη χώρα των θαυμάτων: Περί Ελλήνων στην Ελλάδα", πρώτη δημοσίευση: Ελληνική Επιθεώρηση Πολιτικής Επιστήμης, τεύχ. 1, 1993, στο Κονιόρδος, Σωκράτης (επιμ), Ανθολόγιο. Όψεις της Σύγχρονης Ελληνικής και Ευρωπαϊκής Κοινωνίας, ΕΑΠ, Πάτρα, pp. 217–248.

Voulgaris, G. (2006) 'Κράτος και Κοινωνία Πολιτών στην Ελλάδα', *Ελληνική Επιθεώρηση Πολιτικής Επιστήμης* 28: 5–33.

Zhao, X. and Knobel, P. (2021) 'Face mask wearing during the COVID-19 pandemic: comparing perceptions in China and three European countries', *Translational Behavioural Medicine* 11(6): 1199–1204.

Governmental documents

Greek Government (2020a) Available at: https://COVID19.gov.gr/menoume-asfalis-12-1-apantisis-stis-pio-sychnes-erotisis-gia-ti-chrisi-maskas-apo-ta-pedia/ (Last accessed 28 February 2022).

Greek Government (2020b) Available at: https://COVID19.gov.gr/COVID_map_penalties/(Last accessed 28 February 2022).

Greek Government (2021) Available at: https://COVID19.gov.gr/tag/elliniki-kyvernisi/

Greek National Public Health Organisation (2021) Available at: https://eody.gov. gr/COVID-19-odigies-gia-ti-chrisi-maskas-apo-to-koino/?print=print(Last accessed 28 February 2022).

Greek Parliament (2021) Available at: https://vouliwatch.gr/ask/question/244598c2-a9fb-464b-b251-b2086150ecba (Last accessed 28 February 2022).

Greek Statistical Authority (2021a) Available at: www.statista.com/statistics/1218676/full-COVID-19-vaccination-uptake-in-europe/ (Last accessed 28 February 2022).

Greek Statistical Authority (2021b) Available at: www.statista.com/statistics/1218676/full-COVID-19-vaccination-uptake-in-europe/ (Last accessed 28 February 2022).

Ministry of Health (2021a, March) Available at: www.moh.gov.gr/articles/newspaper/egkyklioi/7419-ypoxrewtikh-xrhsh-maskas-gia-eksyphretoymenoys-polites-poy-eiserxontai-stoys-xwroys-ths-kentrikhs-yphresias-toy-ypoyrgeioy-ygeias (Last accessed 28 February 2022).

Ministry of Health (2021b) Available at: www.moh.gov.gr/articles/newspaper/egkyklioi/7419-ypoxrewtikh-xrhsh-maskas-gia-eksyphretoymenoys-polites-poy-eiserxontai-stoys-xwroys-ths-kentrikhs-yphresias-toy-ypoyrgeioy-ygeias (Last accessed 28 February 2022).

Newspapers

Avgi (2022) Available at: www.avgi.gr/politiki/395641_i-dysareskeia-kata-tis-kybernisis-enteinetai-kai-pagionetai (Last accessed 28 February 2022).

FirstIssue (2021a) Available at: www.protothema.gr/greece/article/1161142/katerini-viral-video-arniton-me-to-paidi-tous-apaitousan-na-bei-i-kori-tous-sto-sholeio-horis-maska-kai-test/ (Last accessed 28 February 2022).

FirstIssue (2021b) Available at: www.protothema.gr/greece/article/1055637/koronoios-enas-stous-tesseris-ellines-den-thelei-na-kanei-to-emvolio-poioi-distazoun-perissotero/ (Last accessed 28 February 2022).

Marine/Commercial (2021a) Available at: www.naftemporiki.gr/story/1773330/apo-deutera-tolockout-gia-tous-anemboliastous-ta-metra (Last accessed 28 February 2022).

Marine/Commercial (2020b) Available at: www.naftemporiki.gr/story/1632052/COVID-19-diadiloseis-stin-europi-kata-ton-perioristikon-metron (Last accessed 28 February 2022).

The Nation (2021) Available at: www.ethnos.gr/ellada/171211_basilakopoylos-xana-ypohreotiki-i-maska-giati-oi-ellines-den-ti-foroysan-poythena (Last accessed 28 February 2022).

The News (2020a) Available at:www.tanea.gr/2009/20/08/greece/koronaios-tesseris-loimoksiologoi-eksigoun-giati-to-kinima-kata-tis-xrisis-tis-maskas-einai-epikindyno/ (Last accessed 28 February 2022).

The News (2020b) Available at: www.tanea.gr/2010/20/27/greece/koronaios-poso-dimofileis-einai-oi-theories-synomosias-gia-ton-koronaio/ (Last accessed 28 February 2022).

The News (2021c) Available at:www.tanea.gr/2012/20/14/greece/kaparesearch-ti-pisteyoun-oi-ellines-gia-to-emvolio-posoi-skopeyoun-na-emvoliastoun/ (Last accessed 28 February 2022).

The Newspaper (2021) Available at: www.iefimerida.gr/ellada/eleghoi-gia-metra-parabaseis-gia-mi-hrisi-maskas (Last accessed 28 February 2022).

The Step (2021a) Available at: www.tovima.gr/2008/21/24/science/maska-giati-ksanaginetai-ypoxreotiki-i-xrisi-tis-o-vasilakopoulos-eksigei/ (Last accessed 28 February 2022).

The Step (2021b) Available at: www.tovima.gr/2005/21/31/society/emvolia-ti-pisteyoun-oi-ellines-gia-to-astrazeneca-poso-fovountai-tis-parenergeies/ (Last accessed 28 February 2022).

Websites

Cityportal (2021) Available at: https://cityportal.gr/poioi-einai-oi-arnites-ellines-aytochthones-ithageneis-poy-moirazoyn-prostima/ (Last accessed 28 February 2022).

cnn.gr (2021) Available at: www.cnn.gr/ellada/story/267970/koronoios-ti-lene-oi-ellines-epistimones-gia-apostaseis-kai-maskes (Last accessed 28 February 2022).

DeutscheWelle.gr (2021a) Available at: www.dw.com/el/ο-κορωνοϊός-είναι-μία-συνωμοσία-των-άθεων/a-55995284 (Last accessed 28 February 2022).

DeutscheWelle.gr (2021b) Available at: www.dw.com/el/γιατί-διστάζουν-γιατροί-και-νοσηλευτές-να-εμβολιαστούν/a-56159025 (Last accessed 28 February 2022).

European Commission (2021a) Available at: https://ec.europa.eu/info/live-work-travel-eu/coronavirus-response/fighting-disinformation/identifying-conspiracy-theories_el (Last accessed 28 February 2022).

European Commission (2021b) Available at: https://ec.europa.eu/info/live-work-travel-eu/coronavirus-response/safe-COVID-19-vaccines-europeans/questions-and-answers-COVID-19-vaccination-eu_el (Last accessed 28 February 2022).

FortuneGreece (2020) Available at: www.fortunegreece.com/photo-gallery/i-pio-treles-theories-sinomosias-gia-ton-COVID-19-pou-diadidonte-pio-grigora-ke-apo-ton-idio-ton-io/ (Last accessed 28 February 2022).

Greek Church (2021) Available at: www.pentapostagma.gr/koinonia/7026314_tha-parameinoyn-meta-tin-pandimia-oi-synitheies-poy-aneptyxan-oi-ellines (Last accessed 28 February 2022).

LabourResistance (2021) Available at: https://ergatikiantistasi.org/tag/κοβιντ-19-ευρωπη/ (Last accessed 28 February 2022).

Lifo (2020a) Available at: https://mikropragmata.lifo.gr/wp-content/uploads/2020/08/IMG_1727-scaled.jpg (Last accessed 28 February 2022).

Lifo (2020b) Available at: https://mikropragmata.lifo.gr/zoi/15-anthropoi-pou-arnountai-na-foresoun-maskes-kai-oi-logoi-gia-afto/ (Last accessed 28 February 2022).

Lifo (2020c) Available at: www.lifo.gr/stiles/pazl-ton-arniton-tis-pandimias (Last accessed 28 February 2022).

Lifo (2021) Available at: www.lifo.gr/now/greece/ereyna-gia-ta-embolia-oi-apantiseis-ton-arniton-kai-ti-tha-toys-allaze-gnomi (Last accessed 28 February 2022).

News 24/7 (2020) Available at: www.news247.gr/20-20/oi-ellines-forane-maska-kai-anisychoyn-gia-tin-tirisi-ton-metron.7645752.html (Last accessed 28 February 2022).

Protagon (2021) Available at: www.protagon.gr/apopseis/tosi-provoli-stous-arnites-tis-maskas-44342120476 (Last accessed 28 February 2022).

Skai News (2020) Available at: www.skai.gr/news/greece/dimoskopisi-skai-maska-psifizoun-oi-ellines-i-stasi-ton-neon-kai-i-anisyxia-stin-attiki (Last accessed 28 February 2022).

TechieChan (2020) Available at: www.techiechan.com/?p=3440 (Last accessed 28 February 2022).

UK Pharmacists Defence Association (2020) Available at: www.the-pda.org/wp-content/uploads/001-Facemask-in-public-EU-Iman-V2.pdf (Last accessed 28 February 2022).

9 COVID-19 in British Columbia, Canada

Health policy responses and social adaptation

Tatsiana Shaban and Emmanuel Brunet-Jailly

9.1 Introduction

The COVID-19 pandemic of 2020 has been called the greatest challenge the world has confronted since World War II (Donahue 2020). In early 2020, the SARS-CoV-2 virus originating in Wuhan, Hubei province, in China started to spread to other countries. On 20 January 2020, the World Health Organization (WHO) found four confirmed cases outside of China. By 11 February 2020, COVID-19[1] had been named. By 11 March, the WHO declared the spread of the COVID-19 a 'pandemic' because the case numbers had reached 118,000 in 114 countries (WHO 2020a, 2020b). Indeed, in March 2020, as cases outside of China grew, so too did the fear of a global pandemic and the realisation that a worldwide emergency was in the making. British Columbia (BC) became, on 28 January 2020, the second Canadian province (after Ontario, ON) to confirm a case of COVID-19 (Schmunk 2020). The first confirmed case involved a patient who had recently returned from Wuhan to Toronto, ON, the most populous city in Canada. Not long after, on 5 March, the first case of community transmission in Canada was reported in BC (Slaughter 2020). As a result of the rapid spread of the infection, the issue of the virus was taken extremely seriously by local, provincial and federal Canadian authorities.

The chapter primarily focuses on government actions and policies developed in response to the outbreak of the virus across British Columbia and briefly across Canada. In so doing, this study covers the period from 28 January 2020, when the first confirmed case was found in BC, until the end of the mass vaccination campaign that reached nearly 80% of the adult population in September 2021. In the first section of this chapter, we detail Canadian federal-provincial relations, drawing from the COVID-19 timeline and outlining certain responses carried out specifically by the BC provincial government.[2] In the second section, we discuss the development from the beginning of the pandemic of public policy, programs and tools introduced by local, provincial and federal authorities. This section provides an analysis of the policy interventions, including the specific mask-wearing recommendation. We discuss the 5 billion (CAD) Provincial Immediate Relief plan to address immediate needs and BC's Restart plan, How to Bring Us Together (Economic Recovery Plan 2020; Restart Plan 2020). In

DOI: 10.4324/9781003244127-10

the third section, we focus upon people's adaptation to COVID-19 in their communities. In particular, we discuss the social patterns related to mask-wearing and cases of discrimination and xenophobia that rose to very high levels during the pandemic.[3]

9.2 COVID-19 timeline in BC through the lenses of federal–provincial relations

On 11 March, 2020, BC had 27 COVID-19 cases. By the end of the month, the BC Centre for Disease Control (BCCDC) had reported 1,000 cases (BCCDC 2020). As the number of cases increased, so did the fear of a global pandemic and understanding that the disease should be dealt with as very serious. Because of the general lack of knowledge on the pandemic, Canadian authorities assumed that their very first and ultimate task was to provide the Canadian public with timely information, i.e. to inform the public about what was going on in the world, across the country and in their community, and to explain, how to best deal with the sudden health risks, including deaths, and recurrent changes (Government of Canada 2020). Concurrently, in Canada, governments assumed that it was important to set up specific rules that helped to educate people and explain what preventive measures and steps could be taken by individuals in their daily lives to increase their safety in the least stressful manner (Desson et al. 2020, pp. 434, 440, 442, 443). As a result, the BC government continually adapted its messages on the situation and, in particular, discussed the state of knowledge on the virus publicly both in Canada and across the world and what this meant for the status of the pandemic in BC. We reflect on this short history by looking at BC's COVID-19 timeline (Nelms 2020) and BC's public policy responses (Henry 2019; Baldrey 2020; BCCDC 2020, 2021a, 2021b; BC Pandemic Provincial Coordination Plan 2020; Government of BC 2020a, 2020b, 2020c, 2020d, 2020e, 2021).

To understand BC's responses, one needs some basic understandings of Canadian federal and provincial relations; these are summed up in Tables 9.1 and 9.2. In brief, the Canadian Constitution of 1867 sets out the division of powers between the federal level (whose seat is in the City of Ottawa, in Ontario) and the ten provinces and three territories. In this Federation, each order of government (federal and provincial) has sovereign powers and authorities derived from the constitution rather than from another level of government. Each level is empowered to deal directly with the citizens in the exercise of its own legislative, executive and taxing powers, and each level of government is directly elected by its citizens.

Historically, according to the Canadian Constitution, health care has been a responsibility shared by both levels of government (Bakvis 2020). The federal government sets and administers national standards for publicly insured health services[4] through the Canada Health Act and provides funding support for provincial and territorial health care services through the Canada Health Transfer (Health Canada 2021). But the primary responsibility for the delivery of health

```
                          ┌─────────────┐
                 ┌────────│  Sovereign  │────────┐
                 │        └─────────────┘        │
        ┌────────────────┐             ┌────────────────┐
        │    Federal     │             │   Provincial   │
        │   Government   │             │   Government   │
        └────────────────┘             └────────────────┘
```

Senate	Governor General	Lieutenant Governor	Legislative Assembly
House of Commons	Prime Minister	Premier	
	Cabinet	Cabinet	
	Ministries	Ministries	
	Territories	Municipal Governments	

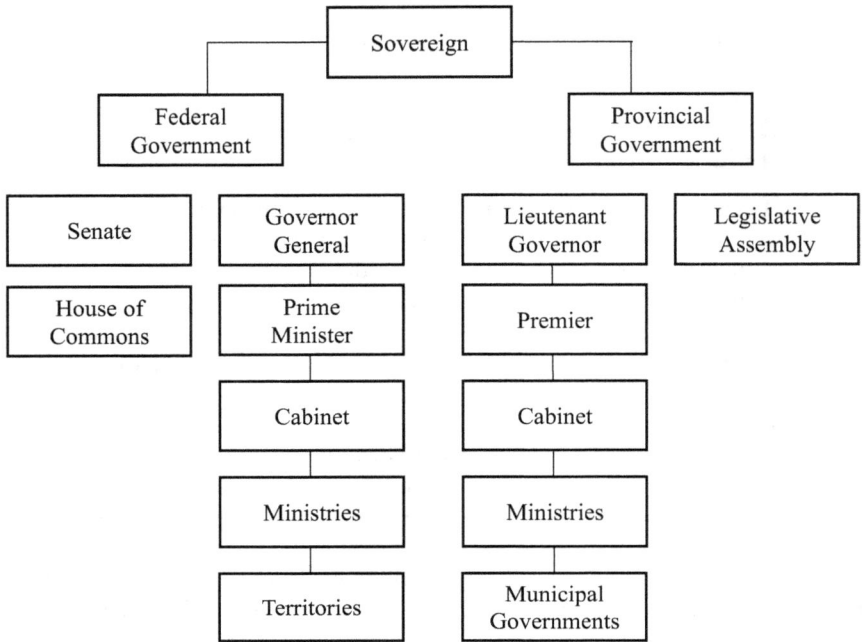

Figure 9.1 Government in Canada
Source: Canada Info (2021)

care services to Canadians falls within provincial and territorial jurisdiction. With $40.37 billion for 2019–20, the Canada Health Transfers are the single largest transfer between federal and provincial/territorial levels of government. They are more than double the second-largest federal transfer regarding economic equalisation, which stands at $19.84 billion. Health transfers are almost three times as much as the Social Transfer – $14.59 billion (Government of Canada 2021a). In addition, the federal government provides health care to specific populations,[5] for example, First Nations on reserve and Inuit communities.

To implement its policies, the Canadian federal department, Health Canada, has divided the country into four great health regions: Atlantic, Quebec, Central and Western Canada (British Columbia is Western Canada). In turn, in BC, there are five regional health authorities (Fraser Health Authority, Interior Health Authority, Northern Health Authority, Vancouver Island Health Authority, Vancouver Coastal Health) and one Provincial Health Services Authority (PHSA). BC's Health Minister, Adrian Dix, and its PHO, Dr. Bonnie Henry, together are responsible for providing equitable and cost-effective health care for people throughout the province (PHSA 2021; Ministry of Health 2021). While the

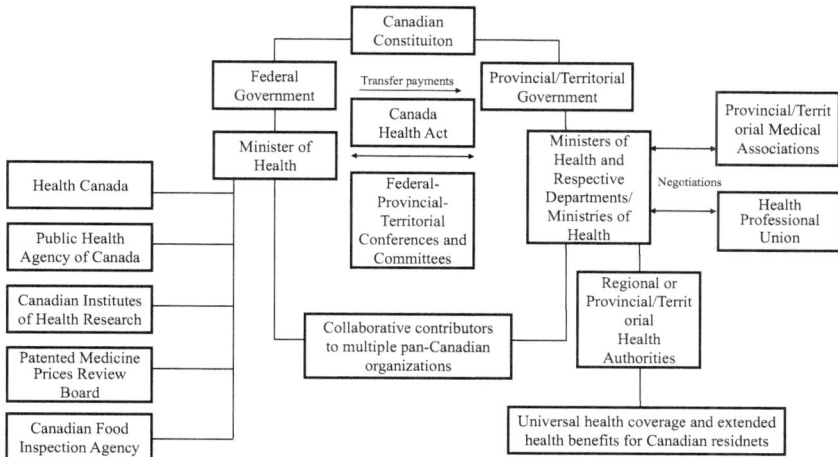

Figure 9.2 Organisation of the health system in Canada
Source: The Commonwealth Fund (2020)

federal government transfers billions of dollars to Canadian provinces, the provinces are responsible for providing similar levels of service across the country.

Health care represents the largest single expenditure item of any provincial government, ranging from 30% to 46% of its budget (Canadian Institute for Health Information 2019). According to a 2012 Environics survey, 81% of Canadians ranked their health-care system as the most important symbol of their Canadian identity, placing health care well above the flag, the anthem and the Charter of Rights and Freedoms. However, when asked about the main cause of problems in the health-care system, a majority (62%) of Canadians pointed to the lack of efficiency in the management of the system. Thus, this perception of inefficiency towers over other problems such as insufficient funding. Indeed, only 26% of Canadians identify lack of funding as a health care problem (The Environics Institute 2012).

Jared Wesley, a political science professor at the University of Alberta and a former director of intergovernmental relations in the Alberta government, called the early part of the pandemic a period of 'emergency federalism', with the current federal liberal Trudeau government taking a leadership role. Wesley said that 'everybody seemed to be in the same boat, rowing in the same direction' (Hall 2021). For instance, in the early stages of the crisis, Prime Minister Trudeau held regular conference calls with all other provincial premiers, who each head a provincial government, to discuss shared priorities. According to Wesley, as the pandemic progressed, the traditional pattern of federal–provincial conflicts reappeared, and the early spirit of cooperation gave way to confrontation. The prime minister and his government had been very reluctant to invoke the Emergencies Act to deal with the national crisis. In the end, in response to the pandemic, each province ended up following its own course, resulting in dramatically different outcomes across the country. Indeed, from its very beginning, Canadian governments and health officials felt scattered and isolated, and overall, governments were slow acting.

During the period from January to March 2020, official pandemic preparations were characterised by a similar kind of miscommunication as had been the case during the severe acute respiratory syndrome (SARS) outbreak of 2003. This general sense of apathy seemed to dominate the wider Canadian health-care system and pointed to systemic dysfunction. For instance, in Ontario, the communication breakdown was so serious that, according to Stephen Maher (2021), by mid-February 2020, more than 15 senior medical officials were holding secret strategy sessions to brainstorm ways to get through to provincial decision-makers.[6] However, as of 30 June 2021, 80% of Canadians reported that their governments handled the pandemic very or somewhat well[7] (Detsky and Bogoch 2020). Unlike in the United States (US), Canadian responses to the coronavirus were not clearly distributed according to party lines, and the Canadian public preserved a form of national consensus on COVID-19. Interestingly, the dominant message which members of parliaments of all parties diffused across the country was that COVID-19 was a crisis and that mainstream expert communities provided the best possible answers (Merkley et al. 2020).

By the end of March 2020, all provinces and territories in Canada (BC, Ontario, Manitoba, New Brunswick, Newfoundland and Labrador, Nova Scotia, Saskatchewan) had declared a state of emergency[8] or a public health emergency (Alberta, Prince Edward Island, and Quebec, Nunavut, the Northwest Territories and Yukon). Once a state of emergency was declared, the declaring level of government could access very broad powers which were prescribed in the legislation (The Public Health Act 2008; The Environics Institute 2020), such as shutting down businesses and other socio-economic activities, suspending many civil liberties (i.e. making it illegal to gather in groups, for instance, larger than a family-hold at home or in an open-air public area). In BC, two policy phases appeared according to two distinct periods or stages: the first phase started at the end of January 2020 and lasted until May 2020, thus, basically lasted as long as the first two waves of COVID-19 and ended when the BC government announced the implementation of a four-phase immunisation campaign, starting with people over 60 years of age[9] in December 2020, and lasting until April 2021. The second stage lasted from May until September 2021, when the government implemented a step-by-step vaccination of nearly all BC residents. We briefly describe those two periods.

British Columbia, which at the outset of the pandemic appeared to be most at risk because of its intense relationships and interconnectivity with Asian countries and communities,[10] actually was able to control the spread of the virus. On 17 March, BC's PHO, Dr. Bonnie Henry, declared a public health emergency, giving herself the power to make verbal-orders to the public that were immediately enforceable, including fining people who ignored public health orders

(Government of BC 2020a). That declaration gave the province extraordinary powers during the crisis, including the ability to restrict travel and to set prices for essential goods like medical supplies and food. According to Emmanuel Brunet-Jailly, BC had relatively successful early interventions and opted for 'buy-in' from the public rather than a more forceful compliance approach (Brunet-Jailly 2020). On 26 March 2020, the BC government announced the list of 'COVID-19 Essential Services' in anticipation of a possible order limiting the operation of businesses to those on the list (BC Government News 2020). Also, the BC Health Minister launched the provincial testing strategy to focus on clustered outbreaks, hospitalised patients and front-line health-care workers (Ministry of Health 2021). The data suggested that physical distancing, travel restrictions, increased testing and contact-tracing capacity helped to slow the spread of the virus by as much as 50% in BC (Detsky and Bogoch 2020). From May to September 2020, BC planned to re-open gradually, starting with parks, jobs/businesses reopening, and students/teachers returning to schools.

According to the provincewide emergency relief plan for businesses and individuals, from 1 May 2020, a financial aid program provided a one-time payment of $1,000 CAD (almost 800 USD) to all those whose work had been affected by COVID-19. Also, as job losses and company shutdowns rattled the economy of the province, the BC government announced spending up to $5 billion CAD to help families and businesses struggling financially through the pandemic (Ministry of Finance 2021). Roughly half of that money was allocated for economic recovery. The emergency relief plan was followed by a Plan to Bring Us Back Together/A Restart Plan/introduced in May 2021. It was a careful plan in which getting vaccinated in four steps was the most important tool. On 2 July 2021, BC eased indoor organised seated gatherings to allow 50% capacity with no masks required. However, experts say the easing of restrictions and reopening of the economy, at a time when the delta variant spread, led to a rise in coronavirus infections, particularly in the province's interior, in areas where vaccination campaigns had very limited success (Alam 2021). Indeed, whereas the alpha variant infected two people on average, according to the Yale School of Public health estimate, the delta variant spread roughly 50% faster, and was 50% more contagious than the original virus (Katella 2021). As a result, the BC government decided to make vaccination[11] against COVID-19 mandatory for workers in long-term care homes and assisted-living facilities (BCCDC 2021b).

9.3 Canadians' adaptation to COVID-19 and mask-wearing as a public policy tool

Today, there is a growing body of evidence (Leung et al. 2020; Brooks and Butler 2021) that well-constructed cloth face coverings are an effective tool in slowing the spread of COVID-19. As of 1 June 2020, nearly 3 in 5 Canadians – 58%[12] – reported that they were regularly wearing face masks when out in public. That was one of the lowest rates of usage of face masks in the Western world. Only 6 of the 25 other countries surveyed reported less take-up of masks: the

United Kingdom (31%), Australia (21%) and the four Scandinavian nations, with Denmark at the very bottom at 3% (YouGOV 2020). Even Americans reported being more likely to wear masks in public than Canadians (Coronavirus Resource Center 2020). According to recent findings from Vox Pop Labs (2020)[13] and the North American COVID-19 Monitor, over time, this rather low percentage of the population increased. However, why were Canadians reluctant to adopt masks?

We believe there are several historical, socio-political and psychological strands of reasons that explain mask-wearing reluctance. At the outset of the pandemic, provincial health officials in BC (but also across Canada and worldwide[14]) were inconsistent in their advice on whether people should wear masks to limit the spread of the disease (Chan et al. 2020). Such a lack of consistency expanded to the debate regarding the spread of the virus by asymptomatic super-spreaders. After months of confusing public messages, the Canadian federal government announced a new rule that within Canada, air travellers had to carry and wear a non-medical mask in order to board a plane (Breen 2020). At the same time, the Public Health Agency of Canada endorsed mask-wearing for the public on a voluntary basis. Indeed, Dr. Theresa Tam, Canada's highest health official and Canada's chief public health officer, said that people who did not have COVID-19 symptoms should wear non-medical masks when in public as 'an additional measure' to protect other people from the pandemic (Government of Canada 2021b). This was the first public admission that COVID's transmission could occur from people who did not feel sick and that the mask could prevent the virus from spreading.

Also, the Canadian prime minister, Justin Trudeau, announced a voluntary new COVID-19 exposure notification app, which became available in some regions in late July 2020. However, Canada's efforts were very unsuccessful when compared with those of, for instance, Taiwan (Wang et al. 2020), Singapore (Wong et al. 2020) and South Korea (Park et al. 2020), which relied much more successfully on modern information-communication technologies to monitor and control the spread of the virus in their communities. Indeed, these countries did not hesitate to integrate travel and health databases, along with information on the rapid test and concurrent contact-tracing results, and were also very successful in implementing mask requirements (Detsky and Bogoch 2020). In sum, in Canada, communication inconsistencies, disorganisation and poor coordination added to the overall lack of clarity, which prevented people from consistently following up on new emerging rules and limited Canadians' abilities to adapt.

Moreover, Canada had a very particular history regarding mask-wearing, which dated back to the period of settlement and the arrival of the first European colonisers and disease outbreaks such as smallpox, cholera, the Spanish flu and much more recently with the 2003 SARS. For instance, during the Spanish flu pandemic that killed more than 50,000 Canadians in 1918, quarantines were also debated by health officials and politicians (Goldenberg 2018). Provinces in Canada and many American cities enforced wearing masks in public (in the US, that was accompanied by libertarian resistance and officials who were sceptical of their efficacy). In the very first months of the Spanish flu pandemic in Canada, some of the first people who wore masks were people with ties to Asia and people who were already accustomed to the practice of wearing masks (Burgess and Horii 2012; Dickin et al. 2020).

Historically, while there were established reasons for normalising mask-wearing in East Asian countries where they were commonly worn, in Canada, the lack of these norms became the greatest cultural barrier. For Canadians, masks evoked panic (Ansari 2020) as well as a stigma – a medical mask meant that you were sick, linking the wearing of the mask with the disease rather than protecting others from oneself – possibly asymptomatic. For instance, BC resident Jong Yun Park told the *Globe and Mail* that he wore a mask whenever he went out in South Korea while visiting when the virus broke out but stopped when returning to Canada. 'If you wear a mask here, people will [consider] you as another patient' (Xu 2020). This cultural misunderstanding and association with the disease rather than with prevention remained a very strong obstacle to mask-wearing.

Furthermore, mask-wearing in Canada happened to be a rather contentious issue due to a record of anti-mask laws across Canada, which made wearing masks illegal during riots or unlawful protests. For instance, the Toronto Transit Commission (TTC) only made face coverings mandatory very late in the pandemic, at the beginning of July 2020. Indeed, the TTC had forbidden its officials from wearing masks until late 2017 (D'Amore 2017). So bus, tram and subway drivers could not wear masks despite air pollution, and it is notable that such a requirement was maintained during the SARS crisis in Toronto throughout 2003 (Hawaleshka 2003). As late as 2013, after several high-profile protests,[15] the Canadian Parliament introduced Bill C-309, which banned the wearing of masks during riots or other unlawful assemblies. It became a criminal offence in Canada, subject to a fine greater than 5,000 CAD (approximately 3,900 USD) or imprisonment of more than 6 months, with very few exceptions (House of Commons 2013). Similarly, in 2017, Quebec passed Bill 62 (anti-face covering law) followed by Bill 21, which prohibited the display of religious symbols by public-sector workers in the work place in order to foster state religious neutrality inside the province (National Assembly of Quebec 2017, 2019). Indeed, the Quebec government expanded this rule to prevent people from receiving certain government services if their face was covered (Boissinot 2017). The law was criticised for being discriminatory and unconstitutional by introducing certain elements of a coercive state (Wells 2017) but was enforced.

Because of this rather recent and counter-intuitive history against mask-wearing, Canada actually had to legalise wearing masks in public. Obviously, some Canadians complained that masks were uncomfortable, unnecessary, harmful to their own health or ineffective. Yet, interestingly, one of the first cases of COVID-19 in Canada was that of a student at Western University who had visited their parents in Wuhan over the Christmas break. On the flight back to Canada, she wore a mask. She self-isolated upon her arrival in Canada, and when she became sick, she showed up at the hospital wearing a mask. As a result, she did not infect anyone else (Taccone 2020). There were also real concerns that masks impede communication for frail elders and the hearing impaired (Novic 2020). Yet today, there is much evidence that such early perceptions have changed. According to Catherine Carstairs from the University of Guelph, 'Not only are we seeing more masks in public, what they denote is also changing, appearing to be a show of solidarity rather than just an act of self-protection', but 'this pandemic has shown how quickly culture can change. As the government continues to adopt new measures, it can transform what masks used to mean and instead of a sign that things are out of control, masks will become a sign of taking back control' (Carstairs 2020). Finally, according to psychology research from the University of Alberta, public acceptance of protective face masks has evolved dramatically in Canada since the beginning of COVID-19 in Canada (Mcmaster 2020). In the face of a serious health threat, Canadians are sensibly following the lead of Asian countries.

9.4 Hate crimes/cases of xenophobia and racism

Due in part to the pandemic outbreak, Canada and BC have not been exempted from the fear of others, with significantly raised levels of racism and xenophobia.[16] Since the coronavirus outbreak began, there have been numerous examples of xenophobia directed towards Asian communities – including verbal harassment, racist statements from individuals and institutions and physical assault. Canada reported a higher number of anti-Asian racism incidents per capita than in the US by more than 100% (Racism Incident Reporting Center 2021). According to the Racism Incident Reporting Center, as of September 2021, there were more than 2,265 reported incidents of anti-Asian racism in Canada: BC continued to report the most incidents per capita of any North American province, state or territory. California was second to BC and led in reports per capita in the US. Both BC and California were homes to historic branches of the Asiatic Exclusion League, a racist organisation advocating for a 'white man's country'. By city, Vancouver reported the highest number of incidents per capita. That was followed by Victoria, Toronto, Burnaby and Richmond: four of the five leading cities for reported anti-Asian incidents are located in BC.

Indeed, during the crisis, underrepresented communities become the focus of much attention and an unfortunate sense of otherness. During the height of the COVID-19 pandemic, Asian communities worried that wearing a mask would make them a target for racism, mainly because of the perception that wearing a mask was perceived as menacing and associated with political extremism or criminality (Xu 2020). Indeed, in the early days of COVID-19, the media featured masked Asian people as illustrations or 'faces' representing the epidemic spreading across the world. As a result, in BC, Asian-looking people wearing masks were verbally and physically attacked (Zine 2020).

A federally funded study conducted by several groups under the umbrella of the Chinese Canadian National Council for Social Justice found that BC had the most reported incidents per capita of any sub-national region in North America (Chinese Canadian National Council for Social Justice 2021). They documented

When was the last time, if ever, the following happend to you in BC?

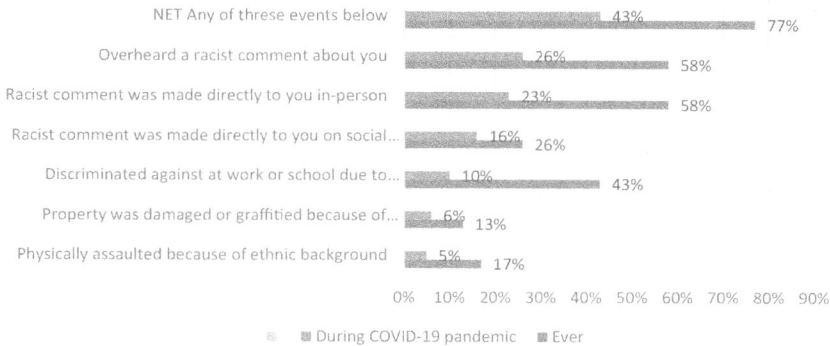

	During COVID-19 pandemic	Ever
NET Any of these events below	43%	77%
Overheard a racist comment about you	26%	58%
Racist comment was made directly to you in-person	23%	58%
Racist comment was made directly to you on social...	16%	26%
Discriminated against at work or school due to...	10%	43%
Property was damaged or graffitied because of...	6%	13%
Physically assaulted because of ethnic background	5%	17%

0% 10% 20% 30% 40% 50% 60% 70% 80% 90%

■ During COVID-19 pandemic   ■ Ever

Figure 9.3 Insights West (2021) survey

more than 1,500 incidents of anti-Asian racism. The president of Vancouver's Chinese Benevolent Association, Fred Kwok, noted that 'Assaults and verbal abuse have intensified, and Chinese people believe if you go to Chinatown you will be attacked'. According to Kwok, many Chinese-owned stores closed as a result, and it took a long time for the police and the city to even say there was a problem (Ballard 2021). A recently released report from the Vancouver Police Department confirmed those issues, showing a 717% increase in hate crimes targeting Asian communities and indeed rising from just 12 incidents in 2019 to 98 in 2020 (Vancouver Police Department 2021). Also, an online survey led by *Insights West* found that 49% of 725 ethnic Asians surveyed in the province of British Columbia (i.e. where Vancouver[17] is located) responded that they had been subjected to racial remarks.

In 1971, Canada became the earliest country to adopt multiculturalism as an official policy. Multiculturalism assumed that diverse ethnic groups were able to co-exist and contribute positively to common society. Today, multiculturalism is very important to most Canadians and defines Canada's image on a global scale (Schertzer et al. 2018). Indeed, Canadian society is complex; after Canadians of European ancestry, Canadians with Asian ancestry comprise the largest and fastest-growing group, roughly 17.7% of the Canadian population (Census 2016). Many ethnic Asian families have been Canadians for generations, with very many descending from people who immigrated during an 1858 Gold Rush or a decade later to work on the country's first transcontinental railway – an enterprise that was integral to BC becoming a part of Canada. However, many experts such as Farid Rohani, who was a board member of Vancouver-based Laurier Institute, an organisation devoted to exploring the pros and cons of multiculturalism (Todd

2014), argued that there were abuses resulting from multiculturalism policy and that misunderstandings of its intentions have led to the creation of societal silos.

BC's Human Rights Commissioner, Kasari Govender, said that COVID-19 led to an increase in both violent and online attacks against marginalised groups across too many communities such as people of Asian, Black, Indigenous, Jewish or Muslim ancestry as well as queer and trans communities; and in her capacity, she launched the BC Commission's first-ever public inquiry into examining the rise in hate-motivated incidents in the province (Cordasko 2021). Also, the BC government now is planning to bring forward anti-racism legislation, with Member of Legislative Assembly Rachna Singh working on a new provincial legislation to address systemic discrimination and hatred.

9.5 Conclusion

In the face of COVID-19, in British Columbia and Canada, overall health policy responses and social reactions seem to have followed the waves of the pandemic and included gradual introduction of social distancing, mask-wearing, contact tracing and quarantining of non-essential travelers. Ultimately, however, social and policy adaptation were presented to the public as being primarily dependent on knowledge and the state of research about the virus on what worked and what did not to limit its spread and, ultimately, vaccination discoveries and campaigns. In sum, there were two policy periods: first, pandemic-spreading-control policy responses dominated. Economic, educational and social activities suffered greatly from adopting social restricting measures. Second, while physical distancing, contact tracing, quarantining and mask-wearing remained mandatory, vaccination campaigns were also swiftly implemented. But while many of those policies were implemented with reasonable success, mask-wearing remained controversial for months and faced many misunderstandings, as illustrated by the rise of verbal and physical violence against Canadians of Asian heritage. While many complained that the government was slow acknowledging the rise of racists responses across the province, the BC human rights commissioner, Govender, is now leading an inquiry which should lead to major legislative changes on two fronts, changes in the criminal and the human rights codes and their concurrent justice processes (Office of the Human Rights Commissioner 2021).

In Canada, mask-wearing turned out to be very contentious; the COVID-19 crisis context brought systemic racism and racial inequities to the centre of the Canadian public discourse. However, on a positive note, in Canada, past pandemics encouraged governments to endorse public health measures and institutionalise necessary changes. Cholera led to the formation of the first public health boards. The Spanish flu was a key factor in the establishment of the federal health department. SARS prompted hospitals to improve their methods of infection control and led to the creation of the Public Health Agency of Canada (Myseum 2020). COVID-19 may result in the improvement of health conditions in senior-care homes and prompted an open discussion regarding the well-being of low-income groups, as well as ethnically diverse Canadian communities, and in BC, in particular, its communities of Asian ancestry.

Notes

1 The WHO announced that respiratory disease caused by the novel coronavirus had been named COVID-19. Officials said the name was chosen to avoid the stigma of associating the illness with any particular country and that other names could be inaccurate.

2 Further detailed information on the government responses is available on the government of British Columbia's website and at McCarthy News's website: COVID-19: Emergency Measures Tracker (Lawson et al. 2021). Lifestreams by Adrian Dix, Minister of Health, and Dr. Bonnie Henry, BC's Provincial Health Officer (PHO) provided regular updates on COVID-19 on YouTube: www.youtube.com/user/Province . . . #Covid19 #CovidBC #coronavirus.

3 In order to collect data for this chapter for the given period of time (between January 2020 and August 2021), we thoroughly monitored provincial and (federal) news that included local and national printed and online newspapers. Also, we watched and analysed guidelines, recommendations, reviews given during online public conferences and briefings (close to 200 briefings in total). Those were presented to the public on a daily and then weekly (monthly) basis for a period of 17 months from January to August 2020 by Adrian Dix, Minister of Health (federal level), and Dr. Bonnie Henry, Provincial Health Officer (PHO). On 20 August, in-person briefings had finished as BC moved into Step 3 of the Restart Plan. Data for policy responses by the government was taken partly from the North American COVID-19 Policy Response Monitor, BC government and Ministry of Health online resources. The cases and data about hate crimes and xenophobia were taken from media and other non-governmental and educational resources that included surveys that monitored people's adaptation to COVID-19 measures or reported by the police in BC.

4 The federal Health Portfolio consists of approximately 12,000 full-time-equivalent employees and an annual budget of over $3.8 billion CAD. It comprises Health Canada, the Public Health Agency of Canada (PHAC), the Canadian Institutes of Health Research, the Patented Medicine Prices Review Board and the Canadian Food Inspection Agency. PHAC may also work with port authorities and border services to monitor individuals entering and exiting the country.

5 In 2019 a new federal government department, Indigenous Services Canada, was created. It funded certain health services for First Nations and Inuit people.

6 The frustration of Ontario doctors reflected a concern expressed by experts across the country during the pandemic, a feeling that the scientists and doctors most qualified to craft a public health response went largely ignored.

7 The poll does not distinguish between federal and provincial governments.

8 Emergency management orders can be made by federal, provincial and municipal levels of government, where they are pre-authorised by legislation (Canadian Civil Liberties Association 2020).

9 BC's immunisation plan phased approach consisted of 4 phases. Phase 1: December 2020 to February 2021; Phase 2: February to April 2021; Phase 3: General population immunisation, April to June 2021; Phase 4: July to September 2021.

10 Vancouver, for instance, had the largest Chinese community in North America.

11 The topic of vaccination (timing and introduction of vaccine passports) is not covered by this chapter.

12 Since the early days of the pandemic, British polling firm YouGov had been surveying people in 29 countries online about their attitudes towards the novel coronavirus and the behaviours they were changing in response to it. Canadians had been surveyed five times, with more than 1,000 respondents each time.

13 'Vox Pop Labs' were founded by academics who specialise in the social and data sciences. A vox pop is a technique used by journalists which consists of

interviewing people at random about their views on a given topic. The number of people interviewed is too small to be a true representation of public opinion; however, their technologies allow them to survey hundreds of thousands of people. And their statistical models allow them to transform these survey data from anecdotal insights into representative statements about the public.

14　The WHO initially recommended that asymptomatic people should only wear a mask if caring for someone with suspected SARS-CoV-2 infection.

15　The Harper government passed the private members bill after the 2010 G20 protests in Toronto and the 2011 Stanley Cup riots in Vancouver.

16　According to an Ipsos poll (Bricker 2020), more Canadians see racism as a serious problem in Canada today than just one year ago: 60% of Canadians think racism is a serious problem, 36% rate it as 'fairly serious', 20% as 'one of the most serious', and 3% as 'the most serious problem facing Canada today'. By contrast, fewer than half (47%) rated racism as a serious problem in 2019 (pre-COVID-19 time).

17　Vancouver is home to North America's largest Chinatown; it surpassed San Francisco in the United States in the last few years. In Metro Vancouver, 43% of residents have an Asian heritage. In Victoria, just 11% of the population has Asian heritage. An analysis of Statistics Canada (2020) reports shows the percentage of those with Asian heritages will continue to grow rapidly across Metro Vancouver, a region that has doubled in population in just 30 years.

References

Alam, H. (2021) 'Delta variant driving 4th wave in BC as associated COVID-19 cases double every 7–10 days: experts'. *CBC News*. Available at: www.cbc.ca/news/canada/british-columbia/delta-variant-doubling-each-week-in-b-c-1.6128945. Accessed September 2021.

Ansari, S. (2020) 'The history of our cultural resistance against masks'. *Opinion, MacLeans*. Available at: www.macleans.ca/opinion/the-history-of-our-cultural-resistance-against-masks/. Accessed September 2021.

Bakvis, H. (2020) 'Federalism and universal healthcare: A question of performance and effectiveness', in Bakvis, H. and Skogstad, G. (eds) *Canadian federalism: Performance, effectiveness, and legitimacy*. 4th ed. Toronto: University of Toronto Press, pp. 310–336.

Baldrey, K. (2020) 'Analysis: How Dr. Bonnie Henry's COVID-19 briefings have become must-see TV'. *Global News*. April 4. Available at: https://globalnews.ca/news/6777833/dr-bonnie-henrys-covid-19-briefings-have-become-must-see-tv/. Accessed August 2021.

Ballard, J. (2021) 'Closing up shop: Vancouver's Chinatown battered by crime, COVID-19 and dirty streets'. *CBC News Vancouver*. Available at: www.cbc.ca/news/canada/british-columbia/vancouver-chinatown-vacancy-crime-vandalism-1.5907997. Accessed September 2021.

BCCDC (British Columbia Centre for Disease Control) (2020) 'Your story, our future: New survey seeks input from British Columbians on the impact of the response to COVID-19'. *News Releases. New Survey*, May 12. Available at: www.bccdc.ca/about/news-stories/news-releases/2020/your-story-our-future-new-survey-seeks-input-from-british-columbians-on-the-impact-of-the-response-to-covid-19. Accessed August 2021.

BCCDC (British Columbia Centre for Disease Control) (2021a) '4 Key ways local governments and Indigenous communities prepare for novel coronavirus

COVID-2019'. *Provincial Coronavirus Response*. Available at: http://www.bccdc.ca/Health-Info-Site/Documents/COVID-19-4-Key-Ways-to-Prepare.pdf. Accessed September 2021.

BCCDC (2021b) 'COVID-19: One year of the pandemic in BC'. *CovidBriefing_20210311*. Available at: http://www.bccdc.ca/Health-Info-Site/Documents/CovidBriefing_20210311.pdf. Accessed August 2021.

BC Government News (2020) 'Province takes unprecedented steps to support COVID-19 response'. *News Release*. Available at: https://news.gov.bc.ca/releases/2020PSSG0020-000568. Accessed August 2021.

BC Pandemic Provincial Coordination Plan (2020) Office of the provincial health officer. *Report*. Available at: https://www2.gov.bc.ca/assets/gov/health/about-bc-s-health-care-system/office-of-the-provincial-health-officer/reports-publications/pandemic-provincial-coordination-plan.pdf. Accessed September 2020.

Boissinot, J. (2017) 'How will Quebec's Bill 62 work? What we know and don't so far'. *The Globe and Mail*. Available at: www.theglobeandmail.com/news/national/quebec-bill-62-explainer/article36700916/. Accessed August 2021.

Breen, K. (2020) 'Health coronavirus: Air travellers required to wear non-medical masks under new rules'. *The Global News*. Available at: https://globalnews.ca/news/6834343/coronavirus-air-travellers-masks/. Accessed August 2021.

Bricker, D. (2020). 'Racism in Canada'. *Ipsos Factum*. National Library of Canada.

Brooks, J.T. and Butler, J.C. (2021) 'Effectiveness of mask wearing to control community spread of SARS-CoV-2'. *JAMA Insights* 325(10): 998–999. doi:10.1001/jama.2021.1505.

Brunet-Jailly, E. (2020) 'International boundaries, borders, and the Coronavirus pandemic: a new era in border policy and public administration research? Commentary in Broucelle, et al. "Beyond Covid-19: five commentaries on reimagining governance for future crisis and resilience"'. *Canadian Public Administration*. https://doi.org/10.1111/capa.12388.

Burgess, A. and Horii, M. (2012) 'Risk, ritual and health responsibilisation: Japan's "Safety Blanket" of surgical face mask-wearing'. *Sociology of Health & Illness* 34(8): 1184–1198. doi: 10.1111/j.1467-9566.2012.01466.

Canada Info (2021) *Government in Canada. Government fact sheet to download*. Available at: www.craigmarlatt.com/canada/images&downloads/downloads_govt_hierarchy.html. Accessed November 2021.

Canadian Civil Liberties Association (2020) *Emergency orders declared across the country*. Available at: https://ccla.org/coronavirus-update-emergency-updates. Accessed August 2021.

Canadian Institute for Health Information (2019) *National health expenditure trends, 1975 to 2019*. Ottawa, ON: CIHI.

Carstairs, C. (2020) 'A brief history of masks from the 17th-century plague to the ongoing coronavirus pandemic'. *The Conversation*. Available at: https://theconversation.com/a-brief-history-of-masks-from-the-17th-century-plague-to-the-ongoing-coronavirus-pandemic-142959. Accessed September 2021.

Census (2016) *Population of Asian Canadian groups*. Statistics Canada. Available at: www.voanews.com/americas/canadas-most-asian-city-faces-surge-hate-crimes. Accessed August 2021.

Chan, A., Lai-yam, Leung, C.C., Lam, T.H. and Cheng, K.K. (2020) *To wear or not to wear: WHO's confusing guidance on masks in the covid-19 pandemic*. London: BMJ Publishing Group. Available at: https://blogs.bmj.com/bmj/2020/03/11/whos-confusing-guidance-masks-covid. Accessed September 2021.

Chinese Canadian National Council for Social Justice (2021) Available at: https://ccncsj.ca/. Accessed October 2021.

Cordasko, L. (2021) 'Rights commissioner launches inquiry into rise in hate amid pandemic'. *Vancouver Sun*. Available at: www.healthing.ca/diseases-and-conditions/coronavirus/rights-commissioner-launches-inquiry-into-rise-in-hate-amid-pandemic/. Accessed September 2021.

Coronavirus Resource Center (2020) *John Hopkins University of Medicine*. Available at: https://coronavirus.jhu.edu/map.html. Accessed 15 September 2021.

D'Amore, R. (2017) 'TTC operators say they were sent home for wearing medical masks'. *CTV Toronto*. Available at: https://toronto.ctvnews.ca/ttc-operators-say-they-were-sent-home-for-wearing-medical-masks-1.3386592. Accessed September 2021.

Desson, Z.D., Weller, E., McMeekin, P. and Ammi, M. (2020) 'An analysis of the policy responses to the COVID-19 pandemic in France, Belgium, and Canada'. *Health Policy and Technology* (9): 430–446.

Detsky, A.S. and Bogoch, I.I. (2020) 'COVID-19 in Canada experience and response'. *JAMA* 324(8): 743–744. doi:10.1001/jama.2020.14033.

Dickin, J., Bailey, P.G. and James-Abra, E. (2020) '1918 Spanish flu in Canada'. *The Canadian Encyclopedia*. Available at: www.thecanadianencyclopedia.ca/en/article/1918-spanish-flu-in-canada?gclid=EAIaIQobChMIlp2d_pn16AIVLv3jBx-2iRAxhEAAYASAAEgLJhfD_BwE. Accessed September 2021.

Donahue, P. (2020) 'Merkel urges unity in biggest challenge since World War II." *Bloomberg News*. Available at: www.bloomberg.com/news/articles/2020-03-18/merkel-urges-solidarity-in-biggest-challenge-since-world-war-ii. Accessed August 2020.

Economic Recovery Plan (2020) *Government of British Columbia*. Available at: https://www2.gov.bc.ca/gov/content/covid-19/economic-recovery. Accessed September 2020.

Goldenberg, S. (2018) *Killer Flu. Library and Archives, Canada*. Available at: www.canadahistory.ca/explore/arts-culture-society/killer-flu. Accessed September 2021.

Government of BC (2020a) 'Province declares state of emergency to support COVID-19 response.' *News R1elease*. Available at: https://news.gov.bc.ca/releases/2020PSSG0017-000511. Accessed August 2020.

Government of BC (2020b) 'COVID-19 action plan: BC's first steps to support people, businesses'. *News Release*, 23 March. Available at: https://news.gov.bc.ca/releases/2020PREM0013-000545. Accessed September 2021.

Government of BC (2020c) *Order of the provincial health officer: Travellers and Employers Order*. 10 April. Available at: https://www2.gov.bc.ca/assets/gov/health/about-bc-s-health-care-system/office-of-the-provincial-health-officer/covid-19/covid-19-pho-order-travellers-employers.pdf.

Government of BC (2020d) *In Plain sight: Addressing indigenous-specific racism and discrimination in BC. HealthCare*. Available at: https://engage.gov.bc.ca/app/uploads/sites/613/2020/11/In-Plain-Sight-Summary-Report.pdf.

Government of BC (2020e) *Technical briefing*. Available at: https://news.gov.bc.ca/files/2020-06-23-Modelling-Technical-Briefing.pdf. Accessed September 2021.

Government of BC (2021) 'BC's response to Covid-19'. *News Release*. Available at: https://www2.gov.bc.ca/gov/content/covid-19/info/response. Accessed August 2021.

Government of Canada (2020) *Coronavirus disease (COVID-19): Outbreak update*. Available at: www.canada.ca/en/public-health/services/diseases/2019-novelcoronavirus-infection.html. March 2020 to September 2021. Accessed August 2021.

Government of Canada (2021a) *Federal transfers to provinces and territories.* Department of Finance Canada. Available at: www.canada.ca/en/department-finance/programs/federal-transfers.html. Accessed August 2021.

Government of Canada (2021b) *Non-medical masks.* Available at: www.canada.ca/en/public-health/services/diseases/2019-novel-coronavirus-infection/prevention-risks/about-non-medical-masks-face-coverings.html. Accessed September 2021.

Hall, C. (2021) 'The House: Can Canadian federalism cope with 21st century threats?' *CBC News.* July 3. Available at: www.cbc.ca/radio/thehouse/federal-provincial-pandemic-climate-change-1.6084889. Accessed August 2021.

Hawaleshka, D. (2003) 'Is this your best defence? As Canadians anguish over how to protect themselves from SARS, health authorities take note of what went wrong'. *Macleans.* Available at: https://archive.macleans.ca/article/2003/4/14/is-this-your-best-defence.

Health Canada (2021) Available at: www.canada.ca/en/health-canada.html. Accessed August 2021.

Henry, B. (2019) 'Canadian pandemic influenza preparedness: Public health measures strategy.' *Canada Communicable Disease Report* 45: 149–163. Available at: www.ncbi.nlm.nih.gov/pmc/articles/PMC6587684/. Accessed August 2021.

House of Commons (2013) Statutes of Canada 2013, Chapter 15, An Act to amend the criminal code (concealment of identity). *Bill C-309.* Available at: www.parl.ca/DocumentViewer/en/41-1/bill/C-309/royal-assent.

Insights West (2021) *Vancouver, BC. Survey.* Available at: www.insightswest.com/about/company/. Accessed September 2021.

Katella, K. (2021) '5 Things to know about the Delta variant'. *Yale Medicine News.* Available at: www.yalemedicine.org/news/5-things-to-know-delta-variant-covid. Accessed October 2021.

Lawson, T., Nathans L., Goldenberg A., Fimiani, M. and Boire-Schwab, D. (2021) 'COVID-19: Emergency measures tracker'. *McCarthy News.* Available at: www.mccarthy.ca/en/insights/articles/covid-19-emergency-measures-tracker. Accessed October 2021.

Leung, N., Chu, D., Shiu, E., Chan, K., McDevitt, J., Hau, B., Yen, H., Li, Y., Ip, D., Peiris, J., Seto, W., Leung, G., Milton, D. and Cowling, B. (2020) 'Respiratory virus shedding in exhaled breath and efficacy of face masks'. *Nature Medicine* (26): 676–680.

Maher, S. (2021) 'Year one: The untold story of the pandemic in Canada: A comprehensive report on the country's mishandling of the crisis of the century.' *Macleans.* Available at: www.macleans.ca/longforms/covid-19-pandemic-canada-year-one/. Accessed August 2021.

Mcmaster, G. (2020) *Public acceptance of protective masks growing in Canada.* Commentary. University of Alberta Medical Press. Available at: https://www.ualberta.ca/folio/2020/07/public-acceptance-of-protective-masks-growing-in-canada.html. Accessed August 2021.

Merkley, E., Bridgman, A., Loewen, P., Owen, T., Ruths, D. and Zhilin, O. (2020) 'A rare moment of cross-Partisan consensus: Elite and public response to the COVID-19 pandemic in Canada'. *Canadian Journal of Political Science* 53(2): 311–318. doi:10.1017/S0008423920000311.

Ministry of Finance (2021) *Budget and fiscal plan 2021/2022 and 2022/2023.* Available at: https://www.bcbudget.gov.bc.ca/2021/pdf/2021_Budget%20and%20Fiscal%20Plan.pdf. Accessed September 2021.

Ministry of Health (2021) *British Columbia*. Available at: http://www2.gov.bc.ca/gov/content/governments/organizational-structure/ministries-organizations/ministries/health. Accessed August 2021.

Myseum. (2020) *The history of pandemics in Canada*. Available at: www.myseumoftoronto.com/programming/pandemics-canada/. Accessed September 2020.

National Assembly of Quebec (2017) *Bill 62, 'An Act to foster adherence to state religious neutrality and, in particular, to provide a framework for religious accommodation requests in certain bodies'*. Quebec: Quebec Official Publisher, The Government of Quebec.

National Assembly of Quebec (2019) *Bill 21, 'An Act Respecting the Laicity of the State'*. Quebec: Quebec Official Publisher, The Government of Quebec.

Nelms, B. (2020) 'The COVID-19 pandemic: A timeline of key events across British Columbia'. *CBC News*, 3 April. Available at: https://www.cbc.ca/news/canada/british-columbia/covid-19-bc-timeline-1.5520943 Accessed August 2021.

Novic, S. (2020) 'Masks are a barrier against the coronavirus. They also pose a major hurdle for deaf people'. *Opinion. The Washington Post*. Available at: www.washingtonpost.com/opinions/2020/07/16/masks-are-barrier-against-virus-they-also-pose-major-hurdle-deaf-people/. Accessed October 2021.

Office of the Human Rights Commissioner (2021) 'BC's human rights commissioner launches province-wide public inquiry into hate in the pandemic'. *News*. Available at: https://bchumanrights.ca/news/b-c-s-human-rights-commissioner-launches-province-wide-public-inquiry-into-hate-in-the-pandemic/. Accessed October 2021.

Park, S., Choi, G.J. and Ko, H. (2020) 'Information technology-based tracing strategy in response to COVID-19 in South Korea – privacy controversies'. *JAMA* 323(21): 2129–2130. doi:10.1001/jama. 2020.6602.

PHSA (Provincial Health Services Authority) (2021) *British Columbia*. Available at: www.phsa.ca/. Accessed September 2021.

Racism Incident Reporting Center (2021) Available at: www.project1907.org/reportingcentre. Accessed September 2021.

Restart Plan (2020) *Government of British Columbia*, 6 May. Available at: https://www2.gov.bc.ca/gov/content/safety/emergency-preparedness-response-recovery/covid-19-provincial-support/bc-restart-plan. Accessed August 2021.

Schertzer, R., McDougall, A. and Skogstad, G. (2018) 'Multilateral collaboration in Canadian Intergovernmental Relations: The role of procedural and reciprocal norms.' *Publius* 48(4): 636–663.

Schmunk, R. (2020) 'Health officials 'confident' first case of coronavirus has been found in B.C'. *CBC News*. Available at: www.cbc.ca/news/canada/british-columbia/coronavirus-bc-updates-1.5442971. Accessed August 2021.

Slaughter, G. (2020) 'Canada confirms first 'community case' of COVID-19: Here's what that means'. *CTV News*, 5 March. Available at: www.ctvnews.ca/health/coronavirus/canada-confirms-first-community-case-of-covid-19-here-s-what-that-means-1.4841249. Accessed August 2020.

Statistics Canada (2020) 'COVID-19 mortality rates in Canada's ethno-cultural neighbourhoods'. *Government of Canada*. Available at: https://www150.statcan.gc.ca/n1/pub/45-28-0001/2020001/article/00079-eng.htm.

Taccone, A. (2020) 'Western University student is fourth coronavirus case in Canada'. *CTV News London*. Available at: https://london.ctvnews.ca/western-university-student-is-fourth-coronavirus-case-in-canada-1.4792371. Accessed September 2021.

The Commonwealth Fund (2020) *International health care system profiles: Canada*. Available at: www.commonwealthfund.org/international-health-policy-center/countries/canada. Accessed January 2022.

The Environics Institute (2012) 'Focus Canada 2012'. *Report*. Available at: www.environicsinstitute.org/projects/project-details/focus-canada-2012. Accessed September 2021.

The Environics Institute (2020) 'Focus Canada – Fall 2020. COVID-19, public policy and government decision-making'. *Final Report*. Available at: https://uploads-ssl.webflow.com/5f931bff6aee7ca287dbada2/60b6b0991fdcf0933027ac91_COVID-19%2C%20public%20policy%20and%20government%20decision-making.pdf. Accessed September 2021.

The Public Health Act (2008) *Victoria BC, Canada*. Available at: www.bclaws.gov.bc.ca/civix/document/id/complete/statreg/08028_01. Accessed 20 August 2021.

Todd (2014) 'Vancouver is the most "Asian" city outside Asia'. *Vancouver Sun*. Available at: https://vancouversun.com/life/vancouver-is-most-asian-city-outside-asia-what-are-the-ramifications. Accessed October 2021.

Vancouver Police Department (2021) 'Year-end 2020. Year-to-Date Key Performance Indicators Report'. *Report to the Vancouver Police Board*. Available at: https://vpd.ca/wp-content/uploads/2021/06/vpd-annual-report-2020.pdf. Accessed September 2021.

Vox Pop Labs (2020). *McMaster University, Hamilton, Ontario*. Available at: https://voxpoplabs.com/about/. Accessed September 2021.

Wang, C.J., Ng, C.Y. and Brook, R.H. (2020) 'Response to COVID-19 in Taiwan: Big data analytics, new technology, and proactive testing'. *JAMA* 323(14): 2129–2130. doi:10.1001/jama.2020.3151.

Wells, P. (2017) 'Why Quebec's Bill 62 is an indefensible mess'. *Macleans*. Available at: www.macleans.ca/politics/ottawa/why-quebecs-bill-62-is-an-indefensible-mess/. Accessed September 2021.

WHO (2020a) 'WHO Director-General's opening remarks at the media briefing on COVID-19-11 March 2020.' Available at: www.who.int/director-general/speeches/detail/who-director-general-s-opening-remarks-at-the-media-briefing-on-covid-19-11-march-2020. Accessed September 2021.

WHO (2020b) 'Coronavirus disease 2019 (COVID-19). Situation report – 51. Data as reported by national authorities by 10am CET 11 March 2020'. Available at: https://www.who.int/docs/default-source/coronaviruse/situation-reports/20200311-sitrep-51-covid-19.pdf. Accessed September 2021.

Wong, J.E.L., Leo, Y.S. and Tan, C.C. (2020) 'COVID-19 in Singapore – Current experience: Critical global issues that require attention and action'. *JAMA* 323(3): 1243–1244. doi:10.1001/jama.2020.2467.

Xu, X. (2020) 'Cultures clash over wearing masks amid virus'. *The Globe and Mail*. Available at: www.theglobeandmail.com/canada/british-columbia/article-cultures-clash-over-wearing-masks-amid-virus/. Accessed August 2021.

YouGov (2020) *Covid-19 monitor. Survey*. Available at: https://business.yougov.com/product/covid-19,UK. Accessed August 2021.

Zine, J. (2020) 'Unmasking the racial politics of the coronavirus pandemic'. *The Conversation*, 3 June. Available at: https://theconversation.com/unmasking-the-racial-politics-of-the-coronavirus-pandemic-139011. Accessed September 2021.

Part II

Asia

10 Preventing the pandemic

Face masks and infectious diseases in Taiwan's modern history

Chen Lihang

This chapter was translated by George Bobyk

10.1 Introduction

During the COVID-19 outbreak, face masks protected people by reducing the possibility of spreading infection. The sudden demand for face masks tested the production capabilities of every nation, and many governments enacted laws that made wearing face masks mandatory. This stimulated a response from the public that often differed between countries. Before the pandemic, few people in Taiwan wore face masks on the streets. The COVID-19 outbreak significantly changed this situation – during the pandemic, nearly everyone wore a face mask. Thus, face masks became a part of people's daily lives. Taiwanese people did not express much opposition to wearing face masks. This is quite different from the scenes of protest seen in the USA. For instance, in March 2021, at least 100 citizens gathered in front of Idaho's General Assembly to protest against policies that made the wearing of face masks mandatory, calling it a violation of citizens' freedom. Protesters in Idaho also set fire to face masks in an act of defiance (*The Guardian*, 2021). Face masks have created some conflicts in Taiwan when people have not followed the rules to collect them, but the number of people dissatisfied at being obliged to wear a face mask has only been a very small minority. Taiwanese people have never come close to forming an 'anti-mask movement' like those seen in the USA. Instead, Taiwanese people have been proactive in requesting the government to come up with an appropriate plan for producing and distributing face masks (Ye, 2021). Why has the situation in Taiwan differed so greatly from that in the USA? One direct reason is the 2003 severe acute respiratory syndrome (SARS) outbreak. Furthermore, I argue that to answer this question, it is necessary to look at the role of face masks in Taiwan's modern history.

10.2 Public hygiene in colonial Taiwan

Face masks started to become widely used in Taiwan during the period of Japanese colonial occupation (1895–1945). This was an important period for the

DOI: 10.4324/9781003244127-12

modernisation of Taiwan's public hygiene. This chapter will start by discussing Taiwan's colonial period, investigating how the Japanese promoted public hygiene in Taiwan, to see what role face masks played in these endeavours.

Taiwan became a Japanese colony in 1895, the same year the Empire of Japan (1868–1947) and Qing China (1644–1912) signed the Treaty of Shimonoseki, where Qing China ceded Taiwan to Japan. Japan used the acquisition of Taiwan as a colonial territory to prove its strength to the West. In March–May 1895, Japan dispatched troops to occupy the island of Taiwan. Finally, by November 1895, Japan had occupied the whole island. The process of occupying Taiwan was anything but straightforward. The moment the Japanese army set foot on the shores of Taiwan, they became embroiled in a bitter battle against numerous diseases, such as dysentery, malaria, cholera and tinea pedis. The Japanese army was so beleaguered by diseases that even the Imperial Guard Regimental Commander Prince Kitashirakawa Yoshihisa (1847–1895) died of disease during the process of occupying Taiwan (Ide, 1937).

Just how miserable was the situation for the Japanese army in Taiwan? Horiuchi Tsuguo (1873–1955) was an Imperial Guard military doctor. From the moment he stepped on the island in 1895, he saw corpses of the Japanese army being sent to the crematorium every day. He noted that there were so many corpses that it was necessary to wrap them up in straw mats and then use a bamboo pole to carry them to the crematorium. The scene reminded him of how two people would use a bamboo pole to carry tuna. In the process of occupying Taiwan, Japan only lost several hundred people in battle, but as many as 4,400 people died of disease (Ide, 1937).

Military doctors of the Japanese army conducted an investigation into the diseases the soldiers died from in Taiwan. This data and knowledge became an important source of information that would eventually improve the ability of the colonial government to tackle the problem of public hygiene in Taiwan. In the eyes of many Japanese people, the architecture of Taiwan's most densely populated areas was graceful, but they were repulsed by the fetid odour of people and livestock living in close proximity, puddles of sewage on the road and mountains of rubbish and excrement. In addition to the city's pungent odours, the Japanese found it difficult to adapt to the dirtiness and humidity, and this environment also concealed manifold hygienic dangers.

Officials dispatched to Taiwan had to adapt not only to Taiwan's local customs but also to the threat of plague, cholera and malaria. In Taiwan, it was common to die from disease. Officials who did not die from disease often just resigned and went home to Japan. Furthermore, even though the Government-General of Taiwan (the institution that Japan used to govern Taiwan) provided better remuneration than in mainland Japan (the salary was 50% higher in Taiwan), many Japanese people feared that a trip to Taiwan would spell their death (Takekoshi, 1905; Wang, 2007).

Japan lacked experience in governing a colony, which created problems for the Japanese government in Taiwan (Sakura, 1961). The differences between the legal systems, local customs and languages posed problems for the new rulers.

Moreover, some Taiwanese people actively resisted the Japanese government, which, in addition to the threat of infectious diseases, was a significant problem. The Government-General of Taiwan made strenuous efforts to stabilise governance and solve the problem of infectious diseases in Taiwan. These measures included the formulation of the Rules for Preventing Infectious Diseases, construction of a water supply and sewage system, implementation of seaport quarantine and traffic regulation, establishment of hospitals and medical research institutions, cultivation of Western medicine to replace traditional Chinese medicine and use of the police and the *baojia* system to promote grassroots hygiene. The Japanese colonial-era *baojia* system was inherited from the Qing dynasty; households were organised into groups that made it much easier for the government to enforce its policies in local society (Hsu, 2004a). These measures enabled the colonial government to control numerous infectious diseases. After 1918, no further cases of plague were reported. By 1920, there were only sporadic cases of smallpox, and cholera disappeared without a trace (Taiwan Centers for Disease Control, 2018a). It was during this period that Taiwan's pre-modern public hygiene began to be modernised.

What role did face masks play in the process of Taiwan's medical modernisation? Face masks were an important part of the Government-General of Taiwan's policies to promote public hygiene: they were one of the commodities mentioned by officials when promoting hygiene education. This chapter will discuss when and how the Government-General of Taiwan promoted the use of face masks to both Japanese people and local Taiwanese people. The Government-General of Taiwan principally used newspapers such as the *Taiwan Daily News* to promote the use of face masks. In addition, some Japanese doctors also submitted articles to magazines; these can be seen in *Taiwan's Women's World* and *The Hygiene Industry's Friend*.

10.3 Making use of face masks: colonial-era hygiene policies

This chapter will introduce and analyse reports and essays about face masks that appeared in colonial-era newspapers, showing how face masks became an important part of Taiwan's colonial-era hygiene policies. The promotion of face masks was an important stage in the modernisation of public hygiene in Taiwan. Reports and essays about face masks appeared prominently in the *Taiwan Daily News*, *Taiwan's Women's World* and *The Hygiene Industry's Friend*. The *Taiwan Daily News* was in operation from 1898 to 1944. It was the Government-General of Taiwan's newspaper for imperial use; it typically supported the stance of the Government-General of Taiwan. Its readers were mainly Japanese people in Taiwan and local Taiwanese elites. In the rest of this chapter, I will discuss the relationship between face masks, infectious diseases and the public's response.

On 21 December 1919, an article appeared in the *Taiwan Daily News* called 'Essential knowledge for preventing influenza'. This article mentions that to prevent influenza, the Taihoku (Taipei) Police Department were using fliers to remind people not to venture to places where groups of people gather, such as theatres, cinemas and sick people's homes. Furthermore, it states that if there are gravely sick people within the household, they should be quarantined alone in a different room to recuperate, and if there are other people who need to care for the sufferer, then the report says:

> If the patient needs people to care for them or be in close proximity, then the carer must use a medical cloth to cover their nose and mouth; moreover, when cleaning the patient's room, they must also prevent dust from dispersing. The patient's nasal fluid and phlegm should be thrown into the toilet, whereas the patient's napkin and bowl of phlegm should be disinfected by being boiled. The patient's bedding and clothes also need to be disinfected in the sunlight . . . in regard to the nose–mouth cover, an absorbent cotton gauze sponge should be used. The patient's family should make sure to promptly use a nose–mouth cover whenever in the vicinity of the patient. If the disease has started to spread within the family, then it's important to disinfect the medical cloth after every use.
>
> (*Taiwan Daily News*, 1919, p. 5)

The newspaper article advises people that a sterile cloth made from absorbent cotton gauze can be used to cover the nose and mouth to protect against infection transmission. Based on the descriptions in the article, the 'nose–mouth cover' is slightly different from a typical modern face mask, but the idea behind them is identical.

In 1918, the Spanish flu caused 25,397 deaths in Taiwan, while infections peaked at 779,523 (Cai, 2013). In the 1920s, the ratio of people who died from a flu infection significantly increased: there were 19,951 deaths from 153,649 infections. Given these numbers, it is not difficult to imagine why numerous articles promoting hygiene appeared in the *Taiwan Daily News*. The 'nose–mouth cover', as it was called in the news report, was promoted by officials during the Spanish flu epidemic to prevent the spread of infection. The newspaper article used the term 'mouth cover' to refer to face masks; however, during that period, it was most common to see face masks being referred to using the Japanese word *masuku* (mask). The Japanese term originates from the English word 'mask'. In Japanese, the word *masuku* has two meanings: a medical face mask and a gas mask. Tsushima Tadao uses this homonym skilfully in a four-panel manga published in the *Taiwan Daily News*. In Tsushima's manga, a concerned mother reads a report in the newspaper about influenza and then immediately tells her children to put on a *masuku*. To the mother's surprise, when her two children appear before her, they are erroneously wearing gas masks instead of face masks (*Taiwan Daily News*, 1938) (see Figure 10.1).

Face masks were not just worn when influenza was spreading. They were also worn when there was poor environmental sanitation. On 23 November 1941, the *Taiwan Daily News* published an article called 'How to use face masks', recommending that people wear face masks whenever in heavily crowded areas, places where there is a great deal of airborne dust and when people exhibit cough

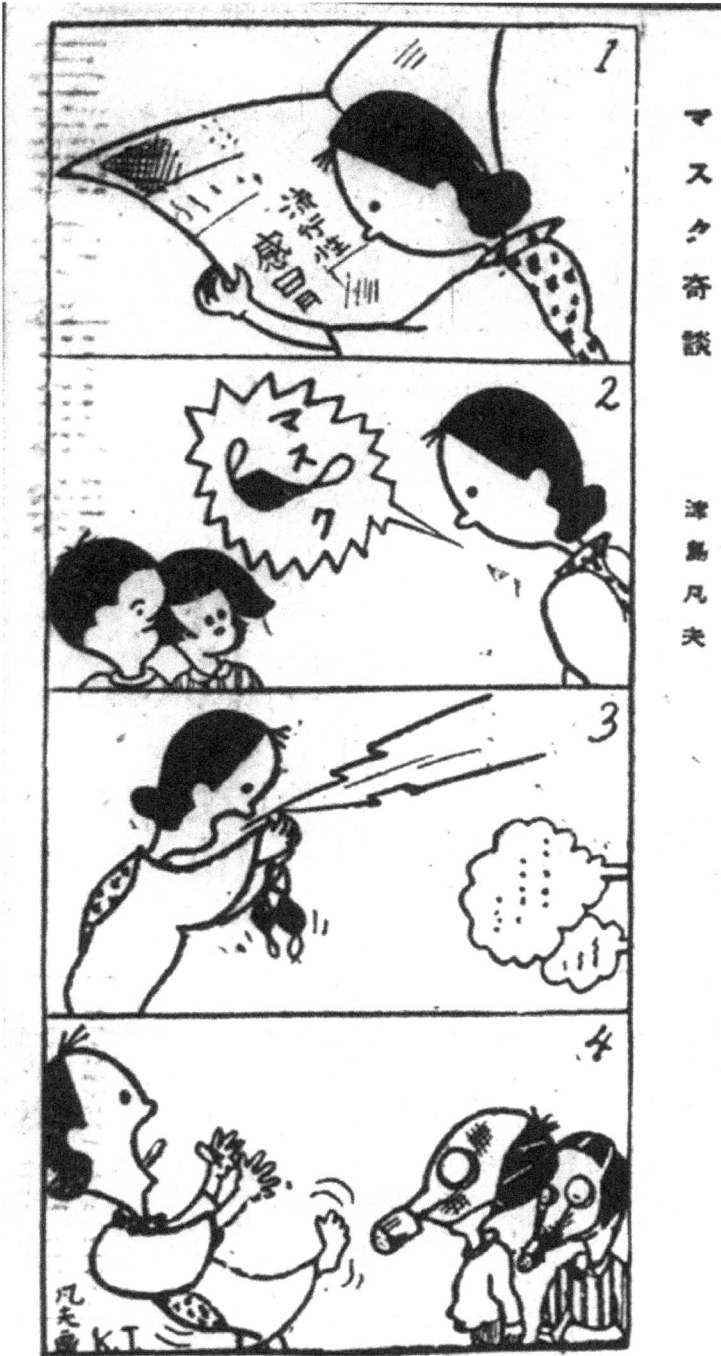

Figure 10.1 A strange tale about masks

symptoms. It is also interesting to note that this article suggests that because it was not very cold in Taiwan, and the roads in Taihoku City (Taipei City) and other cities were orderly and clean, it was not always necessary to wear a face mask (*Taiwan Daily News*, 1941a). This report suggests that when deciding whether to wear a face mask, people should consider the climate and cleanliness of cities in Taiwan as a factor.

Apart from wearing face masks to ward off influenza or when in dirty, crowded places, every time there was an encephalitis epidemic in Taiwan, officials promoted the use of face masks to improve public hygiene. Cerebrospinal meningitis is an epidemic form of meningitis. It is transmitted through air droplets; thus, if there are cerebral meningitis sufferers in the surrounding area, a face mask should be worn.

On 15 January 1941, there were six confirmed cases of cerebrospinal meningitis in Takao City (Kaohsiung City). This shocked the Takao Department of Health because there had only been one case of cerebrospinal meningitis in the previous year. In the short space of a week, there were suddenly six new cases. The Takao Department of Health reminded the city's residents that a face mask must be worn whenever going outside (*Taiwan Daily News*, 1941b). The cerebrospinal meningitis epidemic was not confined to Takao City. According to an earlier report in the *Taiwan Daily News* on 21 March 1935, there were four confirmed cases of cerebrospinal meningitis in Taihoku Prefecture, in an area under the jurisdiction of the North Branch Police Station. Three of the sufferers died from the disease.

For these reasons, the Hygiene Section of the North Branch Police Station took extensive measures to protect people against the epidemic. From 20 March, face masks were provided at the entrances to cinemas and theatres; the aim was to stop the virus from spreading further (*Taiwan Daily News*, 1935a). Moreover, earlier in the same month, Giran (Yilan) District Police Station stipulated that those working at Giran House – a theatre in Giran – must distribute face masks to all people who entered; people within the theatre were also obliged to wear a face mask. Consequently, anyone not wearing a face mask would be made to leave (*Taiwan Daily News*, 1935b). By compelling people who wanted to enter Giran Theatre to wear face masks, the colonial government instilled in people the habit of wearing face masks.

In addition to articles seen in the *Taiwan Daily News*, there were many articles about hygiene education in Taiwan's colonial-era magazines. These magazines show how important face masks were for children's hygiene education. Dr. Sakai Kiyoshi submitted an article to *Taiwan's Women's World* called 'Advice for families with children preparing for middle-school entrance examinations!' (*Sakai*, 1936). Dr Sakai Kiyoshi's essay was written for the parents of children preparing to take the middle-school entrance examination. Dr. Sakai Kiyoshi aimed to warn parents that their child's body would be placed under significant stress while preparing for this 'hellish exam'. The article urges parents to pay particular attention to their child's health, diet and hygiene during this arduous time. Dr. Sakai believed that sleep and exercise were crucial to ensure that the exam did not have a deleterious effect on children's health. At the end of the essay, Dr. Sakai further reminds parents that if there are confirmed cases of influenza, diphtheria or scarlet fever, students should cultivate the habit of wearing face masks when going out and rinse out their mouth when they return home to prevent infection. Aside from students preparing for the middle-school entrance examination, these measures could also help protect infants against contracting viruses since many infants were infected at home. To prevent infants from becoming infected, parents should, therefore, wear a face mask and refrain from getting too close (Obari, 1942).

What was the material and price of face masks promoted in these newspapers and magazines? In reality, face masks were made not only from paper; there were also woollen and leather face masks. The 214th edition of the Nakajima Shoji Corporation's commercial catalogue, published in 1934, shows a selection of advertisements for face masks (see Figure 10.2). Readers could peruse a huge

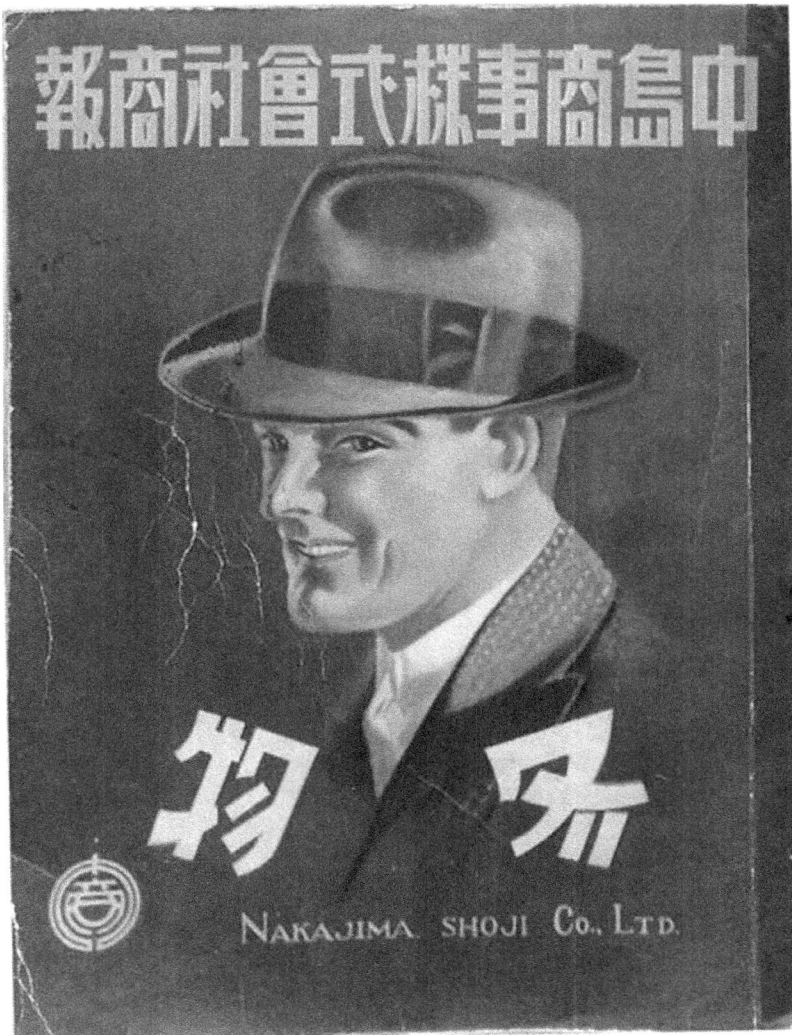

Figure 10.2 Nakajima Shoji Corporation commercial catalogue winter goods

selection of products in the catalogue and purchase products by posting a cheque to the Nakajima Shoji Corporation. These adverts emphasised how face masks could protect against colds and maintain warmth while also being very hygienic, which is very similar to adverts for face masks nowadays (Nakajima Shoji Co., Ltd, 1934). The images printed on the Nakajima Shoji Corporation's catalogue show the different face masks people could purchase at that time.

There were two different types of woollen masks. The first type was a normal woollen face mask; the second type also came with earmuffs, and the price was 90 sen. There were four different grades of woollen face mask with a corresponding price scale ranging from 60 to 95 sen. Woollen face masks, especially the one in the middle of the picture (see Figure 10.3), are very similar in appearance to contemporary face masks.

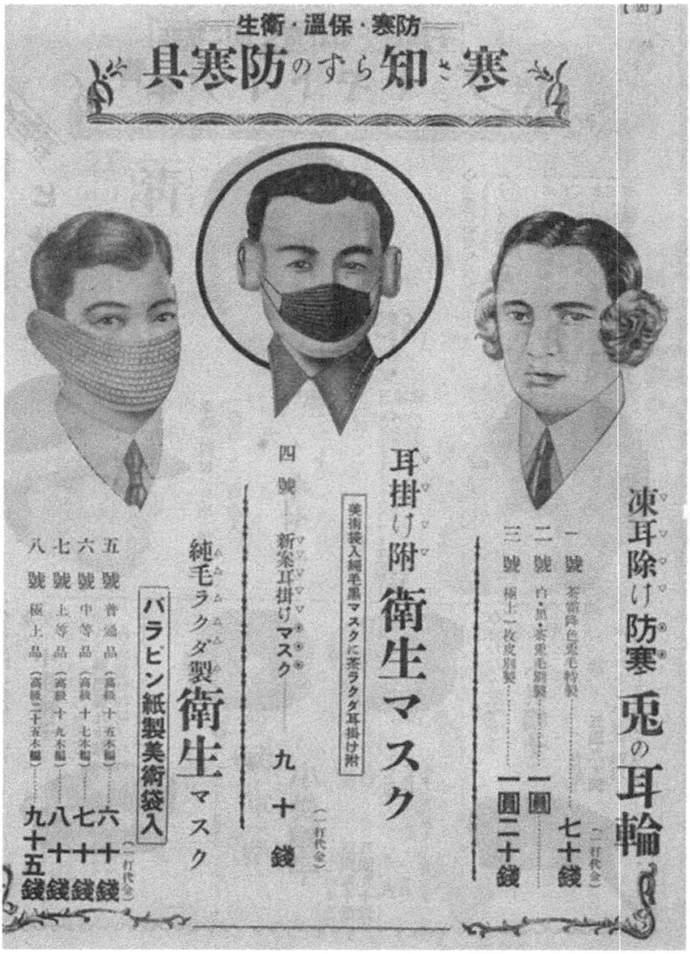

Figure 10.3 Different types of face masks for winter

There were two different types of face masks made of leather: one type was man-made leather (the cheapest could be bought for 58 sen), whereas the most expensive was 1 yen 20 sen. The other type of leather face mask was made using authentic leather; the most expensive was 1 yen 80 sen. Face masks made from leather were in the shape of a rhombus, which is quite dissimilar to the face masks that are popular now (see Figure 10.4).

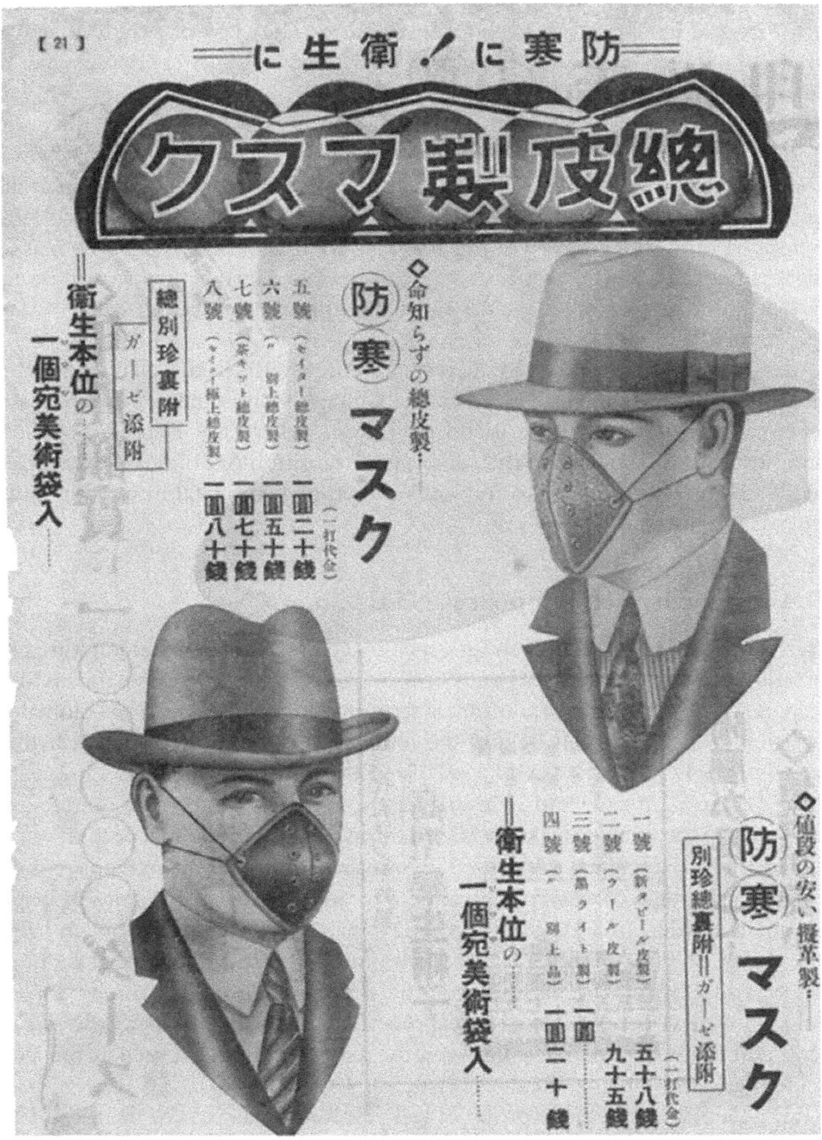

Figure 10.4 Leather face masks in the shape of a rhombus

How did people at the time perceive the price of these face masks? Using the standard salary of vocational school instructors during Taiwan's colonial period, we can gain insight into the relative price of face masks. The commercial catalogue of the Nakajima Shoji Corporation was published in 1934, and the annual salary of instructors at Giran Vocational School in 1934 was between 40 and 70 yen a month. This rough comparison shows how the price of face masks compares to the salary of instructors at Giran Vocational School (Government-General of Taiwan, 1934). It shows that face masks were an expensive commodity for people like vocational school instructors. The class of people that were perhaps more inclined to purchasing face masks were colonial-era doctors like Wu Xinrong (1907–1967), as his diary suggests.

Taiwanese people's colonial-era diaries also provide a great source for understanding how the Japanese colonial-era policies of promoting face masks were adopted by ordinary people. Wu Xinrong was a doctor practising in Tainan during the colonial era. As recorded in his diary, on the morning of 13 March 1939, he hopped onto a rickshaw wearing many layers of clothing and a face mask to visit a patient. There are two probable reasons Wu Xinrong was wearing a face mask on this day: to protect against colds and to prevent infection when examining patients (Wu, 1939).

After World War II (WWII) ended on 15 August 1945, the Nationalist Party (GMD) was subsequently defeated by the Chinese Communist Party and forced to retreat from China to the island of Taiwan, where the Republic of China continues to this day. During the subsequent transition of political power, incremental changes were made to Taiwan's public hygiene, healthcare system and face mask industry.

10.4 Public hygiene in postwar Taiwan

After WWII ended in 1945, Taiwan experienced another historical juncture. The transition of power to the GMD not only impacted politics but also affected how the state would develop its healthcare system and public hygiene. The colonial-era government of Taiwan left behind the foundations of a modern public hygiene system. In 1947, after the GMD took over Taiwan, they formed the Taiwan Provincial Department of Health. Unfortunately, there were outbreaks of numerous diseases thought to have been eradicated during Taiwan's colonial period, such as cholera and malaria. This was caused by insufficient manpower to manage public hygiene, a shortage of materials after the war and a relaxed entry and exit inspection at the border. In addition, the GMD's management of the problem lagged behind that of Taiwan's colonial-era government. The GMD's lack of economic measures supporting the lockdown of the city also caused Taiwanese people to panic. Taiwanese people started to express their dissatisfaction with the government, and there were conflicts between the people and police, such as the Budai Incident and the Xinying Incident (Hsu, 2004b).

Taiwan's postwar hygiene problem was resolved by assistance from the USA. From the 1950s to the 1960s, support from the USA alleviated Taiwan's economic predicament and provided comprehensive plans and policies to improve Taiwan's public hygiene, medical treatment and nutrition. The USA helped set the direction for the development of Taiwan's postwar public hygiene and medical treatment. Furthermore, US aid had a strong effect on the eradication and control of infectious diseases. The US aid supported Taiwan by providing materials such as flour, milk, milk powder and beef; such provision began to change Taiwanese people's eating habits and nutritional intake. From the 1950s to the 1960s, Taiwanese people's physical fitness and ability to fight diseases also improved. The mortality rate of infants, babies and pregnant mothers subsequently decreased. Apart from the US aid, assistance from international organisations and international programmes, such as the World Health Organization, the United Nations Children's Fund and the United Nations Expanded Programme of Technical Assistance, were also instrumental in improving Taiwan's public hygiene and healthcare system.

In 1971, the GMD made the Bureau of Health subordinate to the Executive Yuan, the governmental institution in Taiwan responsible for enforcing the law. This symbolised that the central government placed a greater emphasis on public hygiene policies. From the 1980s to the 1990s, the government successfully promoted a hepatitis B prevention plan and a universal health insurance system, as well as the concept that public hygiene was paramount to a great nation. The idea was to use medical resources as a foundation for Taiwan's foreign diplomacy and internal affairs, demonstrating that Taiwan had reached the standard of an advanced country and strongly supported public hygiene and medical treatment. However, these achievements were constantly tested by new challenges of the times.

10.5 Infectious diseases and the commodification of face masks in postwar Taiwan

What role did face masks play in developing medical treatment and public hygiene in Taiwan's postwar society? We can see that in postwar Taiwan, as the production and sale of face masks became increasingly commodified, Taiwanese people responded by using face masks for purposes that were not explicitly for the prevention of infectious diseases. The primary role of face masks, however, was still preventing the spread of infectious diseases. Shortly after WWII ended, infectious diseases were resurgent in Taiwan.

On 13 May 1946, the 'Weekly pictorial' column in the *Riyuetan Weekly* magazine published a manga depicting an elderly person wearing a face mask. Next to the picture, the text says, 'There was another outbreak of meningitis in Taipei City; citizens all wore face masks to prevent spreading infection. It is now known that the disease has already been extinguished' (Ma, 1946, p. 40). This manga reflects Taipei's 1946 meningitis epidemic. Patients with meningitis suffer from severe headaches, fever and vomiting. In Taiwan, meningitis had two peak periods: the first was 1919–1926, and the second was 1933–1946 (Taiwan Centers for Disease Control, 2018b). Although the peak of meningitis had passed by

1960, from time to time, there were still cases of meningitis in Taiwan. In mid-July 1964, the *United Daily News* reported that several cases of meningitis had appeared in Taipei City. According to this report, the potential risk of infection was greater in crowded public places or in people who felt overly fatigued. The report advised parents to prepare face masks for their children to use when entering and leaving public places to avoid being infected with meningitis (*United Daily News*, 1964). In addition, with the advancement of medicine, although cases of meningitis still occasionally appeared, doctors found that penicillin, antibiotics and anti-inflammatory agents were extremely effective against meningitis, and this reduced the probability of dying from meningitis.

Face masks were also effective against diphtheria and influenza. Diphtheria is a highly contagious and potentially fatal infection that can affect the nose and throat. It is spread by coughs and sneezes or through close contact with someone already infected. In August 1958, more than 20 diphtheria patients were confirmed in Taipei City. Du Shimian, a well-known otolaryngologist, said that it was possible to prevent diphtheria, so parents should always put a face mask on their children when they go out; if their children unfortunately became infected with diphtheria, they should send them to a hospital for isolation and treatment. This shows that there were similarities in the preventive measures taken against diphtheria and meningitis, with the wearing of face masks being a prominent way of inhibiting the spread of infection (Chen, 1958).

In addition to meningitis and diphtheria, face masks were also used to prevent influenza. Nowadays, people think that influenza has long been commonplace, but during the 1950s, this was not the case in Taiwan. In May 1957, influenza gained the attention of the Taiwan Provincial Government. Provincial Chairman Yan Jiagan ordered the Department of Health to provide appropriate prevention and cure. Even pictorial magazines took the influenza epidemic as a theme. One such example is the 'Mischievous little egg' manga in the *Economic Daily News*. The protagonist, 'mischievous little egg', is wearing a comically oversized face mask while saying, 'there are too many people suffering from influenza, so I have to choose this extra-large face mask' (Xiao, 1970, p. 10) (see Figure 10.5).

In addition to the connection between face masks and diseases, face masks were also used to prevent barbers from having unnecessary contact with customers and spreading infection. The Provincial Department of Health issued a general order that 'barbers should not neglect to wear a face mask' (*United Daily News*, 1957, p. 3). In 1969, the Taipei City Bureau of Health launched an inspection of barbershops in Taipei City. Furthermore, the director of the Bureau of Health, Wang Yaodong, called for barbers in Taipei City to wear face masks at work to prevent the spread of infection when shaving customers' faces. Barbershops received the scrutiny of government officials because they were seen as particularly unhygienic places. One of the reasons was because they offered ear-cleaning services, but since the tools used to clean ears were typically not disinfected, they often resulted in customers' ears becoming infected. In addition to calling on barbers to wear face masks, Wang Yaodong also hoped that barbershops would stop providing ear-cleaning services (*United Daily News*, 1969). The emphasis

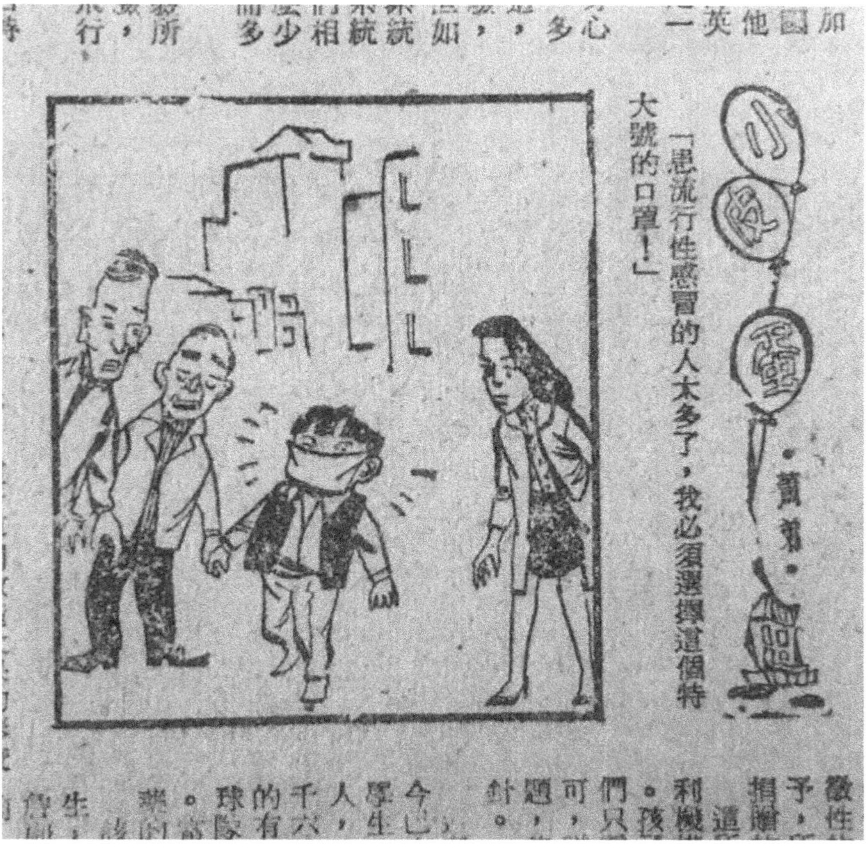

Figure 10.5 Mischievous little egg

the government placed on wearing face masks to prevent infection was a constant in colonial and postwar hygiene policy.

The focus of this chapter will now shift to the production and sale of face masks. In postwar Taiwan, the level of technology used in the production of face masks improved; face masks were no longer just made from leather, wool or paper. From the 1960s to the 1980s, information relating to face masks and their advertisements can be seen in newspapers. Newspapers published many details about the businesses of many well-known factories for producing face masks, such as the Youren Company, the Xinyuan Company, Dixin, Xuanni and Liyou. As face masks became increasingly commodified, their users also started to gradually increase in number. Companies also vied with each other to produce the most appealing and hygienic face masks. This can be seen from the way each company advertised their masks. The face masks produced by the Youren Company were filled with flower oil and green oil, which made their face masks refreshing and comfortable to wear. The Youren Company produced three different types of its 'Liren model' face mask. The prices were all under 20 New Taiwan Dollars (NTD) (*United Daily News*, 1968). The Youren Company face masks were extremely popular. Even though 2,000 face masks were produced daily, they were still unable to meet the demand. The Liren 'dustproof' model face mask was a popular product among motorcycle riders (*Economic Daily News*, 1970a). In addition to being a good companion for motorcycle riders, the Liren model dustproof face mask was also worn by patients, as a report in the *Economic Daily News* mentions:

> This type of face mask is suitable for both motorcycle riders and patients who have been advised by their doctors to wear it. The face mask prevents dust and germs from entering the oral cavity. The face mask uses a rhombus-shaped sponge, the top is soaked in a special medicinal substance, and the edges are inlaid with white plastic. Every face mask is individually wrapped in a white plastic cover, which looks very hygienic. In a typical Western pharmacy, the price is Ten NTD.
>
> (*Economic Daily News*, 1970b, p. 7)

The Youren Company also produced activated-carbon face masks. Activated-carbon face masks are characterised by the use of activated carbon for filtration. The Youren Company also provided this type of face mask to factory workers (*Economic Daily News*, 1972); however, it was not the only company to produce activated-carbon face masks. Another company called Liyou also produced them. Liyou boasted that their face mask would cover everything from the nose to the mouth and provide a high degree of ventilation and was easy to clean. Liyou had its own factory, with a monthly production of more than 72,000 face masks (*Independent Evening News*, 1979).

It is clear that over time the technology involved in producing face masks continued to improve. Moreover, face masks provided the wearer with a degree of privacy. In the case of nurses who spent long hours working in hospitals and interacting with patients, face masks also provided another form of 'protection', as was suggested by a nurse at Taipei University Medical Hospital:

> The main reason most nurses wear a face mask is that they fear spreading germs to others, or for fear of being infected by others and becoming ill. However, Chen Fenyan, a paediatric nurse at Taipei University Medical Hospital, has another reason. She says that, "in addition to avoiding possible droplet infection, when work is very busy or you're in a bad mood, wearing a face mask can also prevent patients from seeing your unpleasant expressions, which could have a negative impact on work".
>
> (Tao, 1987, p. 5)

In postwar Taiwan, the role of face masks was, to some extent, a continuation of the colonial era; they played a pivotal role in preventing the transmission of meningitis and influenza. However, as time passed, the technology used to produce masks continued to improve, making face masks popular among different types of people, such as motorcycle riders and factory workers.

10.6 Conclusion

Face masks have been closely related to social changes and the development of public hygiene in Taiwan. They gradually entered Taiwanese people's daily lives as a result of the hygienic modernisation initiated during the colonial era. They were promoted as a product capable of guarding against colds and preventing the transmission of viruses. Looking at the appearance of face masks, during the colonial era, face masks in a variety of different materials were available for purchase, including paper, leather and wool. In postwar Taiwan, the face mask industry rapidly developed. In 1980, even activated-carbon face masks were available. Today, the production and technology of face masks have naturally continued to improve.

During Taiwan's 2003 SARS epidemic, face masks were an indispensable commodity. Shortly after the outbreak of SARS, when the source and cause of the virus were unclear, the pneumonia-like illness engendered a state of global panic. This was experienced most seriously in China, Hong Kong, Singapore and Vietnam, where the disease was already rampant. By the time the epidemic had grown to four months, Taiwan had experienced several major medical incidents, including the closure of Heping Hospital, 664 confirmed infections and 73 deaths at Renji Hospital. Taiwan was removed from the list of areas affected by SARS on 5 July 2003. People's fears were temporarily assuaged, but the habits of fighting the epidemic were deeply embedded in Taiwanese people's psyche, like quarantining, constant hand-washing, wearing face masks, temperature checks and using alcohol and bleach to disinfect everything. After the epidemic, the government revised the Infectious Disease Prevention and Control Act, the Disease Management Bureau Organisation Act and the Department of Health Organisation Act. Moreover, the government established the National Health Command Centre, which upgraded the national infectious disease prevention and control system. The 2003 SARS epidemic affected and changed Taiwanese people's and the government's understanding of epidemic prevention. This is one reason Taiwan has been able to effectively control the COVID-19 outbreak.

In early 2020, shortly after the COVID-19 outbreak, Taiwan was not producing enough face masks to meet the exponential increase in demand. To guarantee the production of sufficient face masks, the government promulgated a ban on exporting face masks on 24 January 2020. On 6 February the same year, the government formally implemented a system to register the purchase of face masks. Initially, every adult could only purchase two face masks per week. Afterwards, as the production of face masks slowly increased, people could purchase more. During the COVID-19 pandemic, if you walked through the streets of Taiwan, you would see a majority of pedestrians, motorcycle riders, taxi drivers and even roadside shopkeepers wearing face masks. Taiwanese people have reacted in this way because of the lessons learnt from the SARS outbreak. In addition, an indirect reason is the development and promotion of public hygiene during the colonial and postwar eras.

References

Cai, C.H. (2013) 'Influenza and Cholera: A case study of infectious diseases in Taiwan', *Taiwan Studies*, 15(6), pp. 119–170. [in Chinese]

Chen, S.Z. (1958) 'Common knowledge about medicine: preventing diphtheria', *United Daily News*, 2 September, p. 6. [in Chinese]

Economic Daily News. (1970a) 'The dustproof face masks produced by Youren Company are selling very well', *Economic Daily News*, 22 October, p. 8. [in Chinese]

Economic Daily News. (1970b) 'Dustproof face masks', *Economic Daily News*, 14 January, p. 7. [in Chinese]

Economic Daily News. (1972) 'Youren Company supply activated carbon face masks', *Economic Daily News*, 20 November, p. 8. [in Chinese]

Government-General of Taiwan. (1934) *Records of Government-General of Taiwan and its staffers*. Taipei: Government-General of Taiwan. [in Japanese]

Hsu, H.C. (2004a) *Dictionary of Taiwan history*. Taipei: Wenjianhui, p. 544. [published in Chinese]

Hsu, H.C. (2004b) *Dictionary of Taiwan history*. Taipei: Wenjianhui, pp. 246, 959. [in Chinese]

Ide, K. (1937) *A list of achievements governing Taiwan*. Taipei: Taiwan riri baoshe, p. 30. [in Japanese]

Independent Evening News. (1979) 'Activated carbon dustproof face masks', *Independent Evening News*, 31 May, p. 8. [in Chinese]

Ma, G. (1946) 'There was an outbreak of meningitis in Taipei City; citizens all wore face masks to prevent spreading infection. It is now known that the disease has already been extinguished', *Riyuetan Weekly*, 7, p. 40. [in Chinese]

Nakajima Shoji Co., Ltd (1934) 'Nakajima Shooji kabushikigaisha shouhou fuyumono' (Nakajima Shoji Corporation commercial catalogue winter goods), *Nakajima Shoji Co., Ltd*, 214, pp. 20–21. [in Japanese]

Obari, K. (1942) 'Insight into paediatric healthcare', *The Hygiene Industry's Friend*, 163, pp. 38–43.

Sakai, K. (1936) *'Juken junbiki jidou no katei ni fukei kata ni'* (Advice for families with children preparing for middle school entrance examinations!), *Taiwan's Women's World*, 1 March, pp. 124–126.

Sakura, M. (1961) *Various records on Taiwan*. Taipei: Taiwan yinhang jingji yanjiushi, pp. 15, 55. [in Chinese]

Taiwan Centers for Disease Control. (2018a) 'Taiwan Centers for Disease Control's introduction to encephalomyelitis', www.cdc.gov.tw/Category/Page/vbII4z_HYUKVvzQ_tkhAAQ [Accessed 12 May 2021]. [in Chinese]

Taiwan Centers for Disease Control. (2018b) 'Taiwan Centers for Disease Control's introduction to plague', www.cdc.gov.tw/Category/Page/iCortfmEfVKqc-ZMeDdEuDA [Accessed 12 May 2021]. [in Chinese]

Taiwan Daily News. (1919) 'Kanbo yobo shuchi' (Essential knowledge for preventing influenza), *Taiwan Daily News*, 21 December, p. 5.

Taiwan Daily News. (1935a) 'Katsudou shibai nyuujyou ni kami asuku wo shiyou ryuno no man'enkeikou ni kitasyo ga yobou no issaku' (The North Branch Police

Station announces that a mask must be worn when entering movie theatres and theatres in order to prevent the epidemic spreading), *Taiwan Daily News*, 21 March, p. 7. [in Japanese]

Taiwan Daily News. (1935b) 'Masuku wo senumono ha gekijiyou kara taikyo wo meisu Girankai no ryuno booatsujin' (Anybody that is not wearing a mask will be asked to leave the theatre, checks will be carried out in Giran), *Taiwan Daily News*, 9 March, p. 3. [in Japanese]

Taiwan Daily News. (1938) 'Masuku kidan' (A strange tale about masks), *Taiwan Daily News*, 17 January, p. 3. [in Japanese]

Taiwan Daily News. (1941a) 'Masuku no mochiikata' (How to wear a mask), *Taiwan Daily News*, 23 November, p. 4. [in Japanese]

Taiwan Daily News. (1941b) 'Gaishutsu ni ha masuku Takao shinai ni ryuno hatsusei' (Because of the outbreak in cerebrospinal meningitis, a face mask must be worn in Takao City whenever going outside), *Taiwan Daily News*, 15 January, p. 4. [in Japanese]

Takekoshi, Y. (1905) *A record of governing Taiwan*. Tokyo: Hakubunkan, pp. 15–16. [in Japanese]

Tao, Y.W. (1987) 'The reason for wearing a face mask', *Min Sheng Daily*, 25 October, p. 5. [in Chinese]

The Guardian. (2021) '"Here fire, you hungry?" Idaho Covid protesters burn masks in front of capitol', *The Guardian*, 6 March. www.theguardian.com/world/2021/mar/06/idaho-covid-protesters-burn-masks-state-capitol [Accessed 30 June 2021].

United Daily News. (1957) 'Chairman Yan pays special attention to influenza: orders the Department of Health to quickly establish laws to provide a prevention and cure. Education Department issues order of schools intensify prevention measures', *United Daily News*, 15 May, p. 3. [in Chinese]

United Daily News. (1964) 'Cases of epidemic meningitis were discovered in Taipei City; in addition, several cases of patients suffering from purulent meningitis were also found. The Department of Health is awaiting a detailed report', *United Daily News*, 17 July, p. 3. [in Chinese]

United Daily News. (1968) 'The Liren model dustproof face masks are cool, refreshing and not stuffy', *United Daily News*, 10 April, p. 4. [in Chinese]

United Daily News. (1969) 'Barber shops are unhygienic, Department of Health orders for things to improve, and implores barbers to wear a face mask', *United Daily News*, 25 November, p. 6. [in Chinese]

Wang, H.Y. (2007) 'The material lives of Japanese in Taiwan during the Japanese colonial period'. PhD thesis. National Taiwan Normal University, pp. 28–29. [in Chinese]

Wu, X.R. (1939) 'The diary of Wu Xinrong', 13 January 1939, The archives of the Institute of Taiwan History Academia Sinica, http://taco.ith.sinica.edu.tw/tdk/ [Accessed 6 February 2020]. [in Japanese]

Xiao, D. (1970) 'Mischievous little egg', *Economic Daily News*, 8 January, p. 10. [in Chinese]

Ye, M. (2021) 'Compared to people in Europe and America, why do Taiwanese people seem more willing to wear face masks?], *The News Lens*, www.thenewslens.com/article/151132?fbclid=IwAR1f4xEUsNYUhRSZBAdVcqT5LLS1TAKKdXVTOEecKOGPAguhw3saXDfUO2s [Accessed 5 September 2021]. [in Chinese]

11 Social values and mask-wearing behaviour during the COVID-19 pandemic in Japan

Masahisa Endo and Gento Kato

11.1 Introduction

Japan has been relatively successful in controlling COVID-19 infections. Compared to other developed countries, it has experienced a low number of infections and deaths in relation to population. One explanation for this result may involve the lack of resistance to mask-wearing among Japanese citizens. While some countries made mask-wearing mandatory, the Japanese government never even considered doing so. The COVID-19 outbreak in Wuhan had an immediate impact not on infection or immigration restrictions but on the sale of masks in Japan, where stocks were quickly depleted. Citizens began wearing masks voluntarily right at the beginning of the pandemic.

Even before the pandemic, mask-wearing was more common in Japan than in other countries. With a history dating back to the Spanish flu, mask-wearing in Japan has been described as 'a routine practice against a range of health threats' (Burgess and Horii 2012; 1184). Masks are a common preventive measure, used to protect people from influenza and hay fever. Additionally, in recent years, people without symptoms have been observed wearing masks, a phenomenon known as 'fake mask (*date masuku*)' among young people. Women sometimes wear masks to hide the fact that they aren't wearing makeup or even because they think it is fashionable (*Asahi Shimbun* 22 Feb, 2020).

However, as the introductory chapter notes, not all Japanese people wear masks, and some are opposed to wearing masks. During the pandemic, it became difficult for people to avoid wearing masks in public spaces, where services could be denied to unmasked customers. Passengers without masks were arrested on airplanes on grounds that they could endanger the safety of others. In response to such situations, about a thousand people demonstrated against mandatory mask-wearing in January 2022.

What are the factors that shape mask-wearing behaviour during a pandemic in a country where many people routinely wear masks? This chapter examines mask-wearing behaviour in Japan, with a particular focus on political factors. The next section examines the government's mask policy during the early stages of the pandemic. The third section investigates the factors that encouraged people to wear masks. Section 11.4 presents the data, while Section 11.5 interprets the results of our analysis.

DOI: 10.4324/9781003244127-13

11.2 Mask policies in Japan

In contrast to other countries, where masks were required in public places, Japan never made mask-wearing mandatory – nor did it even consider such measures. However, although the Japanese government lacked a clear policy, mask-wearing became widespread during the pandemic.

Since the beginning of the COVID-19 outbreak in Wuhan in January 2020, several mask-related issues have been reported in Japan. First, the Japanese government paid little attention to quarantine measures during this period, focusing instead on protecting Japanese citizens living in and returning from Wuhan. Although mask-wearing was already standard practice in China, the Japanese Ministry of Health, Labour and Welfare (MHLW) recommended masks only for people returning from Wuhan with symptoms such as coughing and fever and not for all Japanese citizens returning from Wuhan.

Second, the shortage of masks in China affected mask inventories in Japan. Japan was dependent on imported masks from China, which produced nearly 70% of Japanese stock. As the mask shortage worsened in China, many Chinese tourists in Japan purchased large quantities of masks before returning home. Starting in mid-January, when the first cases of COVID-19 were confirmed in Japan, demand also increased among Japanese people, and mask orders surged, leading to a domestic shortage.

Third, despite the shortage of masks, Japan sent masks to China; on 28 January, the Japanese government sent a government-chartered plane to Wuhan to help Japanese citizens leave the city. In addition to protective clothing, the plane was loaded with masks for the Chinese government. Japanese companies and local governments also sent stockpiled masks to China. According to the Chinese Embassy in Japan, a total of 2.72 million masks were sent to China prior to 10 February, 2020. Chinese social-networking sites welcomed the influx of Japanese masks.

Japan became seriously concerned about the spread of COVID-19 on 3 February, 2020, when the cruise ship *Diamond Princess* arrived at the port of Yokohama. Discovering that there were infected passengers on board, the Japanese government took measures to combat COVID-19 by refusing to allow the passengers or crew to disembark. Subsequently, the number of infected people gradually increased, requiring Japan to implement urgent countermeasures.

At this stage, the MHLW did not emphasise mask-wearing as a recommended preventive measure. Instead, it advised people to disinfect their hands by washing them with soap or using alcohol-based disinfectants. The MHLW even posted on its website the following message: 'the effectiveness of wearing masks in outdoor areas is not well recognised unless the area is very crowded'. When measures were initially being implemented to curb infection on the *Diamond Princess*, some passengers and crew members were reportedly seen walking around without masks.

However, the fact that mask-wearing was not mandated did not prevent Japanese people from wearing masks. Although the Japanese government and MHLW did not require it, mask-wearing gradually became the norm throughout Japanese society. As the initial outbreak in Japan was thought to be tourism related, a debate over wearing masks first emerged in the tourism industry. In February, industry associations called for masks to be worn in department stores and taxis to control infection among service providers who came into contact with unspecified numbers of people. Although mask-wearing had never been a common practice in customer-service contexts, it gradually became standard practice to wear masks in public places.

The demand for masks continued to increase in February, when the existing mask stocks were exhausted. Lines formed at pharmacies, masks were bought up, and the resale of masks at high prices on the internet became an object of public concern. Masks disappeared from store shelves; the shortage of masks in nursing care, medical care, and public transportation, where they were badly needed, became an urgent issue.

Facing public complaints about the shortage of masks, the Japanese government responded by subsidising companies to increase mask production, promoting domestic manufacturers instead of relying on imports from China. The government also decided to ship domestically produced masks to medical institutions in advance. In early March, the government distributed masks to several cities and towns in Hokkaido, where the infection had spread, and released 2.5 million masks held in reserve. It also took steps to prohibit the resale of masks at prices higher than the original purchase price. However, voters did not express strong approval of these measures, with 67% of respondents to an *Asahi Shimbun* poll in mid-March rating the government's efforts to address the mask shortage as 'not sufficient'.

On 1 April, when the declared state of emergency was becoming a reality and tensions were mounting over the spread of COVID-19, the government suddenly announced that it would extend the distribution of masks to nursing homes and elementary and junior high schools by giving two cloth masks (commonly known as *Abenomasks*) to every household in the country. These reusable cloth masks were intended to reduce demand, making it easier for medical institutions to obtain surgical masks. However, the policy was heavily criticised from the outset, in part because cloth masks were considered somewhat ineffective in preventing infection. At this point, people had hoped for cash benefits and were disappointed to receive masks instead.

Distribution of the *Abenomasks* began in mid-April in some parts of Tokyo. The process did not go smoothly, as there were problems with quality and inspections. Since the supply problems were corrected by May, many people no longer needed cloth masks by the time they were delivered. For this reason, the distribution of *Abenomasks* is remembered as a failed policy (Asia Pacific Initiative 2021, 286).

From the outset of the pandemic, the government did not promote mask-wearing to prevent COVID-19 infection. However, it cannot be said that the government considered mask-wearing unnecessary. For example, in late March, the government cited mask-wearing by students at elementary and junior high schools as a precondition for ending school closures, imposed at the end of February. In other words, the government did view mask-wearing as a useful measure for controlling the spread of COVID-19.

While the government did not actively promote mask-wearing or make the practice mandatory, mask-wearing as a means of preventing infection became widespread in Japanese society during the pandemic. When Japan and China simultaneously experienced a shortage of masks, demand for masks increased quickly in Japan, where people showed little resistance to mask-wearing. Although the government did not promote mask-wearing vigorously, it did play a role in regulating supply and demand during the first half of 2020.

11.3 Mask-wearing behaviour in Japan

Social psychologists who examined the use of masks during the pandemic have generally focused on two mechanisms. First, people wear masks to prevent themselves and others from becoming infected (Sakakibara and Ozono 2020, 2021). Second, people wear masks because they perceive it to be a norm – it is necessary to wear a mask because other people do (Nakayachi et al. 2020). Studies have suggested that the first mechanism has a greater impact over time, as the infection continues to spread (Sakakibara and Ozono 2021).

While these studies have attempted to directly measure the psychological motivations that lead people to mask, this chapter focuses on the types of people who choose to wear a mask. In particular, it explores the extent to which political factors influenced this phenomenon in Japan. As US studies have shown, masking can be associated with political ideology or partisanship; differences in behaviour can also be reflected in the political process (Pew Research Center 2020; Mahalik et al. 2022).

This chapter examines three political factors. The first involves ideological conflicts among voters. One possible hypothesis is that conservatives, like American Republicans, do not wear masks. This is because conservative ideology is associated with masculine values (Winter 2010). Since Japanese ideology is primarily concerned with foreign policy and constitutional debates, we would also like to examine social values. Social values are beliefs regarding the diversity as well as changing nature of society, and in the case of Japan, they are discussed particularly in terms of family forms and institutions. Japan's social values, which are always discussed in analyses of policy opinion (even in recent years), can be divided into traditional family-centred values and liberal values that allow same-sex marriage and separate surnames for married couples. It is thus hypothesised that people with more traditional values are less likely to wear masks.

Second, trust in political actors can influence mask use. In countries that made mask-wearing mandatory, people who trusted the government were more likely to follow its instructions and wear masks. In other words, trust in those who make and implement policies will manifest as direction-following behaviour. In Japan, however, mask-wearing was never required. More to the point, medical experts took the initiative in promoting Japan's COVID-19 control measures, with politicians appearing to play a relatively small role.[1] We, therefore, hypothesise that, in Japan, trust in government actors did not lead to mask-wearing behaviour. Instead, trust in medical professionals influenced mask-wearing.

Third, political knowledge may also influence mask-wearing. People who have more political knowledge are better at collecting and processing various types of political information. Such information can help them understand the effectiveness of various COVID-19 measures. We therefore hypothesise that people with more political knowledge are more likely to wear masks.

Moreover, the key variables listed (ideology, social values, trust in political actors, and political knowledge) may be related to age and sex; for this reason, our analysis controls for these effects.

11.4 Data

To explore mask-wearing behaviours during the pandemic in Japan, we conducted a web survey on 17–18 March 2021.[2] This period fell at the very end of the second state of emergency, which began on 8 January and ended on 21 March 2021. Although we used the Rakuten Insight Inc. Survey Panel to collect responses, resulting in a less representative sample than those produced by traditional survey modes, the respondents were sampled in proportion to the population in terms of age and sex. Among those who completed the survey, we excluded respondents who appeared to be survey satisficers. To identify satisficers, we used the questions to check whether respondents had read each question carefully. We also excluded respondents who answered all questions about COVID-19 behaviours in the same way. Data from 1,882 respondents were included in the analysis.

The dependent variable was the response to a question about the extent to which participants intended to wear masks in public spaces for the next six months. The question covered a range of intended COVID-19-related behaviours. The exact wording was as follows: 'I would like to ask you about the next six months. How many of each of the following actions do you expect to perform?' The nine actions were presented in the following order: going out to crowded places, practicing social distancing, going out or travelling, wearing masks in public spaces, covering one's mouth while coughing, using hand sanitizer, touching one's face or eyes with unwashed hands, shaking hands or hugging people and disinfecting personal surfaces properly. For each question, the response options were always, frequently, sometimes, seldom and never.

Both OLS and logit were used to test the hypothesis in the following section. The five-point response options ranged from 'never' to 'always', and OLS was used to simplify the interpretation of results. We also relied on a logit model with a dummy variable, which took the value 1 to mean 'always' and 0 for all other responses, since dependent-variable responses skewed towards 'always', as will be shown later. The results showed no significant difference between the two models.

The independent variables were ideology, social value, trust in political actors and political knowledge. In relation to ideology, respondents chose a political position between 0 (very liberal/left-wing) and 10 (very conservative/right-wing) to describe their own political views. To determine social values, we asked whether the respondents agreed or disagreed with the idea that married couples should be legally allowed to have separate surnames. A high social-value score meant that they favoured this idea. Other questions ascertained whether the respondents approved or disapproved of various policy issues; a factor analysis extracted axes of social value, with separate surnames for married couples and same-sex marriage, in particular, showing large factor loadings. However, the present analysis focused on a single question to simplify interpretation.

The question about trust in a person or organisation was asked as a query about general trust, not trust in the specific issue of COVID-19. Nevertheless, although this question was placed before the COVID-19 related questions, it is undeniable that actors involved with COVID-19 are being evaluated from such a perspective at the time the web survey was carried out. Here, while Prime Minister Yoshihide Suga and the Ministry of Health, Labor and Welfare are taken as government actors, questions for medical experts are also used. A large value means a higher level of trust.

To measure political knowledge, we noted how many of the six politics-related questions were answered correctly. All of the questions had four possible responses. Three involved institutional knowledge of the judicial system, cabinet responsibilities and Upper House terms. For the questions involving knowledge of particular actors, the respondents had to identify the positions of three politicians (Minister of Land, Infrastructure, Transport and Tourism Kazuyoshi Akaba, Minister of Health, Labour and Welfare Norihisa Tamura, and Chief Cabinet Secretary Katsunobu Kato).

The control variables included COVID-19 infection experiences, levels of concern about COVID-19, expected COVID-19-related situations and sociodemographic variables. People who had already experienced actual (or even suspected) COVID-19 infections might be more cautious and more likely to wear masks. The dummy variable was 1 if the respondent had been infected with a verified or suspected case of COVID-19 and 0 otherwise. Those who had suspected infections but received negative PCR test results were classified as 1 for this dummy variable. People were also expected to be more cautious if they were surrounded by others who had been infected. A dummy variable, therefore, took 1 if someone close to the respondent (a family member, relative, friend, or colleague) had been infected and 0 otherwise.

It seemed natural for concerned people to wear masks, even if no one around them was infected. Since we also asked the respondents how worried they were at the time, this factor was used as a control variable in the analysis. A larger value indicated a higher level of concern.

Expected future COVID-19 situations could influence whether people choose to wear masks in the future. The survey asked respondents how they thought the COVID-19 infection situation would develop over the next six months and whether they thought some events were likely to occur. We focused on whether respondents expected a COVID-19 vaccine to be developed, produced and made widely available. At the time of the survey, in March 2021, the vaccination program had not yet taken shape. We also focused on whether the probability of being newly infected with COVID-19 was likely to drop significantly. In both cases, a large value indicated that people considered this highly likely. Such people would not be wearing masks.

As for sociodemographic variables, conventional variables such as sex, age and education were included in the analysis. The reference group for age included people in their 20s. The dummy for marital status and children was also included here, since the presence of more family members could wear masks from mask fear of infection.[3]

11.5 Analysis

Table 11.1 presents the distribution of responses on mask-wearing. In March 2021, when the second emergency declaration was on the horizon, people expected to continue wearing masks in daily life in the near future. In fact, 86.4% of respondents believed that they would always wear masks. By contrast, only 2.0% of the respondents said that they would 'seldom' or 'never' wear masks.

Figure 11.1 presents the distribution of COVID-19-related intentions for the next six months. Among these, wearing a mask was the most common response. Using hand sanitizer and covering the mouth when coughing were equally common responses, indicating an increase in hygiene awareness. A much lower percentage chose social distancing, another central measure in Japan. The frequency dropped significantly for behaviours that people were advised to avoid, such as touching the face or eyes with unwashed hands, going out and travelling and shaking hands or hugging people.

Table 11.2 presents the results of the regression and logit analysis. The dependent variable is the intention to wear a mask; the higher the value, the more often the respondent reported wearing a mask. The OLS and logit results are much the same for both.

No relationship was found between conservative ideology and mask-wearing. Unlike in the US, the usual political conflicts did not affect mask-wearing in Japan. Instead, from a social-value perspective, people with more traditional

Table 11.1 Wearing masks in public spaces for the next six months

Always	86.4%
Frequently	8.0%
Sometimes	3.6%
Seldom	1.4%
Never	0.6%
N	1882

Source: web survey carried out in March 2021

COVID-19-related behavioural intentions for the next six months

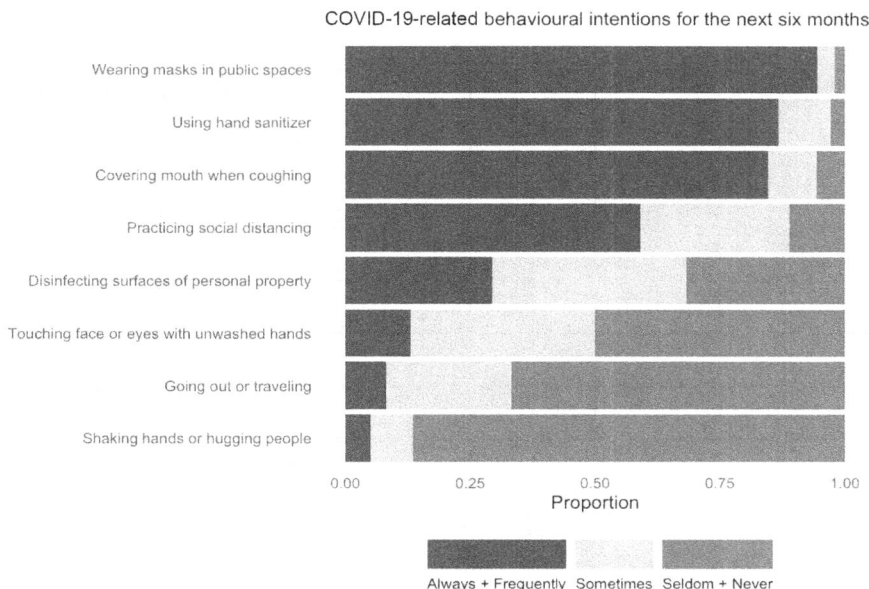

Figure 11.1 COVID-19-related behavioural intentions for the next six months

Source: web survey carried out in March 2021

Table 11.2 Explaining the intention to wear a mask in Japan

	OLS			Logit		
(Intercept)	4.031	(0.099)	***	−1.088	(0.465)	*
Ideology	0.087	(0.093)		0.352	(0.453)	
Social value	0.212	(0.058)	***	0.961	(0.277)	***
Trust in PM Suga	0.047	(0.066)		0.127	(0.325)	
Trust in MHLW	−0.080	(0.073)		−0.416	(0.359)	
Trust in medical experts	0.217	(0.070)	**	0.617	(0.334)	+
Political knowledge	0.189	(0.064)	**	0.911	(0.310)	**
Experience or suspected COVID-19 infections	0.001	(0.048)		0.046	(0.249)	
Experience of infections around respondents	0.042	(0.050)		0.367	(0.278)	
Concerns about COVID-19	0.305	(0.055)	***	1.395	(0.264)	***
Expectation of vaccine availability	0.263	(0.064)	***	1.233	(0.311)	***
Expectation of a drop in infection rate	−0.112	(0.058)	+	−0.499	(0.287)	+

(*Continued*)

Table 11.2 (Continued)

	OLS			Logit		
Female	0.133	(0.032)	***	0.726	(0.164)	***
Age (30s)	−0.071	(0.057)		−0.297	(0.302)	
Age (40s)	−0.090	(0.056)		−0.380	(0.293)	
Age (50s)	−0.171	(0.058)	**	−0.686	(0.296)	*
Age (60s)	−0.136	(0.061)	*	−0.602	(0.315)	+
Age (70s)	−0.200	(0.065)	**	−0.941	(0.328)	**
Married	0.031	(0.040)		0.124	(0.201)	
Having kids	0.039	(0.041)		0.010	(0.206)	
College education	0.015	(0.032)		0.077	(0.157)	
R^2		0.078				
Adj. R^2		0.068				
AIC					1297.99	
BIC					1412.33	
Log Likelihood					−628	
N		1711			1711	

*** $p < 0.001$; ** $p < 0.01$; * $p < 0.05$; + $p < 0.1$

Predictor values are rescaled to 0–1 range.

Source: web survey carried out in March 2021

values avoided wearing masks. It is important to note that social values continued to have an effect, even after controlling for age and sex. Perhaps traditional family-centred values were influenced by a masculinity orientation.

Regarding trust in political actors, trust in PM Suga and the MHLW did not encourage mask-wearing. However, trust in medical experts did lead to mask-wearing. It can thus be inferred that trust in the medical experts implementing COVID-19 measures in Japan is more likely to be associated with COVID-19-prevention behaviour. On the flip side, this finding also suggests that distrust in medical professionals is associated with anti-COVID-19-prevention measures.

These results confirm the hypothesis that more political knowledge leads to mask-wearing. It is interesting to note that political knowledge actually influences mask-wearing, a traditional, pervasive method of prevention that is not difficult to implement.

Figure 11.2 shows the change in the value of the three key variables (social value, trust in medical experts and political knowledge) and the average of the predicted probabilities of intending to always wear a mask, based on the logit model. The circles indicate the mean predicted probability, while the thick line indicates a 90% confidence interval and the thin line indicates a 95% confidence interval. The magnitude of the regression-analysis coefficients indicates that these three variables have a significant impact: in relation to social value, the most traditional attitude has a probability of about 80%, while the most liberal attitude has a probability of more than 90%. For trust in experts, the probability is less than

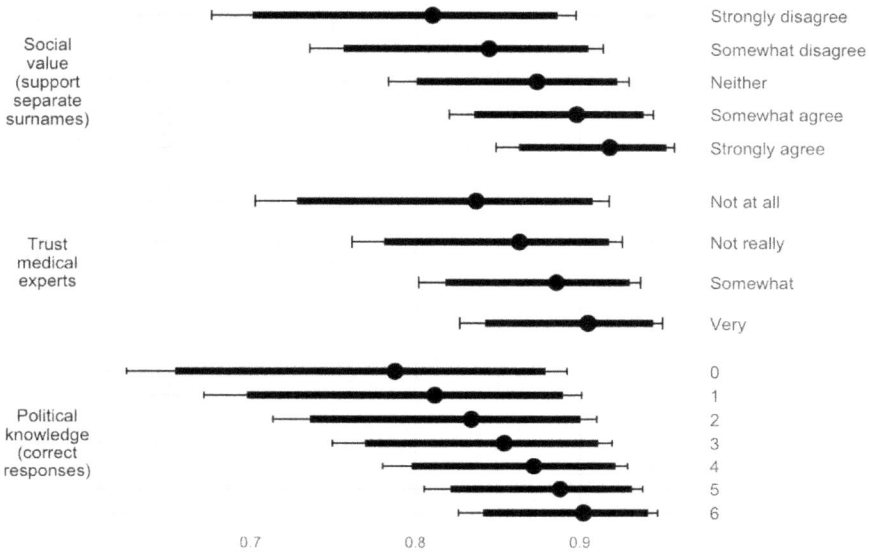

Figure 11.2 Average predicted probability of the intention to always wear a mask (with 90% and 95% confidence intervals)

Source: web survey carried out in March 2021

85% for those who have no trust at all but more than 90% for those who have a great deal of trust. Political knowledge is below 80% at the lowest level and above 90% at the highest level.

Looking at the control variables, it is clear that infection experience has no effect on mask-wearing. However, the more worried people are, the more likely they are to wear masks. In addition, the more people expect a vaccine to be available soon, the more likely they are to wear masks. This suggests that the more enthusiastic people are about controlling COVID-19 and getting a vaccine, the more likely they are to wear masks. By contrast, the more optimistic people are about the likelihood that the infection rate will decrease significantly (e.g. by 10%), the less likely they are to wear masks.

Among the sociodemographic variables, more women wear masks, as in the U.S (Mahalik et al. 2022). In addition, people in their 50s and older are less likely to wear masks than people in their 20s. Given that elderly people are more concerned about infection, it may seem surprising that younger people are more likely to wear masks. While political knowledge has an impact, the degree of education does not. Although we predicted that having a family would make people more likely to wear masks, being married and having children were not associated with mask-wearing intention.

11.6 Conclusion

This chapter outlines Japan's mask policy and investigates the types of people who intend to wear masks, with a focus on political factors. Prior to the pandemic, Japanese people were not resistant to wearing masks. Soon after the outbreak in Wuhan, the demand for masks increased enormously. As a consequence, the government did not need to make masks mandatory. Instead, it functioned as a regulator of mask demand and supply in the domestic market. Some people created controversy by refusing to wear masks at the city council or on airplanes, and an aversion to mask-wearing, linked to anti-vaccine and conspiracy theories, did surface in the form of anti-mask demonstrations, but on a very small scale.

In the March 2021 survey, a fairly large percentage of respondents said that they would continue to wear masks for the next six months. This analysis of mask-wearing also reveals that the intention to wear a mask was shaped by social values rather than the left-right ideologies. Trust in medical professionals, as opposed to the prime minister or MHLW, was linked to COVID-19-related behaviour. This implies that medical professionals strongly influenced the COVID-19 response because they were fully involved in responding to the pandemic. It also suggests that, when medical professionals lose public trust, COVID-19 countermeasures will not be successful. The relationship between political knowledge and mask-wearing indicates a high information load related to COVID-19 measures in a context in which information is updated on a daily basis. Discovering the best way to communicate information may be a challenge for future governments.

One limitation of this study is that it does not include the urban–rural index as a control variable. As rural areas are less densely populated, people may choose not to mask outside, making it important to control for urban and rural locations. This could not be done here because the survey did not ask for a place of residence. However, we did include some proxy variables, such as 'the infection status of people around you', which was relevant because the infection situation was more severe in urban areas in March 2021. In this case, the infection status of close people had no effect.

Notes

1 Instead of focusing on mask-wearing, Japan's basic COVID-19 policy measures encouraged people to avoid the '3Cs' (crowded places, close-contact settings and confined and enclosed spaces). Based on an expert analysis of infection routes, the policy aimed to control infection by eliminating clusters of mass infection. Experts, rather than government officials, developed the framework of Japan's COVID-19 countermeasures. They also appeared on TV regularly, calling for a drastic reduction in human-to-human contact.
2 This survey was supported by JSPS KAKENHI Grant Number 19H00584.
3 All independent and control variables are rescaled from 0 to 1 to compare the magnitude of their effect on each other.

References

*Asahi Shimbun (*22 Feb, 2020) 'Koron, Masuku Izon Shakai' (Opinions, Mask Dependent Society), retrieved from Asahi Shimbun Cross-Search (Kikuzo II visual).

Asia Pacific Initiative. (2021) 'Shingata Korona Taiou Minkan Rinji Chosakai Chosa Kensyo Hokokusho' [The Independent Investigation Commission on the Japanese Government's Response to COVID-19]. Tokyo: Discover 21, Inc.

Burgess, A. and Horii, M. (2012) 'Risk, ritual and health responsibilisation: Japan's "Safety Blanket" of surgical face mask-wearing', *Sociology of Health & Illness*, 34(8), 1184–1198.

Mahalik, J. R., Di Bianca, M. and Harris, M. P. (2022) 'Men's attitudes towards mask-wearing during COVID-19: Understanding the complexities of mask-ulinity', *Journal of Health Psychology*, 27(5), 1187–1204.

Nakayachi, K., Ozaki, T., Shibata, Y. and Yokoi, R. (2020) 'Why do Japanese people use masks against COVID-19, even though masks are unlikely to offer protection from infection?', *Frontiers in Psychology*, 11, 1918. https://doi.org/10.3389/fpsyg.2020.01918

Pew Research Center. (2020) 'Republicans, democrats move even further apart in coronavirus concerns', *Pew Research Center.* www.pewresearch.org/politics/2020/06/25/republicans-democrats-move-evenfurther-apart-in-coronavirus-concerns/

Sakakibara, R. and Ozono, H. (2020) 'Psychological research on the COVID-19 crisis in Japan: Focusing on infection preventive behaviors, future prospects, and information dissemination behaviors', *PsyArXiv*. July 13. https://doi.org/10.31234/osf.io/97zye

Sakakibara, R. and Ozono, H. (2021) 'Hitobito ga Masuku wo Chakuyousuru Riyu toha: Kokunai Kenkyu no Tsuishi to Risaachikuesuchon no Kensyo [Why do people wear a mask? A replication of previous studies and examination]', *The Japanese Journal of Psychology*, 92(5), 332–338.

Winter, N. J. G. (2010) 'Masculine republicans and feminine democrats: Gender and Americans' explicit and implicit images of the political parties'. *Political Behavior*, 32, 587–618.

12 COVID-19 infection control in China

The Chinese crisis-management system and mask mandates

Hongyi Liu

12.1 Introduction

Since January 2020, the rapid spread of the COVID-19 pandemic has had a huge impact on the international community. As of February 2022, the pandemic had already taken more than 5.7 million lives worldwide, proving once again the importance of effective disease-control measures. COVID-19 was first detected in China, and until February 2020, most COVID-19 cases were found there. Thereafter, however, China created a rapid disease-control system and quickly popularised infection-control measures such as mask-wearing. As a result, the numbers of infections and deaths in China have remained relatively low, so that in numeric terms, it can be said that the country has successfully contained the pandemic. Particularly, as COVID-19 spread throughout the world, the disease-control achievements of the Chinese government remained unique among the world's major powers. This fact raises the following questions: What sort of crisis-management system did the Chinese government create amid the spread of COVID-19? Why was it relatively smooth for the Chinese government to popularise mask-wearing? Finally, what were the effectiveness and issues of this governance in terms of the crisis-management system and process of mask popularisation?

Until now, the uniqueness of China's crisis management and security has often been interpreted based on its centralised regime. During the COVID-19 pandemic, in particular, China's disease-control measures were very different from those instituted in Western countries and were met with considerable criticism (Meng 2020; Yuan 2020). However, virtually no other political regime with a central government wielding great power actually contained the spread of infection as did China. Therefore, the concrete policies and logic of the Chinese government should be analysed rather than dismissed as the results of a centralised regime. This study analyses the relationship between China's central and local governments and between local governments and grassroots in terms of policy implementation and sharing of responsibilities. The term 'grassroots' (Chinese: 基层 *jiceng*) used in this study means 'a primary organisation in Chinese politics' and designates party organisations in enterprises, rural areas, government organs, schools, research institutes, communities, social organisations among others (Hishida 2010; National Congress of the Communist Party of China 2017).

DOI: 10.4324/9781003244127-14

Unlike the central and local governments, grassroots played a concrete role in governance during the COVID-19 pandemic and are thus just as worthy of attention.

Furthermore, as COVID-19 spread worldwide, many local communities in East Asia, unlike those in Europe and America, showed relatively little opposition to the popularisation of masks among ordinary citizens. In Japan and South Korea, for example, the public cooperated in mask-wearing, keeping the number of infections low throughout the pandemic (Horii 2012; Fisher and Choe 2020). This might lead us to believe that China, like its culturally close neighbours Japan and South Korea, has a mask-wearing culture. In fact, however, unlike its neighbouring country Japan, China did not adopt the hygiene practice of mask-wearing until its COVID-19 outbreak despite experiencing multiple epidemics of other diseases. This is clear from the fact that at the outset of the COVID-19 outbreak in China, most families did not have masks prepared, leading to a period of overwhelming mask shortage and panic buying. Rather, lack of hygiene practices and low standards of living within Chinese society have been shown to be directly linked to the COVID-19 outbreak (Ding et al. 2020). We must thus interpret the success of Chinese mask mandates based on the policies implemented since 2020.

The purpose of this study is therefore to investigate the Chinese government's crisis-management system and the process by which it popularised mask-wearing during the COVID-19 pandemic. Moreover, this study evaluates the effectiveness of and issues with this crisis-management system and mask popularisation. To that end, this study reviews the outbreak of COVID-19 in China in January 2020 and summarises the policy and response of the Chinese government. I further discuss the reactions of the Chinese society and citizens at the time of these arrangements, covering mainly Chinese state-run media such as newspapers. The reason state-run media reports are covered more than online public opinion is that the Chinese government has long been considered to use software and filters to control online public opinion (Brady 2008), and content unfavourable to the Chinese government tends to be deleted. On the other side, although it is common to think of Chinese newspapers as aligned with government propaganda, following market reforms, Chinese newspapers actually have an aspect of catering to public opinion (Stockmann 2011). According to the analysis conducted by Zhu (2020), during the 2020 COVID-19 outbreak, there were overwhelming dissenting voices in China's online society that, for a time, the government was unable to control. Therefore, it is very likely that some online content from that time has already been deleted, whereas newspapers catering to public opinion have some value as sources in that they objectively record the situation of society at that time.

12.2 The Chinese public-health crisis-management system through the lens of COVID-19

12.2.1 *The Chinese crisis-management system seen in 'wartime state' declarations*

In January 2020, COVID-19 began to spread in and around Hubei Province. China's central government responded swiftly despite the irresponsible actions and responses of local officials in the early stages of the outbreak, which caused them to miss the optimal time to take infection-control measures. Under the supervision of the central government, from 24 January 2020, medical teams from around the country were dispatched to Wuhan City, and in only ten days from 24 January, temporary hospitals were built for those in quarantine and those with minor symptoms. From 25 January, all communities of Wuhan, with a combined population of more than 12 million, were simultaneously placed under a lockdown, and food and essential supplies were procured and distributed by the government. The outcomes of this strategy, as claimed by the Chinese government's propaganda, may be viewed as an example of China's unifying force and capacity for mobilisation. In other words, China's centralised administrative framework and strong mobilisation capacity ensured the effectiveness of the crisis-management system during the COVID-19 outbreak.

However, since April 2020, the number of new infections remained low throughout China, limiting the opportunities for the centralised administrative framework to showcase its effectiveness. In this context, the declaration of a 'wartime state' by various local governments may be cited as the typical crisis-management system in China. Since February 2020, the declaration of a 'wartime state' in China has not actually been accompanied by wartime control. Instead, in most cases, it is limited to enhancing existing disease-control measures. 'Wartime state' and 'state of emergency' were originally declared by the authority of the People's Congress (and its Standing Committee) and the State Council, respectively (The Central Government of the People's Republic of China 2018). Therefore, there was no legal basis to declare a 'wartime state' during the COVID-19 outbreak, and in substance, this was nothing more than a sort of crisis-management system. Nevertheless, since May 2020, 'wartime state' was frequently used while infection had been virtually contained throughout the country. Specifically, in July 2020, Vice-Premier of the State Council of the People's Republic of China Sun Chunlan said during an inspection that 'When a (COVID-19) case is confirmed, all administrative divisions must immediately enter a wartime state', thus reflecting the Chinese government's stance on the matter (The People's Daily 2020). Table 12.1 presents the cases of 'wartime state' declarations in China since the onset of the COVID-19 pandemic.

Thus, looking at 'wartime state' declarations in China between February 2020 and January 2021, the following two characteristics can be identified in the Chinese crisis-management system as it pertains to the relationship between the central and local level. First, the official announcements in the COVID-19 crisis-management system were mostly made by local governments. Although the authority to declare a 'wartime state' or a 'state of emergency' actually belongs to the central government, the 'wartime state' declared by the Chinese government during the COVID-19 pandemic was different. COVID-19 was an exceptional situation in China, and the central government could undoubtedly have declared a 'wartime state' or a 'state of emergency'. Thus, the central government actually delegated the power to declare a 'wartime state' to local governments, a decision that in a sense symbolises their autonomy.

Table 12.1 Major cases of 'wartime state' declarations since the onset of the COVID-19 pandemic in China (revised and corrected from Liu (2021, pp. 4–5))

Target of 'Wartime State'	Time of Declaring a 'Wartime State'	Scale of Local Population	Number of New Infections at the Time of Declaration	Subject of Declaration	Primary Measures
Zhangwan District, Shiyan City, Hubei Province	12 February 2020	415,000	536	Zhangwan district government	Full lockdown, forced quarantine of residents (stay at home)
Shulan City, Jilin Province	11 May 2020	608,000	13	Jilin provincial government	Contact tracing and quarantine, partial lockdown
Fengtai District, Beijing City)	13 June 2020	2.025 million	5	Fengtai district government	Epidemiological study, contact tracing and quarantine, expanding polymerase chain reaction (PCR) test subjects
Mentougou District, Beijing City	15 June 2020	344,000	106 (throughout Beijing City)	Mentougou district government	Epidemiological study, contact tracing and quarantine
Chaoyang District, Beijing City	15 June 2020	3.473 million	106 (throughout Beijing City)	Chaoyang district government	Epidemiological study, partial lockdown
Daxing District, Beijing City	15 June 2020	1.712 million	106 (throughout Beijing City)	Beijing city government	Epidemiological study, contact tracing and quarantine
Urumqi City, Xinjiang Uygur Autonomous Regions	16 July 2020	3.552 million	17	Uygur autonomous regional government	Epidemiological study, recommending PCR testing for all residents
Yunnan Province	19 September 2020	48.583 million	0	Yunnan provincial government	Enhancing quarantine measures in airport and remote areas, reviewing grassroots-management system

(*Continued*)

Table 12.1 (Continued)

Target of 'Wartime State'	Time of Declaring a 'Wartime State'	Scale of Local Population	Number of New Infections at the Time of Declaration	Subject of Declaration	Primary Measures
Qingdao City, Shandong Province	13 October 2020	10.072 million	6	Qingdao city government	Review of disease-control system, epidemiological study, recommending PCR testing for all residents
Dalian City, Liaoning Province	20 December 2020	5.987 million	2	Dalian city government	Epidemiological study, recommending PCR testing for all residents
Shunyi District, Beijing City	26 December 2020	1.228 million	2	Shunyi district government	Epidemiological study, recommending PCR testing for all residents
Shenyang City, Liaoning Province	30 December 2020	8.322 million	2	Shenyang city government	Epidemiological study, recommending PCR testing for all residents
Heihe City, Heilongjiang Province	2 January 2021	1.581 million	4	Heihe city government	Epidemiological study, recommending PCR testing for all residents
Shijiazhuang City, Hebei Province	3 January 2021	11.031 million	4	Shijiazhuang city government	Enhancement of existing disease-control measures, recommending PCR testing for all residents

Second, the conditions for declaring a 'wartime state' were not standardised in terms of the target areas and concrete measures to be taken and varied widely between regions. For example, in all regions that declared a 'wartime state' in or after September 2020, the number of new infections was less than ten. Doubts remain regarding the necessity of entire regions with populations numbering in millions entering a 'wartime state' in response to extremely small numbers of new cases without further subdivision based on alert levels. The ease of declaring a 'wartime state' also resulted in cases where grassroots and the public were unnecessarily impacted by disease-control measures.

Thus, in the COVID-19 disease-control system, while the central government wielded great power, local governments also maintained some autonomy. This may have been meant to elicit a swift response by local authorities, who had a better understanding of the situation on the ground. Their flexible response might have played a role in the tendency to declare a 'wartime state' during COVID-19 outbreaks. However, delegating this power to local authorities simultaneously implied making them responsible for any failure to prevent infection. There were numerous cases of local officials being removed from their positions during the COVID-19 pandemic due to disease-control failures, whereas no central leaders took responsibility in the same way. This may be regarded as an example of how central and local authorities specify their responsibilities and roles. Ultimately, this shifting of blame was directly linked to overreactions by local authorities and often led to grassroots and the public being unnecessarily impacted by disease-control measures.

As explained, during the COVID-19 epidemic, China's central government delegated both authority and responsibility to local governments, causing local governments to react with unnecessary 'wartime state' declarations and to shift the responsibility for disease control to the grassroots. Simultaneously, local governments shifting responsibility to grassroots sometimes led grassroots to overreact and avoid responsibility as well. For example, in January 2022, amid an outbreak in Xi'an City, a pregnant woman was denied admission to the hospital for failure to undergo a nucleic acid test (PCR test) and later had a miscarriage. At first glance, this tragic incident may be attributed to the irresponsible actions of those in charge at the grassroots. However, looking at the larger context, the more likely reason is that local governments took excessive disease-control measures and placed the responsibility for new infections on grassroots, which in turn shifted this responsibility to the general public. Thus, since the latter half of 2020, the responsibility for disease control during COVID-19 outbreaks substantially shifted from the central government to local governments and from local governments to the grassroots. Because the people are the final link in this chain of responsibility, in this case, the issue of shifting responsibility ultimately had a negative impact on the general public.

In general, in the early stages of the COVID-19 pandemic, the Chinese government's centralised administrative framework played a considerable role in resolving the outbreak. Then, after successfully containing the epidemic, the 'wartime state' showed some effectiveness in China's disease control. However, due to the lack of institutionalised basis, the authority to declare a 'wartime state' and the responsibility that accompanies such authority was shifted from the central to the local level, leading local governments to take excessive measures and further shift the responsibility to grassroots. From the vantage point of the COVID-19 crisis-management system, this gives us a glimpse of the multilayered hierarchical relationships existing in Chinese politics, from centre to the grassroots.

12.2.2 Effectiveness and issues of the Chinese crisis-management system

The relationship between the central and local levels in Chinese politics has been described as a 'centralised' system in which, while local authorities maintain some discretionary power, the central government wields great authority overall (Nakagane 1979; Amako 2018). After the COVID-19 outbreak, this political system played a substantial role in China's disease-control measures. Needless to say, China could at once mobilise in its entirety owing to its centralised administrative framework, creating a comprehensive system to contain the epidemic. Nevertheless, local authorities maintained some autonomy in declaring a 'wartime state', and responsibility was undeniably shifted from the central to the local level and from the local to the grassroots level. The central government shifting responsibility for outbreaks to local authorities posed the risk that these authorities would take unnecessary disease-control measures and further shift responsibility to grassroots.

In general, in crisis management, the Chinese political system took a form that gave some autonomy to local authorities, even as the central government continued to wield tremendous power. Within such a system, on one hand, centralisation makes it easier to take effective action against a major crisis, while on the other, it leaves some autonomy to local authorities and allows them to make flexible decisions. However, that aim was a bit too idealistic in some respects. In practice, giving power to local authorities may have led local governments to shift responsibility further down the hierarchy rather than taking flexible decisions on the ground. Conversely, in a centralised system in which the centre wields enormous power, there is also the risk that local authorities will hide or fail to report issues until they are discovered by the central government. In other words, we may identify a dilemma in the Chinese crisis-management system, as some of its outcomes are contrary to the expectations underpinning its current structure.

12.3 The process of mask popularisation in China during the COVID-19 pandemic

12.3.1 Mask shortage and panic buying at the start of the epidemic

From the end of 2019, reports and information on the 'pneumonia of unknown cause' in Wuhan circulated on social networking sites, causing alarm among ordinary citizens of Wuhan. At the time, a trend of buying masks was already visible in the city. Especially from January 2020, as the infection spread rapidly, the lack of confirmed information on how to combat the new disease left many Chinese citizens in a state of panic. On 25 January 2020, after the lockdown was implemented in Wuhan, an overwhelming shortage of medical supplies including masks was reported (Wang and Zhang 2020). As a result, people all over the country began to purchase large quantities of masks as a disease-prevention measure. From 24 January, however, mask factories and subsidiaries throughout China had already been placed under the control of the Chinese government, making masks difficult to find (Wang 2020). Moreover, the beginning of the COVID-19 outbreak coincided exactly with the Chinese New Year holidays, and many mask factories were closed for that reason. Thus, government control, absence of a custom of mask-wearing among citizens, high demand coupled with low production output, panic buying and other factors led to a sudden spike in the price of single-use masks and difficulties in acquiring them. It was reported that masks with a production cost of 0.3 yuan (about 0.05 USD), priced at 0.6 yuan (about 0.1 USD) until 23 January, had increased to 2 yuan (about 0.3 USD) by 28 January (The Beijing News 2020). On 28 January, in Hubei Province, there were reports of a pharmacy being fined by the government for selling masks originally priced at 0.6 yuan for 1 yuan (about 0.15 USD). In response to the news, many took to the internet, stating, 'That price is more than reasonable' or 'Here they are being sold for 5 Yuan a piece' (The Paper 2020).

It has been estimated that, during its COVID-19 epidemic, China consumed at least 10 to 15 million masks per day (Da et al. 2020). To meet the demand for masks, the Chinese government mobilised mask factories to the fullest extent possible and converted production lines that originally manufactured other products into mask production lines. To that end, there was also a tendency to grant manufacturing licences in a short time (Zou 2020). Nevertheless, the production volume of factories throughout China, totalling 8 million pieces on 29 January and 12 million pieces on 2 February, was insufficient to keep up with demand at the time. In that context, a crucial role was played by imports of masks from abroad. However, after the World Health Organization declared COVID-19 a 'Public Health Emergency of International Concern' on 30 January 2020, even importing masks from abroad became difficult. Furthermore, although the Chinese government had taken control of most medical supplies at the time, the whereabouts and specific means of distribution of these resources were not made public. The shortage of information available in the early stages of the epidemic was a factor causing anxiety in the public.

Thus, while the mask shortage had a strong impact on ordinary Chinese people, masks themselves became an object of great concern and interest among the general public, so that some joked about the phrase 'Do you have a mask?' becoming an everyday greeting (He 2020). In other words, the initial lack of information and mask shortage were a crucial opportunity to make the importance of masks known to the Chinese public at the time. This surely made a significant contribution to the popularisation of mask-wearing in China.

12.3.2 *Promotion of mask popularisation by the Chinese government*

In the early stages of the COVID-19 outbreak, confirmed information about the 'new disease' was scarce, causing significant alarm and inconvenience among healthcare workers and the public. In response to this, at the end of January 2020, the Chinese Centre for Disease Control and Prevention published a 'COVID-19 guidebook for the public'. This guidebook explained precautions for wearing masks, the necessity of wearing masks in public facilities and more. In conjunction with this, in early February, many local transit systems and public facilities in China began performing temperature checks and requiring masks to enter the premises.

While the Chinese government went to great efforts to promote mask popularisation, this endeavour was limited by several factors. First, amid an overwhelming mask shortage, many people were unable to obtain masks at all. Specifically, rural areas of China, unlike cities, were unprepared for mask popularisation in terms of institutions, resources and hygiene awareness. Even in early February, when infection was rampant throughout the country, many rural areas lagged behind in mask popularisation, with disease-control measures in some communities consisting merely of repeating the blanket recommendation for residents to not leave their homes (You 2020). Thus, in the early stages of mask popularisation, nationwide rules about mask-wearing were comparatively lax.

Furthermore, a lot of information on masks was circulating at the time, and even the government did not have all the information right. For example, on 4 February 2020, the Guangdong Provincial Centre for Disease Prevention and Control compiled a guidebook on mask-wearing. This guidebook stated, 'If you can't find a mask, use a piece of cloth to cover your nose and mouth' and 'When absolutely necessary, masks may be reused'. The next day, however, the same centre issued a second version of the guidebook and announced discontinuation of use of the first version. In the second version, it was stated that 'Cotton masks, sponge masks and activated charcoal masks are not effective in preventing viral infection', and the line about reusing masks was removed.

Additionally, because many regions of China were in lockdown at the time, traditional promotional campaigns including posters and newspapers were limited. Therefore, the process of mask popularisation in China made effective use of the power of online influencers. For instance, Dr Zhong Nanshan, Dr Zhang Wenhong and other physicians working on the front lines against COVID-19 were frequently featured in the media and were very popular with the general public. On 24 February, Fudan University held the class 'COVID-19 Prevention and Control', which was live-streamed on the video site Bilibili. Dr Zhang Wenhong, who is also a professor at Fudan University Medical College, taught precautions about mask-wearing and other disease-control measures. According to news reports, the livestreaming was very popular, attracting an audience of more than 100,000 (Zhang and Sun 2020). Meanwhile, video-sharing sites and apps were also used as means to popularise mask-wearing. As of today, in

February 2022, Dr Zhang Wenhong's follower count on Douyin (the Chinese TikTok) has reached 2.1 million.

12.3.3 China's policy to maintain mask-wearing in public places after infection was contained

The Chinese government introduced mask mandates not only during outbreaks but even after the infection had been contained. This strategy is particularly worthy of attention, as its effects have lasted until today, in 2022. During the COVID-19 pandemic, the Chinese government responded to an act of not wearing a mask with a recommendation instead of mandating. However, by giving facilities greater power to enforce mask-wearing, it created a mechanism for the resolution of problems between facilities and individuals.

On 7 February 2020, an incident was reported in Shanghai in which a man not wearing a mask argued with a station employee at an underground ticket gate and was then detained by the Public Security Department. This was reported in the Chinese media as the first instance of a crime due to not wearing a mask in Shanghai during the pandemic (Sohu 2020). Incidentally, while we might tend to focus on the man 'being detained for not wearing a mask', it is also reported that 'despite being denied entrance by station staff, [the man] attempted to force his way through and assaulted the staff'. Several similar incidents occurred throughout China during the COVID-19 pandemic, with sanctions mostly pursuant to the Public Security Administration Punishment Law of the People's Republic of China enacted in 2006. The relevant articles of the Law are quoted as follows:

> Art. 2 A person who commits one of the following acts shall receive a warning or a fine up to 200 Yuan. If the illegal act is serious, they shall incur detention for at least 5 and up to 10 days, and a fine of up to 500 Yuan. . . .
> *(2) disturbing the public order at stations, harbours, wharves, airports, shopping malls, parks, exhibition halls and other public places. (3) disturbing the public order on buses, trams, trains, boats, aeroplanes and other means of public transportation . . .*
> Art. 50 A person who commits one of the following acts shall receive a warning or a fine up to 200 Yuan. If the illegal act is serious, they shall incur detention for at least 5 and up to 10 days and a fine of up to 500 Yuan. *(1) refusing to comply with the regulations or decisions issued by the People's Government during a state of emergency. (2) obstructing state institution employees from carrying out their duties in accordance with the law* (continued).
>
> (The Central Government of the People's Republic of
> China 2005, emphasis mine)

Thus, the provisions of the Public Security Administration Punishment Law, which constituted the grounds for sanctions against not wearing a mask, appear to be relatively ambiguous. While a mask mandate was indeed imposed by the Chinese government, as described, the State Council, which has the authority to declare a 'state of emergency', did not actually do so after the COVID-19 outbreak. Therefore, the 'regulations or decisions issued by the People's Government during a state of emergency' mentioned in Art. 50 (1) are, in fact, not applicable to mandating masks in public places. Meanwhile, most public-facility employees are not state public servants, and them prompting people to wear masks does not qualify as 'state institution employees . . . carrying out their duties in accordance with the law' mentioned in Art. 50 (2). Furthermore, not wearing a mask by itself can hardly be characterised as an act of 'disturbing the public order' as per Art. 23 (2). In view of this, in the current Chinese system, there is ambiguity regarding whether failing to wear a mask in a public place constitutes a violation of the law, and it is somewhat difficult to impose sanctions simply for not wearing a mask.

In other words, until the existing law is amended, there are no legal grounds to enforce mask-wearing, and such enforcement as it is in effect is a form of asking for the public's understanding and cooperation. It has been noted that the extent of public cooperation in disease-control measures is largely determined by the degree of public trust in the government (Han et al. 2021). In fact, as COVID-19 spread to the world, trust in governments decreased, and many citizens became uncooperative with disease-control measures. In contrast, China's success in popularising infection-control measures is evidence of its institutional superiority in the COVID-19 pandemic. In view of this, it can be said that China's disease-control measures, despite the lack of institutional grounds, proved comparatively effective because Chinese people had considerable trust in the government.

However, comprehensive public understanding of disease-control policies is expected to require thorough explanations coupled with a substantial amount of work. In this case, government institutions alone struggle in their response. In the case of China, grassroots were effectively mobilised and served to assist government institutions during the pandemic. For example, resident committee leaders and employees of various public facilities took on the role of urging mask-wearing and other disease-control measures in their everyday lives. Furthermore, as described, grassroots took on a more substantial role because local governments shifted the responsibility for disease control to them. Because of this shift of responsibility, when members of the public were initially uncooperative with mask-wearing norms, that became a conflict not between 'the government and the public' but between 'employees and the public'. Therefore, looking at society overall, public discontent tended to not focus on a single target, and relatively little was directed at the government. Moreover, dispatching the Public Security Department only when people actually took uncooperative attitudes towards mask-wearing and argued with employees, rather than having it demand mask-wearing from the start, was a useful strategy to save public resources during the pandemic. To sum, it would have been extremely difficult to quickly popularise masks in China were it not for the efforts of grassroots.

Considering these facts, a unique logic can be found in the Chinese government's enforcement and management of mask-wearing. Although China's existing law includes multiple provisions that are relevant for mask-wearing, all of their standards are ambiguous, and doubts remain regarding whether they qualify as legal grounds for a mask mandate. Thus, the Chinese government's requirement of mask-wearing to use public facilities served, in practice, as a mechanism to seek the public's cooperation. This mechanism proved highly effective on the ground owing to Chinese people's trust in the government and the efforts of the grassroots. Thus, mask-wearing ultimately became prevalent in the lives of Chinese people, and it is now characterised as an integral part of everyday life.

12.4 Case study: mask-wearing policies in Shanghai

During the pandemic, Shanghai was on the frontlines against COVID-19, as the city receives 40% of China's international flights and welcomes many new entrants every day. In spite of that, Shanghai's disease-control accomplishments are considered excellent, by far surpassing those of any other city in China (China Central Television 2021). This study outlines disease-control measures in Shanghai with a focus on mask-wearing and examines their characteristics. A representative example among them is the 'Notice on wearing masks and conducting temperature checks at public places' announced on 8 February 2020 by the Shanghai COVID-19 Prevention and Control Task Force. The notice contained the following provisions.

> 1. Those who enter harbours, stations, long-distance bus stations, underground stations, medical institutions, shopping malls, supermarkets and other public places in Shanghai, or board any public transportation, must wear a mask and cooperate with a temperature check. Those who fail to cooperate will be denied entrance by the staff.
> 2. Those who, by failing to comply with the present notice, disturb the public order, endanger public safety or obstruct state institution employees from carrying out their duties shall be punished in accordance with the law.
> (continued)

In comparison with the provisions of the central government, which were limited to advice and recommendations, Shanghai's notice made mask-wearing mandatory in public places, undeniably raising the hurdle of disease-control measures. However, the definition of 'public place' and the scope of the 'law' on which the sanctions are based are ambiguous, such that in practice, some facilities may have applied these provisions unnecessarily. As mentioned, creating a system such as this requires the understanding and cooperation of citizens and the mobilisation of grassroots. Accordingly, Shanghai swiftly arranged its own disease-control system and mobilised grassroots. For example, it has been reported that by 12 February 2020, temperature-checking equipment had been put in place in all 412 stations of the Shanghai underground, and station staff had been deployed to perform temperature checks and demand mask-wearing at the ticket gates of each station (Liu 2020).

As for disease-control measures by grassroots in Shanghai, this study references the disease-control rules for employees of China Mobile Communications Corporation (hereinafter abbreviated to China Mobile) to analyse the attitudes towards mask-wearing in the grassroots controlled by the Chinese Communist Party. China Mobile is a Chinese state-owned mobile communications company, and it is the largest mobile network carrier in the world. In February 2020, the China Mobile Shanghai Branch sent the following notice to all employees.

> Notice to the employees of the China Mobile Shanghai Branch (February 2020)
> 1. We call for safety and hygiene awareness by all employees. Thoroughly implement individual protective measures, wash your hands frequently, be hygiene conscious, avoid poorly ventilated indoor spaces and crowded public places, and wear a mask correctly when you leave your home.
> 2. Employees should commute on foot or by car. Avoid public transit as much as possible to prevent infection during your commute.
> 3. Employees must always check their temperature before coming to work. Employees with a body temperature of 37.5°C or higher should quarantine at home.
> 4. Littering of used alcohol pads is forbidden. Do not mix disinfectant with acidic substances.

Considering this notice, it is clear that the disease-control measures implemented by Shanghai's grassroots, including state-owned companies, were even stricter than those announced by the Shanghai municipal government. For example, while Shanghai City's notice mandated mask-wearing in 'public places', China Mobile's rules said to 'wear a mask . . . when you leave your home'. This may be due to the fact that the local government left the operation of disease control, as well as the responsibility for any failures, to grassroots. This point appears to be consistent with the shifting of responsibility from local governments to grassroots described earlier.

Subsequently, in January 2022, the China Mobile Shanghai Branch sent the following notice to all employees.

> Notice to the employees of the China Mobile Shanghai Branch (January 2022)
> 1. Rules for employees travelling outside Shanghai
> (1) Employees are forbidden to travel to (or through) a foreign country without authorisation. You should avoid travelling to areas within the country that have a medium to high risk of infection and avoid unnecessary travel in general.
> (2) When leaving Shanghai, employees must report their travel information and personal health information in advance and obtain authorisation from their department manager.
> (3) When leaving Shanghai, employees must implement thorough hygiene and safety measures and are strictly required to report any relevant symptoms or travel through high-risk areas. If the area you are visiting becomes high

risk, postpone your return to Shanghai until the high-risk status has been lifted.

(4) Employees must undergo a PCR test within 48 hours of returning to Shanghai and submit a negative result before re-entering the workplace. Employees should then monitor their own health for one week, perform daily temperature checks, avoid crowded places, and wear a mask correctly.

(5) Each department must register employees' travel conditions and check employees' safety conditions and PCR test results before they return to the workplace. . ..

4. Employees should be very careful about their personal health. You should wear a mask correctly, maintain social distancing and be conscious of personal hygiene. No more than ten persons should be eating together. Banquets whose participants occupy more than five tables should be reported to the relevant resident committee.

(continued)

As of January 2022, two years after the outbreak of COVID-19, the pandemic has not shown signs of a conclusion. Simultaneously, it is notable that disease-control measures in the Chinese grassroots have not been relaxed, and strict restrictions continue. A particularly representative example of this is employees being forbidden to travel outside their own region without authorisation. In practice, travel restrictions such as these are imposed not only by state-owned companies but by most government institutions and national education institutions throughout China as well. Such a strict system in party-controlled grassroots, such as state-owned companies, government institutions etc., is made possible by the mobilisation capacity and organisational power of grassroots organisations. Looking at China Mobile's notice, for instance, it is clear that there are personnel responsible for checking employees' travel and health conditions. Thus, we can conjecture that this mechanism seeks employees' understanding by having the responsible personnel provide individual explanations when employees express any questions or complaints about the rules, as opposed to simply demanding that employees comply with disease-control measures.

12.5 Effectiveness and issues of Chinese mask-wearing popularisation policies

The previous section outlined the process by which mask-wearing was popularised in China. Within that process, the effectiveness of Chinese policies to popularise mask-wearing may be summarised in the following four points.

First, under a centralised administrative framework, government control succeeded in promoting the production of crucial supplies. Because the Chinese government placed masks and other medical supplies under its own control, mask production quickly got on the right track, eventually contributing to the early popularisation of masks in China.

Second, although the information disclosed in the early stages of the outbreak was scarce, the Chinese government utilised its own authority combined with tools such as video-sharing sites to disseminate correct information on mask-wearing, informing citizens of the need to wear masks while easing their anxiety at the same time.

Third, during the COVID-19 outbreak, the Chinese government effectively mobilised grassroots and gained public cooperation in mask mandates based on the pillar of public trust.

Fourth, despite the issues and costs discussed in what follows, China's popularisation of effective disease-control measures, starting with the quick adoption of a mask mandate, and its success in containing the infection serve as good evidence to support the superiority of the Chinese political system. Specifically, the contrast with the rapid rise in the number of cases abroad must contribute greatly to the legitimacy of the Chinese government.

Conversely, three problems can be found in China's policies to popularise mask-wearing. First, amid the COVID-19 outbreak of January 2020, the Chinese government controlled medical supplies including masks; however, the way medical supplies were managed and distributed under government control was not made public, causing growing suspicion among the public.

Second, while the Chinese government mobilised grassroots to the fullest extent possible, the persistence of the COVID-19 pandemic means that the costs of this governance and grassroots mobilisation are likely to rise, eventually becoming a financial burden.

Third, there are significant discrepancies between the mask-wearing regulations of local governments and those of grassroots, and the possibility that grassroots may be introducing unnecessary measures cannot be ignored. Moreover, as discussed, public trust in the government is the key to disease-control measures, but the shifting of responsibility from local authorities to grassroots, along with the related problems, runs the risk of eroding that trust.

12.6 Conclusion

From the perspective of China, COVID-19 has been a sort of 'litmus test' revealing the effectiveness and issues of the Chinese crisis-management system. In the early stages of the COVID-19 outbreak, the Chinese government arranged effective disease-control measures by harnessing the extraordinary unifying power and mobilisation capacity of its central government. After the initial outbreak was contained, however, issues in the Chinese crisis-management system emerged. Due to a dilemma concerning the relationship between central and local authorities, the central government gave autonomy to the local governments, leading, however, to excessive disease-control measures and shifting of responsibility by local governments, with the risk of negative consequences in the lives of the general public.

Meanwhile, looking at the process of mask popularisation in China soon after the outbreak of COVID-19, perspectives attributing China's success in popularising and mandating masks entirely to its centralised system of government appear unconvincing. The same is true for interpretations attributing this success to Chinese people's habits and mask-wearing culture. In fact, China's success was likely the result of effective mechanisms created by the government, public cooperation stemming from trust in the government, and the mobilisation of grassroots leaders and employees. Particularly crucial among these factors was government authority, which was directly linked to public trust and grassroots' capacity for mobilisation. Even in a political society like that of China, government authority and power essentially originate from public approval and support. Therefore, government authority can certainly contribute to effective disease-control measures; nevertheless, abuse of authority and excessive responsibility shifting ultimately weaken government authority. Considering the experience of COVID-19, mask-wearing may be viewed as an indicator of the government's mobilisation capacity and unifying power and of the degree of trust in the government.

References

Amako, S. (2018) *Chugoku Seiji no Shakai Taisei [Social Regime of Chinese Politics]*, Tokyo: Iwanami Shoten.

Brady, A.M. (2008) *Marketing Dictatorship: Propaganda and Thought Work in Contemporary China*, Lanham, MD: Rowman & Littlefield Publishers.

China Central Television (2021) Buzuo Quanyuan Jiance, Fabu Butiren, Shanghai Fangyi Ruhezuodao Wuzhanshi [Without Testing all Citizens, and Do not Mention Specific Person on Press Conference, How Shanghai Achieved 'No Wartime' in Epidemic Prevention], 31 January, viewed 10 February 2022, https://news.cctv.com/2021/01/31/ARTIfH2rzeT32b2cJX9SXVNt210131.shtml

Da, X., Dong, B.L. and Xu, J.F. (2020) 'Gongxu liangduan rushou, pojie kouzhao kunjun [Start at both sides of supply and demand to solve the dilemma of mask]', *Caijing Magazine*, 6 February. [published in Chinese].

Ding, L., Cai, W., Ding, J.Q., Zhang, X.X., Cai, Y., Shi, J.W., Liang, Q.M., Zhang, L.F., Sun, L.Z., Qu, J.M., Jiang, F., and Chen, G.Q. (2020) 'An interim review of lessons from the novel coronavirus (SARS-CoV-2) outbreak in China', *Scientia Sinica Vitea*, 50(3), pp. 247–257 [published in Chinese].

Fisher, M. and Choe. S.H. (2020) 'How South Korea flattened the curve', *The New York Times*, 23 March, viewed 10 February 2022, www.nytimes.com/2020/03/23/world/asia/coronavirus-south-korea-flatten-curve.html.

Han, Q., Zheng, B., Cristea, M., Agostini, M., Bélanger, J.J., Gützkow, B., Kreienkamp, J. and Leander, N.P. (2021) 'Trust in government regarding COVID-19 and its associations with preventive health behaviour and prosocial behaviour during the pandemic: a cross-sectional and longitudinal study', *Psychological Medicine*, 1–11. doi:10.1017/S0033291721001306.

He, J.W. (2020) 'Kouzhaode feichang jiafa: richanliang huojiang liangyi, renghui duanque haishi baohe? [The extraordinary addition of masks: daily output may reach 200 million, will there be a shortage or saturation?]', *Southern Weekly*, 22 February [published in Chinese].

Hishida, M. (2010) *Chuugoku Kisou karano Gabanansu [Governance from the Chinese Grassroot]*, Tokyo: Hosei University Press.

Horii, M. (2012) *Masuku to Nihonjin [Mask and Japanese]*, Tokyo: Shumei University Press.

Liu, H.Y. (2021) 'Shingata Koronauirusu Kansenshou wo Meguru Chuugoku Seifu no Taiou: Senjijyoutai no Hatsurei to sono Mondaiten [Response of the Chinese government to the new coronavirus outbreak: Announcement of wartime state and its problems]'. *Waseda Daigaku Shagakuken Ronshuu [The Waseda Journal of Social Sciences]*, 38, pp. 1–10.

Liu, Z.H. (2020) 'Fugong Dierzhou, Jizhe Zoufang Shanghai Ditie Gongjiao Chuzuche, Shinei Gonggongjiaotong Anquanma [In the second week of resumption of work, I visited metro, bus, and taxi in Shanghai: is public transportation safe?]', *Xinmin Weekly*, 17 February [published in Chinese].

Meng, J.G. (2020) 'To tame coronavirus, Mao-style social control blankets China', *The New York Times*, 15 February, viewed 10 February 2022, www.nytimes.com/2020/02/15/business/china-coronavirus-lockdown.html.

Nakagane, K. (1979) 'Chuugoku: shakaishugi keizai seido no kouzou to tenkai [China: structure and development of socialist economic system]', in M. Iwata (ed.), *Gendai Shakaishugi [Modern Socialism]*, Tokyo: Toyo Keizai Shinpo.

National Congress of the Communist Party of China. (2017) *Constitution of the Communist Party of China*, Beijing: People's Press [published in Chinese].

Sohu (2020) 'Shanghai shouli budai kouzhao qiangchuang ditie beixingju [First administrative attachment case in Shanghai due to forcibly breaking into the subway without wearing a mask]', *Sohu News*, 8 February, viewed 10 February 2022, www.sohu.com/a/371455789_255783.

Stockmann, D. (2011) 'Race to the bottom: Media marketization and increasing negativity toward the United States in China', *Political Communication* 28(3), pp. 268–290.

The Beijing News (2020) 'Zhiji feiyan: youren tunhuo yongxianjin jiaoyi, xianshang duanhuo xianxia duangong [Approaching the pandemic: some people hoard goods and use cash to trade, online and offline supply is cut off]', *Beijing News*, 28 January [published in Chinese].

The Central Government of the People's Republic of China (2005) 'Public security administration punishment law of the People's Republic of China', viewed 10 February 2022, www.gov.cn/ziliao/flfg/2005-08/29/content_27130.htm

The Central Government of the People's Republic of China (2018) 'Constitution of People's Republic of China, viewed 10 February 2022, www.gov.cn/guoqing/2018-03/22/content_5276318.htm

The Paper (2020) 'Kouzhao Jinjiazhi 6mao Fan 1 yuan Beifa? Guanfang Huiyingle [A pharmacy was fined for selling mask priced 0.6 yuan for 1 yuan? Here is the official response], *The Paper*, 13 February [published in Chinese].

The People's Daily (2020) 'Haobu fangsong zhuahao changtaihua yiqing fangkong jianjue fangzhi yiqing fantan [Do not relax and pay attention to normalizing epidemic prevention and control, resolutely prevent the epidemic rebounding]', *The People's Daily*, 29 July [published in Chinese].

Wang, H.Y. (2020) 'Kouzhao Channeng Quanqiu Guoban, Weihe Haishi Yizhao Nanqiu? [The production capacity of masks in China accounts for more than half of the world, why is it still hard to get a mask?]', *Sanlian Lifeweek Magazine*, 3 February [published in Chinese].

Wang, Y.Q. and Zhang, J.Y. (2020) Wuhan Zhiwai Hubei Duodi Yiyong Wuzi Gaoji: Kouzhao Zuique, Genben Maibudao [Medical supplies in Hubei outside Wuhan are in emergency: masks are the most in short supply and cannot be bought at all], *Beijing News*, 27 January [published in Chinese].

You, D.N. (2020) 'Fengbaoyan Zhongde Xiangyang: Yige Putong Jiatingde Fengbi Shenghuo [Xiangyang in the eye of the storm: the quarantined life of an ordinary family]', *Nan Feng Chuang*, 3 February [published in Chinese].

Yuan, L. (2020) 'In coronavirus fight, China sidelines an ally: Its own people', *The New York Times*, 18 February, viewed 10 February 2022, www.nytimes.com/2020/02/18/business/china-coronavirus-charity-supplies.html.

Zhang, H. and Sun, Y.Z. (2020) 'Fudan Xinguanfeiyan Fangkong Diyike, Zhang Wenhong Jianglesha [Fudan's first lesson of new coronavirus prevention, what did Zhang Wenhong say]', *The Paper*, 24 February [published in Chinese].

Zhu, J.R. (2020) 'Afutakorona no Chuugoku Seiji Shakai: Kikoetekita Zenshin no Jihibiki [After corona's Chinese political society: the sound of progress]', in Contemporary China Research Base (ed.), *Korona Ikou no Higashi Ajia Hendou no Rikigaku [Dynamics of East Asia after corona]*, University of Tokyo, Tokyo: University of Tokyo Press.

Zou, J. (2020) 'Shanghai Kangyi Yishenglingxia, Lianzuodoufu Dedou Luqile Xiuzi [Under the order to fight the epidemic in Shanghai, even the tofu maker get started]', *The Paper*, 15 February [published in Chinese].

13 Public mask-wearing behaviour and perception towards COVID-19 intervention policies in Thailand

A mixed-methods study

Upalat Korwatanasakul and Sivarin Lertpusit

13.1 Background

All countries have been hit hard by the ongoing coronavirus disease 2019 (COVID-19) pandemic since the first quarter of 2020, posing significant challenges to global public health systems. As of 20 August 2021, the World Health Organization (WHO) reported 210 million confirmed cases of COVID-19 and 4.4 million deaths due to COVID-19 worldwide. Several countries implemented a series of lockdowns and restrictions to prevent the spread of COVID-19 and therefore faced a trade-off between preventing a health emergency and avoiding financial and economic crisis (Intarakumnerd and Korwatanasakul 2020).

In early 2020, COVID-19 quickly spread to Thailand, as the country is a leading business and travel destination for Chinese people due to its proximity to China. According to the WHO (2021), on 13 January 2020, Thailand became the first country outside China to report confirmed cases. As of 21 November 2021, officials had confirmed approximately two million cumulative cases and 20,305 cumulative deaths (WHO 2021). Thailand successfully controlled the COVID-19 situation as evidenced by its significantly low daily confirmed cases and deaths in the single to double digits throughout 2020.

13.1.1 COVID-19 timeline

Thailand has experienced three waves of COVID-19 outbreaks, with the fourth wave starting in June 2021. Several transmission clusters, the largest of which was the Lumpinee Boxing Stadium cluster, triggered Thailand's first wave of COVID-19. The government successfully mitigated it by declaring a state of emergency, suspending all commercial international flights and implementing lockdown measures.

Despite inbound travel restrictions, the government failed to control national borders, resulting in the second wave in December 2020. Officials discovered that infected illegal migrant workers had crossed the Myanmar–Thailand border

DOI: 10.4324/9781003244127-15

from Tachileik to Mae Sai District, a district located in the northern area of Thailand. Several weeks later, an outbreak occurred in the Burmese migrant worker community in Samut Sakhon, a province near Bangkok, contributing to widespread COVID-19 in Bangkok and the metropolitan area. Consequently, the daily new confirmed COVID-19 cases rose to three digits in January 2021. Nevertheless, the government was able to swiftly flatten the COVID-19 curve with strict lockdown measures at the beginning of February 2021.

Despite implementing several health and containment measures, Thailand experienced a third peak soon thereafter, in April 2021, thanks to clusters in the entertainment district in Bangkok. Moreover, the movement of people across provinces during the long Songkran holiday season worsened the situation, causing the daily confirmed cases to exceed four digits for the first time. The fourth wave took shape as COVID-19 cases had been rising since April. The overcapacity of hospitals and the closure of construction worker camps in Bangkok and the metropolitan area forced workers to migrate back to their hometowns. Thus, these two incidents catalysed the fourth wave and the infection across Thailand.

13.1.2 Government policy measures in response to COVID-19

Thailand has been implementing strict containment measures since the first wave of the COVID-19 outbreak. These measures include quarantines and confinement; travel bans and restrictions; closure of schools, universities and public places; cancellation of public events; and obligatory shutdown of economic activities (OECD 2021).

Despite the strict containment measures, the COVID-19 situation in Thailand has worsened over time due to the inexplicably slow and insufficient vaccine rollout. The government came under sharp criticism for its handling of vaccine procurement, particularly in terms of vaccine choices. Thailand relied mainly on Sinovac and AstraZeneca vaccines and opted not to import mRNA vaccines such as Pfizer-BioNTech and Moderna. Nevertheless, the government revised its vaccine policy to secure as many vaccines as possible, regardless of their characteristics, responding to the high number of daily confirmed cases and deaths. As with other countries, Thailand's vaccination policy prioritised front-line healthcare personnel and long-term-care-facility residents, people with high-risk medical conditions and those aged 60 years and older. On 1st July 2021, the government expanded the vaccination coverage to people aged 18 to 59 years. The coverage is still minimal due to the insufficient volume of vaccines. As of 28 August 2021, the number of cumulative vaccine doses administered in Bangkok and Thailand was approximately 7.9 million and 26 million, respectively (Bangkok Metropolitan Administration 2021). Within Bangkok, 6.3 million persons had received the first dose, while 1.4 million persons had received the second shot.

A face mask policy was also a significant factor in preventing the spread of COVID-19. Initially, face mask policies mainly involved control of domestic face mask supply and price, in response to the excessive demand for face masks during the first COVID-19 wave. According to a 2016 survey of the Health Service

Support Department (2016), only 19% of the survey sample usually wore a face mask when having a cold or flu, demonstrating inadequate understanding of public health and infectious diseases protection among Thai people. In addition, a 2019 survey by Tultrairatana and Phansuea (2021) found that more than half of the survey sample (54.3%) did not wear a facial mask in response to air pollution. Since Thai people did not have a habit of wearing face masks, especially for preventing infectious diseases, before the COVID-19 outbreak, the domestic supply of face masks was meagre, which reflected their low demand. The scarcity of face mask supply led to a distortedly high price during the COVID-19 pandemic. To guarantee equal access for the public, the government listed face masks as regulated products under the Government Gazette on 4 February 2020 (Department of Internal Trade 2020). The definition of face masks covers medical masks, disposable masks for industry and disposable dust masks.

Furthermore, the government enforced a face mask law to control the public behaviour of mask-wearing. Initially, the government asked for public cooperation for mask-wearing in public spaces, particularly areas with high infection rates, for example, Bangkok. On 7 June 2021, the government announced the National Communicable Disease Committee's Regulation regarding the Violation of Disease Control Preventive Measures to enforce public mask-wearing in response to the fourth wave (The Secretariat of the Cabinet 2021). The law states that properly wearing masks in public places, public transportation and private passenger cars with more than one passenger is fully mandatory for every individual. Those who violate the law are subject to a fine of up to 20,000 baht (approximately 600 USD). The law also applies to improper mask-wearing behaviours, in other words, wearing a mask under a chin and leaving a nose or mouth uncovered. In addition to the mask-wearing law, the Department of Health (Ministry of Public Health) encouraged the public to wear masks within their residence to prevent infection among family members, believed to be the leading cause of the COVID-19 surge.

This chapter combines quantitative and qualitative analyses to examine the public's mask-wearing behaviour and its rationales, with a particular interest in the relationship between mask-wearing behaviour and public trust and perception towards the government's policy responses. It is structured as follows. Section 13.2 discusses research methods, quantitative analyses and qualitative analyses, focusing on the Bangkok area, and describes the data used in the study. Section 13.3 presents the findings based on the mixed-methods analysis. Section 13.4 concludes and provides policy implications.

13.2 Research method

This study uses a mixed-methods analysis based on the systematic integration of quantitative and qualitative data, allowing for more comprehensive and synergetic utilisation of the data. First, the study uses quantitative analysis to assess general patterns of the public's mask-wearing behaviour and perception towards the government's mask-wearing policy measures. Furthermore, a follow-up qualitative analysis through interviews validates and contextualises the quantitative results and identifies the motivations and rationale behind the observed behaviour and perception. Both quantitative and qualitative analyses focus primarily on the public's mask-wearing behaviours in Bangkok, the centre of the COVID-19 outbreaks.

13.2.1 *Quantitative analysis*

The quantitative method used in this chapter is descriptive statistics, employing two secondary data sources, namely, the structured observation of mask-wearing behaviour (AiMASK) and the survey of public health behaviours to prevent COVID-19 infection (Anamai Poll). AiMASK is a structured observation conducted by the National Research Council of Thailand's (NRCT) Artificial Intelligence System to Assess Mask-Wearing Behaviour Project. The main objective of this structured observation is to collect information on the public's mask-wearing behaviours in Bangkok. It employs artificial intelligence technology to detect mask-wearing behaviours and reports daily on the collected statistics by area. The observation covers 30 areas around Bangkok in eight types of public places: convenience stores, commercial banks, inside and outside market areas, bus stops, crossing bridges, department stores and pavements. The observed sample varies daily, ranging from 7,000 to 12,000 persons.

The second data source is the Anamai Poll conducted monthly by the Department of Health. The data used in this chapter are from the 12th and 13th Anamai Poll, covering 21 June–16 July 2021 and 19 July–20 August 2021. The survey aims to proactively observe people's behaviour around COVID-19 prevention measures and use the data as input for health management and policy measures against the COVID-19 pandemic. The Department of Health carries out a monthly online survey within a specific time period. The survey is open to all individuals in different provinces and regions across Thailand. The survey consists of four sections: basic information (i.e. sex, age, residential area and occupation); preventive actions to reduce the risk of COVID-19 infection; concerns regarding the current COVID-19 situation; and specific issues for each period, for example, mask-wearing behaviours within a residence. The data from the 12th and 13th Anamai Poll cover 10,432 and 6,087 observations, respectively. Table 13.1 provides summary statistics of the observations in Bangkok and Thailand.

One possible caveat to the Anamai Poll data concerns the sampling bias. The sample is possibly biased towards specific groups in the population due to a self-selection problem, for example, different abilities to access the Internet and different interests in participating in the survey among others. However, this study employs qualitative analysis to validate and cross-check the results from the quantitative analysis, which is the main advantage of the mixed-methods analysis used in this chapter.

Table 13.1 Summary statistics of the 12th and 13th Anamai Poll, 2021

Poll	12th Anamai Poll		13th Anamai Poll	
Period	21 June–16 July		19 July–20 August	
Bangkok				
Sex				
Female	238	83.2%	196	81.3%
Male	48	16.8%	45	18.7%
Age				
Below 15	1	0.3%	3	1.2%
15–24	8	2.8%	12	5.0%
25–44	126	44.1%	89	36.9%
45–59	115	40.2%	107	44.4%
60 and over	36	12.6%	30	12.4%
Occupation				
Public officer	105	36.7%	101	41.9%
Farmer	1	0.3%	0	0.0%
Village health volunteer	2	0.7%	1	0.4%
Freelance and business owner	35	12.2%	34	14.1%
Private officer	81	28.3%	47	19.5%
Student	6	2.1%	10	4.1%
Housewife	16	5.6%	10	4.1%
Retiree	14	4.9%	16	6.6%
Retailer (market)	8	2.8%	4	1.7%
Other	7	2.4%	6	2.5%
Unemployed	11	3.8%	12	5.0%
Total		286		241
Thailand				
Sex				
Female	8,117	77.8%	4,633	76.1%
Male	2,315	22.2%	1,454	23.9%
Age				
Below 15	118	1.1%	45	0.7%
15–24	469	4.5%	357	5.9%
25–44	3,464	33.2%	2,150	35.3%
45–59	4,918	47.1%	2,807	46.1%
60 and over	1,463	14.0%	728	12.0%
Occupation				
Public officer	3,285	31.5%	1,631	26.8%
Farmer	2,172	20.8%	1,268	20.8%
Village health volunteer	2,099	20.1%	1,120	18.4%
Freelance and business owner	1,088	10.4%	808	13.3%
Private officer	505	4.8%	350	5.7%
Student	391	3.7%	157	2.6%
Housewife	260	2.5%	183	3.0%
Retiree	229	2.2%	112	1.8%
Retailer (market)	187	1.8%	298	4.9%
Other	111	1.1%	31	0.5%
Unemployed	105	1.0%	129	2.1%
Total		10,432		6,087

Source: Authors, based on the 12th and 13th Anamai Poll survey data (Department of Health 2021)

13.2.2 *Qualitative analysis*

This study conducts qualitative in-depth interviews with Thai people living in Bangkok. It uses an interpretivist approach to determine the mask-wearing behaviours, motivations and perception towards the government's mask-wearing policy measures. The approach helps us understand the social world through the perspectives of research participants and their experiences embedded within broader socio-political structures (Bryman 2016). The inclusion criteria for the recruitment of participants are age and residence area. The informants must live in Bangkok and belong to one of the following age groups: 25 and under, 26 to 55 years old and 56 and above.

The sample is selected through a purposive sampling method, relying on researchers' judgement about the informants' representativeness. The purposive sampling method guarantees the heterogeneity of the sample in terms of age and occupation to better illustrate public opinion. The interviews consist of ten informants, two of whom are under 26 years old, six of whom are between ages 26 and 55 and two of whom are over 55 years old. Their occupations include graphic designer, merchant, teacher, fitness trainer, house cleaner, student, restaurant worker and job seeker.

The semi-structured interview follows the survey questionnaire of the Anamai Poll, providing an opportunity to validate and augment the findings from the quantitative analysis. The interview also includes additional questions about motivations and perceptions around mask-wearing behaviours and the government's face mask policies. Each semi-structured in-depth interview lasts 45 to 60 minutes and is conducted online. The interview period is 16–26 July 2021.

3. Public behaviour and perception of mask-wearing: a mixed-methods analysis

This section presents the findings from the mixed-methods analysis. It discusses general trends of mask-wearing behaviours and perceptions towards face mask policies derived from the quantitative observation and survey data. In addition, the qualitative results supplement and expand the discussion of the quantitative analysis while presenting a new set of findings that do not show up in the quantitative data.

13.3.1 *Mask-wearing behaviours*

Before the COVID-19 outbreak, almost all participants wore face masks to protect them from air pollution such as fine particulate matter (PM2.5), indicating a public health concern. However, only two participants reported wearing a face mask to reduce the risks of flu infection, implying low health consciousness in terms of infectious diseases. The results are consistent with the previous findings of the Health Service Support Department (2016) and Tultrairatana and Phansuea (2021), presented in Section 13.1.2.

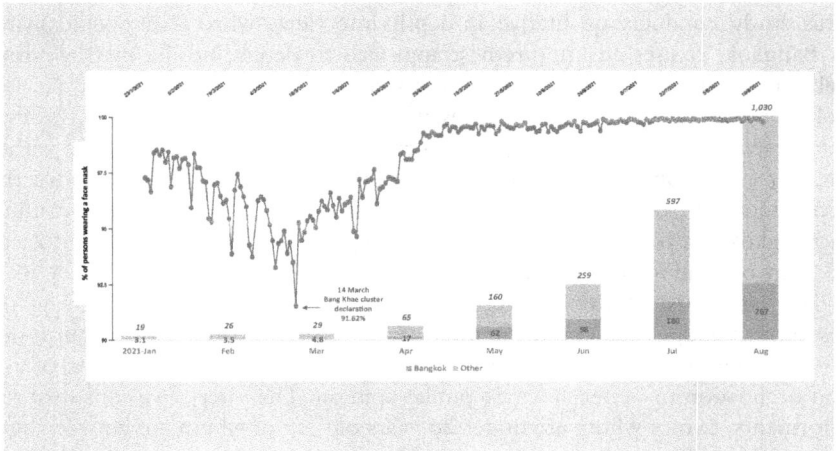

Figure 13.1 Number of confirmed cases and mask-wearing behaviour (as of 21 August 2021; unit: thousands of cases and percentage)

Notes: the numbers in italic = total confirmed cases in Thailand; the numbers at the bottom = confirmed cases in Bangkok; the line chart shows a percentage of persons wearing a face mask.

Source: Authors, based on the data of AiMASK (National Research Council of Thailand 2021) and DDC OpenData (Department of Disease Control 2021d).

After the COVID-19 outbreak, the interview participants' attitudes towards mask-wearing and public health concerns changed. All participants reported regularly wearing face masks in public places. Figure 13.1 shows the number of confirmed cases and mask-wearing behaviours in Bangkok, based on the quantitative AiMASK data. During January to August 2021, more than 90% of the sample wore a face mask correctly in public places (illustrated by the line chart). Notably, more than 99.5% wore a face mask in public places during June–August 2021 to respond to the sharp rise in the number of daily confirmed cases in this period (presented by the bar chart). Thus, the quantitative and qualitative findings are consistent.

Nevertheless, Figure 13.1 also shows a downward trend of mask-wearing in public places from January to March 2021, corresponding to the early third wave. The public might have felt less worried about the COVID-19 situation due to the low number of daily confirmed cases after the strict lockdown in February. On 14 March 2021, the Bangkok Metropolitan Administration found a new COVID-19 cluster in Bang Khae, a district in Bangkok, and locked down six fresh markets in the area (Thai PBS News 2021). The declaration raised public awareness and concern about the high infection risk and, in turn, encouraged people to resume proper mask-wearing behaviour. Hence, the percentage of people correctly wearing face masks sharply rose right after the announcement of the Bang Khae cluster.

Therefore, the mask-wearing behaviour possibly depends on two factors: a degree of health impact and public awareness and concern. Before the COVID-19 outbreak, few people wore face masks as a preventive action or wore them properly since they had low consciousness of infectious diseases such as the flu (Health Service Support Department 2016). However, Thai people quickly adopted mask-wearing behaviour after the COVID-19 outbreak, possibly because COVID-19 has a significantly higher health impact than the flu. In addition, public awareness and concern also play an essential role in determining mask-wearing behaviour among Thai people, reflected in the changes in mask-wearing behaviours in response to the number of daily COVID-19 confirmed cases in different time periods (Figure 13.1).

In contrast to the AiMASK data, whose scope is limited to only major public areas, the Anamai Poll data allows broader and deeper coverage of analysis, one of which is a community-level analysis. During 21 June–20 August 2021, approximately 66% of the survey participants observed that everyone in their community wore a face mask properly, whereas 27% of the participants reported seeing people in their neighbourhoods wearing face masks incorrectly. In the same period, 7% stated that only a few people or no one in their community wore a face mask. Thus, in general, the results are consistent with those of the AiMASK observation and the in-depth interviews.

Furthermore, the Anamai Poll provides mask-wearing behaviour statistics for a more extensive set of public places. According to Figure 13.2, people are strict about wearing a face mask in convenience stores (95% of the observations), department stores (94%), markets (93%), hospitals (93%), meeting centres (92%) and transportation (90 %). However, fitness centres (68%), gambling spots (casino, cockpit and games centre: 73% in total) and nurseries (76%) are the public places where most people relax their mask-wearing behaviours, in other words, sometimes wearing a mask or sometimes not wearing a mask. Reinforcing the results of the Anamai Poll, the interviewees advised that they usually wear face masks in public places, particularly those where no food or drink is consumed. In contrast, they take off their face masks at restaurants, nightclubs, public places for sports activities and open-air recreation areas. The rationales for their relaxed mask-wearing behaviour involve physical and psychological reasons.

> Wee (21 years old): 'When running or playing football, I do not wear a mask. It is hard to breathe. It is a physical matter'.
> Ed (44 years old): 'I went to the seaside to relieve my stress. There were few people at the beach. So, I think it was okay not to use a face mask'.
> Muk (22 years old): 'I took off my mask when I went to a pub because I had to eat, drink and socialise with friends. Wearing a mask is strange'.

The interviews also reveal the differences in mask-wearing behaviours among different age groups. Older generations tend to be more risk averse and avoid going to public places, as they are more vulnerable to COVID-19. In contrast, younger generations are more reckless. They tend to hang out in public spaces and take off their face masks when socialising.

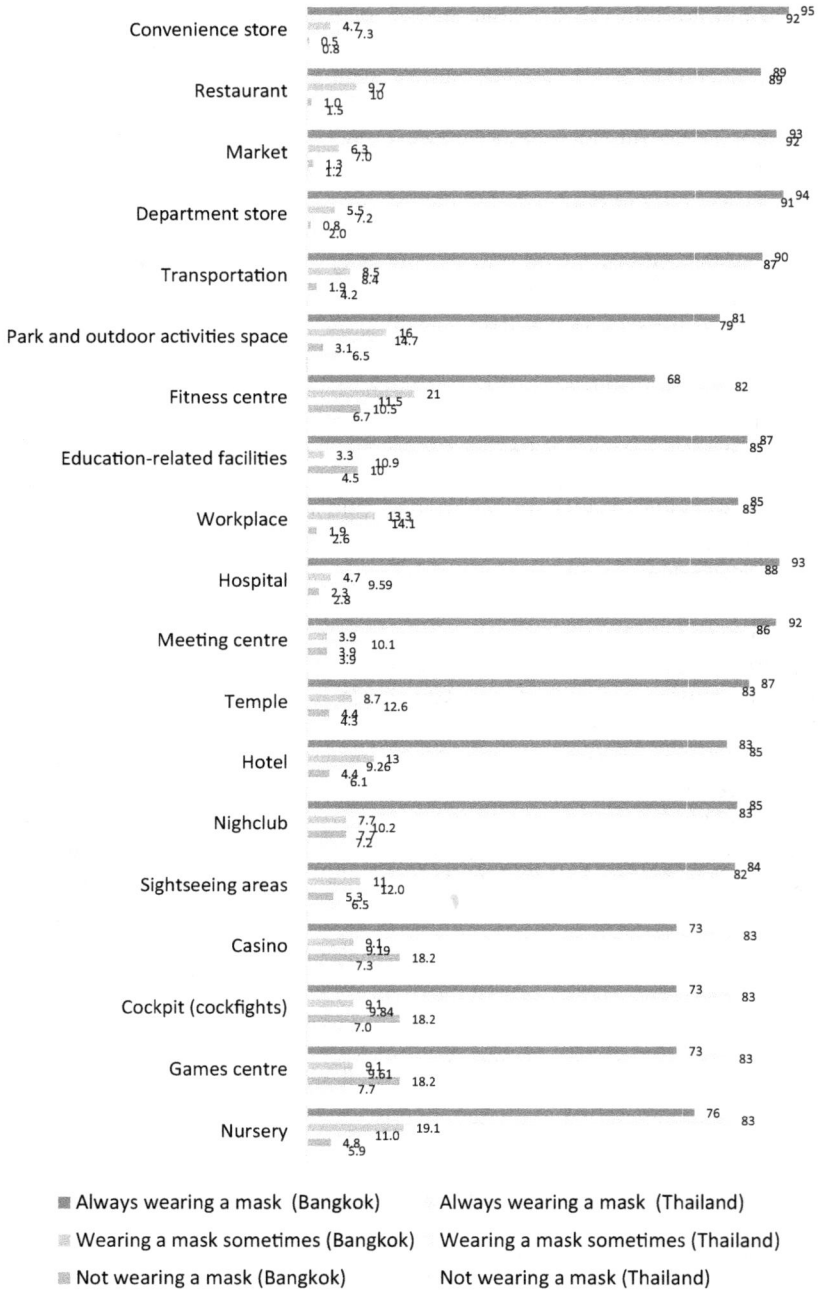

Figure 13.2 Mask-wearing behaviour by public place, 2021 (%)
Source: Authors, based on the 13th Anamai Poll survey data (Department of Health 2021)

Muk (22 years old): 'I went to a national park. I didn't think it was necessary to wear a mask in uncrowded and open spaces. Because I drink and talk at a nightclub, it is natural that we do not put masks on'.

Dream (27 years old): 'I don't wear a face mask in pubs and restaurants. I go there to drink and fulfil our social lives'.

Suree (66 years old): 'I still have to go out to sell lottery tickets, but I wear a two-layer mask, hand gloves and a face shield'.

13.3.2 Rationales behind the mask-wearing behaviours

As noted by all interview participants, preventive actions are the priority under the COVID-19 pandemic, particularly when the vaccine rollouts are inexplicably slow and insufficient. The first vaccines were delivered to Thailand in late February 2021, most of which were given to public health personnel (Department of Disease Control 2021a). The rate of fully vaccinated people was 10% on 28 August 2021 and reached 44% on 3 November 2021 (Department of Disease Control 2021b, 2021c). The participants primarily worry about their own health and that of their family members. Therefore, they choose the cheapest, easiest and most effective preventive action, that is, mask-wearing, to reduce the probability of COVID-19 infection and transmission among their family members. Regardless of the government's face mask policies, they wear face masks in public places because of their confidence in the efficacy of masks, social pressure and social norms reflected by different age groups.

First, all participants reported their confidence in the efficacy of face masks due to the scientific evidence adduced by the international and academic communities. They learned about the benefits and were given instructions about mask-wearing from various sources, but not governmental agencies, indicating the low public trust and negative public perception towards the government's communication and perhaps management under the COVID-19 situation.

Second, mask-wearing behaviours are also explained by social pressure. Thai society has a strong sense of community and a socially oriented culture. Therefore, social pressure and mainstream social behaviours influence individual practices (Embree 1950). Almost all interview participants (eight out of ten) revealed that social pressure caused stress and partially forced them to wear masks. In other words, regardless of age, occupation and educational background, the participants addressed a similar impact from social peer pressure.

Nuch (43 years old): 'Community pressures have a huge impact on my consideration. Sometimes, I forget to bring a face mask. I must buy a new one as soon as possible because of the social pressure. We also must have a social responsibility. So, wearing a face mask is a common way to show social responsibility'.

Every member of society is both a subject and an object of social pressure and stress. For instance, the participants put social pressure on people who do not wear face masks in public areas by staring at them, checking their own face masks and spraying alcohol. Most of the interviewees stated that they would leave the place afterwards, whereas two interviewees would inform a person in charge of the area to deal with such people. One participant firmly said that she would directly tell them to wear masks properly.

> Suree (66 years old): 'When I saw people who did not wear a face mask, I approached and asked them to wear one. I also strongly support the face mask policy that fines people who do not wear face masks properly'.

Finally, social norms reflected by different age groups potentially affect mask-wearing behaviour. Among the interview participants, younger and older generations appeared to exhibit different social norms. Even though all participants agreed on the necessity of mask-wearing in public places, the younger generations said it should not be legally mandatory. They believe that mask-wearing is their choice, but people should be socially responsible amid the pandemic. The mask-wearing policy, implemented on 7 June 2021, imposes a fine on those who do not wear a face mask in public areas, limiting individual freedom. Four participants (Muk (22 years old), Wee (21 years old), Tam (29 years old) and Dream (27 years old)) indicated that the state should not intervene in the public's decision-making. However, the older generations view collective social safety as the priority and freedom as a mere excuse for selfishness during the crisis.

> Suree (66 years old): 'Wearing a face mask is for our community. It is not a choice. You become "a risk" for others if you deny wearing a face mask. It is your right not to wear a face mask in a normal situation, but it is not a personal matter under the pandemic'.

13.3.3 Public perceptions towards the government's policies in response to the COVID-19 pandemic

Generally, most interviewees do not trust or are not confident in the government's general policy responses and communication. Instead of following the official organisations, they get information on COVID-19 from other sources. The interviewees indicated that they had received information concerning COVID-19 from social influencers, for example, medical doctors, newscasters, social activists and mass media, such as the Standard, Channel 3, Workpoint and Thai PBS. However, family members are the primary source of COVID-19 knowledge for the interview group aged 56 and above. Regardless of generation, no interviewees mentioned official government agencies as their source of COVID-19 information, implying that public trust towards the government's communication under the COVID-19 crisis was poor. Furthermore, the younger generation reveals negative perceptions towards the government communication scheme and its degree of trustworthiness.

> Tam (29 years old): 'I do not follow the state agencies and the government official press releases. I do not believe in that information because the

government does not show sincerity to the public. The information is still questionable. Somehow, the presented data is not important to the public'.

Sasi (31 years old): 'Mostly, I follow well-known news agencies to learn about COVID-19 and update information that I should know to prevent myself from infection. News reporters somehow provide multidimensional data from various credible sources. Information from the government alone is not sufficient'.

The government measures encouraged the public to wear masks within their residence as the number of infected cases and deaths from COVID-19 has dramatically increased since June 2021. Figure 13.3 illustrates the discrepancy between public behaviour and perception of mask-wearing at home. Approximately 90% of the observations favour the policy (10.9% disagreed with the policy of wearing a mask at home). However, half of them find the policy impractical and hard to follow, while only one-third always wears a face mask at home.

Similarly, the interview results show that all informants realise the benefits of mask-wearing at home but decline to follow the measure, which they consider impractical for physical and psychological reasons. Home is a safe zone where people, in general, feel the most relaxed physically and mentally. Moreover, the participants do not believe that mask-wearing alone prevents COVID-19 transmission at home.

Ed (44 years old): 'I don't think mask-wearing at home would help to prevent the infection. First, I cannot put on a mask all the time. My house is my

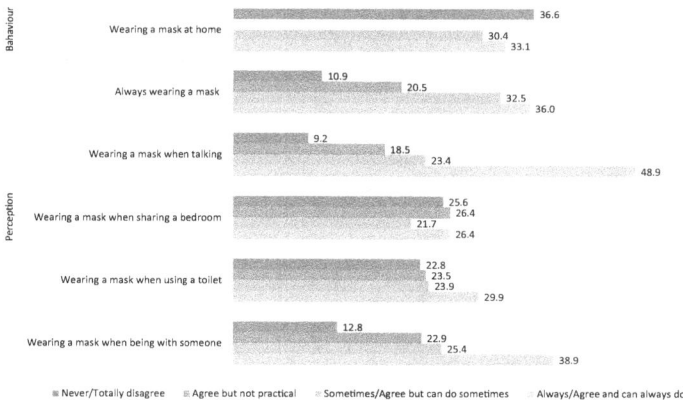

Figure 13.3 Discrepancies between public behaviour and perception of mask-wearing at residence, 2021

Note: Regarding behaviour, respondents were asked to answer either 'Never', 'Sometimes' or 'Always'. In contrast, regarding perception, respondents were asked to answer either 'Totally disagree', 'Agree but not practical', 'Agree but can do sometimes' and 'Agree and can always do'.

Source: Authors, based on the 13th Anamai Poll survey data (Department of Health 2021).

workplace to prepare ingredients to cook. I have to scrape coconuts, stir the rice with coconut milk, and wrap desserts. My job needs physical strength, which naturally needs an adequate oxygen flow. How can I strictly put the mask on all the time?'

Dream (27 years old): 'It is not necessary to put a mask on in a house. I don't think it works because the disease spreads everywhere. My family has our meals together. We use the same toilet. Wearing a mask itself is not enough to control the infection at home'.

Tam (29 years old): 'My house is a safe zone for my family and myself. It will be too stressful to wear a mask in the house'.

Furthermore, the interview participants were confident in their family members. The participants reported that they knew the behaviour of their family members through constant and proper communication and observation. As a result, family members formed interpersonal trust within a family context, supporting the idea of social trustworthiness. In contrast, wearing a mask at home may cause insecurity and worries among family members. It is not a common practice and is against the concept of family in Thai culture that prioritises interpersonal trust (Department of Women's Affairs and Family Development 2021; Soratana et al. 2019).

Social trustworthiness implies interpersonal trust or limited trust among family members and friends, which directs the members to behave in a beneficial way towards other members. Moreover, their behaviour is socially committed without legal enforcement (Kwon 2019). This concept may also explain why people observed relaxed mask-wearing behaviours in their community, as presented in Section 13.3.1.

Muk (22 years old): 'Naturally, we (family members) should trust each other. I trust my family members' behaviour. We all share the information on the COVID-19. Hence, I am confident that they have proper behaviour and have good hygiene'.

Nok (35 years old): 'If my family members contact any risk cases, they will inform and protect us. We trust each other, and I don't think wearing a mask in a house is necessary'.

13.4 Conclusion and policy implications

This chapter explains mask-wearing behaviours and motivations among the Thai population and discusses their perceptions of the government's policy responses to the COVID-19 crisis. On the basis of the analysis, the factors that shape mask-wearing behaviours include a degree of health impact, public awareness and concern, social trustworthiness, age (related to health impact) and activities performed in specific public places. The analysis also finds that self-protection (preventive action), social pressure and social norms reflected by different age groups are the fundamental motivations behind mask-wearing behaviours. Understanding the factors and the incentives behind mask-wearing behaviours helps authorities formulate better policy measures directly relevant to a specific target group, such as age cohort, community and public place. However, correct policy measures without public trust often lead to failures. Therefore, the government may employ strategies such as indirect communications and community mechanisms to help in delivering its policy measures to the public, which currently has low trust and negative perception towards the government's communication and management. For instance, communications through social influencers possibly help in delivering intended information and messages to the public, while using community mechanisms may help with monitoring the mask-wearing behaviours at the micro level.

References

Bangkok Metropolitan Administration (2021) *Covid-19, BMA*, viewed 28 August 2021, <www.bangkok.go.th/covid19>.

Bryman, A. (2016) *Social Research Methods*, 5th edn, Oxford University Press.

Department of Disease Control (2021a) *Report on Vaccination*, 1 January, Department of Disease Control, Ministry of Public Health, viewed 4 November 2021, <https://ddc.moph.go.th/vaccine-covid19/getFiles/10/1620103984990.pdf>.

Department of Disease Control (2021b) *Report on Vaccination*, 28 August, Department of Disease Control, Ministry of Public Health, viewed 4 November 2021, <https://ddc.moph.go.th/vaccine-covid19/getFiles/10/1630221091457.pdf>.

Department of Disease Control (2021c) *Report on Vaccination*, 3 November, Department of Disease Control, Ministry of Public Health, viewed 4 November 2021, <https://ddc.moph.go.th/vaccine-covid19/getFiles/10/1620103984990.pdf>.

Department of Disease Control (2021d) *DDC Open Data*, Department of Disease Control, Ministry of Public Health, viewed 18 August 2021, <https://ddc.moph.go.th/viralpneumonia/>.

Department of Health (2021) *Anamai Poll*, Department of Health, Ministry of Public Health, viewed 18 August 2021, <https://sites.google.com/view/hia-surveillance/anamai-poll-covid/%E0%B8%84%E0%B8%A3%E0%B8%87%E0%B8%97-1>.

Department of Internal Trade (2020) *Announcement of Department of Internal Trade*, Department of Internal Trade, Ministry of Commerce, viewed 18 August 2021, <www.dit.go.th/Content.aspx?m=12&c=27793>.

Department of Women's Affairs and Family Development (2021) *Open Data Portal for Family Strength 2020*, Department of Women's Affairs and Family Development, Ministry of Social Development and Human Security, viewed 11 November 2021, <https://opendata.nesdc.go.th/dataset/family?id=f4217c0c-8a0c-445d-9711-39ca6440b9f2&is_fullscreen=1>.

Embree, J.F. (1950) 'Thailand-A Loosely Structured Social System,' *American Anthropologist*, vol. 52, no. 2, pp. 181–193.

Health Service Support Department (2016) *Thai People Do Not Usually Wear Mask*, Health Service Support Department, Ministry of Public Health, viewed 22 August 2021, <https://hss.moph.go.th/show_topic.php?id=694>.

Intarakumnerd, P. and Korwatanasakul, U. (2020) 'Business Impacts and Government Supports for Firms' Upgrading and Innovation under COVID-19 in Southeast Asia,' *STEPI S&T Policy Journal*, vol. 3, no. 2, pp. 21–53.

Kwon, O.Y. (2019) 'Social Trust: Its Concepts, Determinants, Roles, and Raising Ways,' in Kwon, O.Y. (ed.), *Social Trust and Economic Development; The Case of South Korea*, Edward Elgar Publishing.

National Research Council of Thailand (NRCT) (2021) *AiMASK*, National Research Council of Thailand, viewed 18 August 2021, <https://aimask.aiat.or.th/>.

Organisation for Economic Co-operation and Development (OECD) (2021) *Tackling Coronavirus (COVID-19)*, Organisation for Economic Co-operation and Development, viewed 18 August 2021, <www.oecd.org/coronavirus/country-policy-tracker/>.

Soratana, N., Ratana-Ubol, A. and Kimpee, P. (2019) 'Family Strengths and Thai Context: Characteristics of Family Strengths, Factors and Ways of Promoting Life-long Learning,' *University of Management and Technology Journal*, vol. 16, no. 2, pp. 428–437, viewed 18 November 2021, <https://so06.tci-thaijo.org/index.php/umt-poly/article/view/232171/159741>.

Thai PBS News (2021) *"Bang Kae Cluster" 224 Infected End Up Three Days Lock Down*, Thai PBS News Agency, viewed 8 November 2021, <https://news.thaipbs.or.th/content/302438>.

The Secretariat of the Cabinet (2021) *National Communicable Disease Committee's Regulation Regarding Violation on Disease Control Preventive Measures*, The Secretariat of the Cabinet, viewed 8 November 2021, <www.ratchakitcha.soc.go.th/DATA/PDF/2564/E/122/T_0004.PDF>.

Tultrairatana, S. and Phansuea, P. (2021) 'Symptoms Related to Air Pollution, Mask-Wearing and Associated Factors: A Cross-Sectional Study among OPD Pollution Clinic Patients in Bangkok, Thailand,' *Journal of Health Research*, viewed 11 November 2021, <https://doi.org/10.1108/JHR-11-2020-0548>.

World Health Organization (2021) *Coronavirus disease (COVID-19)*. World Health Organization, viewed 20 August 2021, <www.who.int/news-room/q-a-detail/coronavirus-disease-covid-19-masks>.

14 The consciousness of public actions concerning the COVID-19 in Cambodia

Yuko Shimazaki

14.1 Introduction

The coronavirus disease 2019 (COVID-19) outbreak has overwhelmed the world on an unprecedented scale. People have been left with no choice but to adjust to changes in their ways of life, including socialisation. The pandemic has been faced in complex ways with various emotions, such as confusion, fear, anger, distress and sorrow, including the hope that this crisis will be over. Since the beginning of the pandemic, the Cambodian government has taken actions to control the situation. However, the responses of the Cambodians to the measures of the government widely differ according to political, social and cultural backgrounds, which subtly influence one another. Thus, this chapter intends to illustrate the measures undertaken by the Cambodian government thus far, the reactions of the people towards such measures and the extent to which such measures have been effective. As such, many types of attitudes amongst the people of Cambodia towards the immediate impacts of COVID-19 were observed.

14.2 Political system and authoritarian politics in Cambodia

Prime Minister Hun Sen and the Cambodian People's Party (CPP) have been in influence for 28 years since the first national election supervised by the United Nations Transitional Authority in Cambodia (UNTAC) in 1993, which secured electoral success in 2003, 2008 and 2018. During these years, Cambodia has achieved huge economic growth because of international development assistance and foreign investment. From 2004 to 2007, economic growth reached a rate of more than 10%, where gross domestic product increased by up to 7% per year on average during the period from the subprime mortgage crisis in the United States to the outbreak of COVID-19. At the same time, disapproval of the CPP one-party rule has remarkably increased. Rapidly attracting support, Cambodia National Rescue Party (CNRP) of the largest opposition party made a breakthrough in the 2013 national election and the 2017 local elections. The increased support for the CNRP eventually proved to be a threat to the CPP, which began exerting pressure on CNRP members and their right to freedom of speech.

DOI: 10.4324/9781003244127-16

In September 2017, the Cambodian authorities charged CNRP leader Kem Sokha with treason. Furthermore, the dissolution of the party was ordered on the suspicion of a coup, where 118 top executive members were forbidden to engage in any political activity (Amnesty International 2019). After the 2018 election, the government announced that individuals who helped Sam Rainsy, the opposition leader, to return to Cambodia from his exile in France would be charged with treason. Afterwards, approximately 57 members of the CNRP were detained, whereas 105 were prosecuted between August and November 2019 (Amnesty International 2019; Human Rights Watch 2018). Allegedly, the oppression of the opposition party may have played a part in the tactics of the CPP to win the 2018 election.

In 2017, the government suppressed mass media that were critical of the government. One of such cases occurred in September 2017, where the *Cambodian Daily*, an English-language daily paper, has published for 24 years, starting soon after the civil war, was forced into discontinuation and was fined 6.3 million USD. The discontinuation led to great shock at home and abroad. The international society severely criticised the Cambodian government for violating freedom of speech. The Ministry of Foreign Affairs of Cambodia officially denied the charge. However, according to Human Rights Watch, discontinuing the *Cambodian Daily* was only one of the cases in which the expression of mass media regarding the disapproval of the government was forced into closure. Moreover, the Voice of America and the Cambodian office of Radio Free Asia were also put under pressure (Human Rights Watch 2018). Journalists critical of the government were arrested. Human rights organisations inside and outside of the country closely observed the ongoing situation, where the government exercised rigid control over freedom of the press.

14.2.1 Freedom of speech in Cambodia

When UNTAC was established in Cambodia after the civil war, the nation worked on forming its national governance and received international aid and cooperation, which were closely related to the concept of human rights and democracy. If inhumane or undemocratic behaviours were exhibited, then the nation could have been sanctioned. However, Cambodia of today is shifting its economic system from that based on international aid to that giving importance to public and private investments. The Cambodian government maintains diplomatic relations mainly with China, whose amount of overseas direct investment in Cambodia is the largest, which gave China a significant political influence. According to the Council for the Development of Cambodia, the largest share was derived from a Chinese investment of 2.75 billion USD (Council for the Development of Cambodia n.d.) in 2019. Consequently, Cambodia has adopted a more pro-China attitude. Therefore, the financial importance of Western countries has become weak.

The situation regarding freedom of speech and human rights has worsened, which has drawn international criticism. According to Freedom House, the *degree of freedom* in Cambodia was assessed as *Not Free*, with a score of 24 out of 100, which is as low as that of Myanmar (Global Freedom Status 2021). The extent of freedom in 210 countries and regions was examined on the basis of access to political rights and civil liberty (Global Freedom Status 2021). Under the category of access to political rights, Cambodia obtained a score of 5 out of a total score of 40. The global index of the degree of democracy placed Cambodia in the 152nd rank out of 176 countries (Global Freedom Status 2021).

In terms of COVID-19 in Cambodia and the regulation of freedom of speech and freedom of the press, Human Rights Watch (2020) reported that 17 individuals were arrested and detained for four months (between the end of January 2020 and 24 May 2021) for spreading *fake news*. These individuals were charged with agitation, conspiracy and spreading of disinformation under criminal law. The organisation said that 'this is a violation of free speech and a violation of human rights'. This report clearly mentioned that the arrests included four party members and supporters of the opposition party.

14.3 COVID-19 in Cambodia – measures by the government

COVID-19 was first detected in Cambodia in 2020. The spread of the virus was sufficiently contained to avoid overwhelming the capacity of the healthcare system. Consequently, the impact of the delta variant of COVID-19 was minimal, whereas the government immediately restricted the movement of the people. In fact, however, the government found difficulty in taking precautionary measures because of the insufficiency of its medical capacity. In framing the measures against COVID-19, Cambodia received Official Development Aid and support from international organisations, such as the World Health Organization (WHO), the World Bank and other agencies of the United Nations (UN).

These international organisations developed support activities in liaison with the Ministry of Health. To conform to the COVID-19 guidelines established by the WHO, the Ministry of Health conducts PCR tests, surveys of cases and tracing of persons required to undergo quarantine (WHO 2020b). The guidelines for Cambodia were as follows: incident management and planning, surveillance and risk assessment, laboratory management and support, clinical management and health care services, infection prevention and control, non-pharmaceutical public health measures, risk communication and points of entry and operational logistics. Particularly, the WHO worked closely with the Ministry of Health and published the 'Cambodia, Coronavirus Disease 2019 (COVID-19) Situation Report', which covers the latest situation and is updated weekly.

Although the situation was changing on a daily basis, the Cambodian government began to implement administrative and legal measures with less international intervention at the same time to consolidate its authority. The government passed bills that clearly reflected its firm decision-making. The provisions can be divided into two periods, namely the first period at the early stage of infection and the second, when another impact came, which was 18 months after the first detected case of COVID-19.

14.3.1 *The first period: provision for COVID-19*

According to the WHO, the first positive case of COVID-19 was confirmed in Cambodia in January 2020. The first case was a Chinese male who travelled from Wuhan to Preah Sihanouk province in the south of Cambodia (WHO 2020a). At the time, although many other countries began to enforce immigration restrictions, Cambodia actually failed to restrict immigration from China given its political influence on the country.

In March 2020, another positive case was confirmed domestically – a Cambodian living in Siem Reap province who was in close contact with a Japanese with COVID-19 staying in Cambodia (8 March 2020) (Chheng 2020). Following the confirmation, the government eventually set to work on COVID-19, which led to the immediate closure of all schools in the province. On 16 March, the government ordered the forced closure of schools across the country (Ministry of Education, Youth and Sport [MoEYS] 2020).

Afterwards, a ban on religious events and activities and on social meetings and gatherings was implemented on a daily basis. Entertainment facilities, such as theatres, museums, nightclubs and karaokes, were also closed. By the end of the month, all casinos were closed. During the early stage, Cambodia employed internal and external measures to reduce the movement of people by enforcing restrictions on entry and embarkation to and from specific countries. Moreover, Prime Minister Hun Sen imposed a ban on travelling to Europe, the United States and Iran, which was posted on his Facebook page on 15 March. Moreover, borders between Thailand and Cambodia were closed (Royal Government Spokesperson Unit 2020). Lastly, the government issued an official announcement on restrictions for entry by air travel.

Restrictions on immigration included the suspension of the issuance of tourist visa, e-visa and arrival visa, which are available at the airport at the time of arrival; acquisition of visa from the Cambodian Embassy abroad or the Cambodian consulate general in advance of embarkation; presentation of health certificate or proof of a negative COVID-19 test produced by the health authorities of one's country 72 hour prior to departure to Cambodia; presentation of a certificate of insurance, which states a coverage amount of 5,000 USD; medical examination and screening upon entry to Cambodia; and lastly, observance of instructions for isolation and quarantine and measures for containing COVID-19, which are issued by the Ministry of Health of Cambodia. These instructions were posted on the website at the end of March 2020.

Within one month, the Cambodian government responded to the situation without delay. On 30 March, Prime Minister Hun Sen sent a message via Facebook saying that the government was preparing a new bill that placed severe restrictions on movement as part of its measures to contain the spread of COVID-19. Afterwards, the government issued an order that prohibited movement between Phnom Penh and other provinces and between administrative districts (Royal Government of Cambodia 2020).

On 17 April, this was set up concretely and agreed as the draft law in the Senate. On 27 April, ten days after the agreement in the Senate, 'the Constitutional

Council of Cambodia approved unanimously as the draft law on State of Emergency' (Rinith 2020a, 2020b; Sokhean 2020). Setting this new law helped to consolidate the power of the government to control the situation. At the time when the law was enacted, the cumulative total cases of COVID-19 in Cambodia were much fewer than those in other countries.

14.3.2 *The second period: mask mandate and strengthening of penal regulations*

In February 2021, one year after the first case was confirmed, another surge of COVID-19 cases occurred. The Cambodian government implemented more stringent measures to control the situation and reinforced the penal codes, such as Cabinet Ordinance No. 37 entitled the 'Law on Preventive Measures Against the Spread of COVID-19 and other Severe and Dangerous Contagious Diseases', which was issued on 12 March. The regulation was binding, such that individuals who violated the provisions should pay a penalty. The law consisted of 18 articles, which included a mask mandate in places designated by the Ministry of Health and specimen collection for PCR testing as required by Cambodian authorities. Offenders were liable to pay a fine.

As stated by the Ministry of Labour and Vocational Training, the minimum wage in Cambodia was 192 USD per month (Prakas No. 303/20KB/Br.K.Kh.L). However, as of 12 March 2021, under the new Cambodian legal provisions, anyone without a face mask or who disregards a warning to wear face masks will be fined from 200,000 riels (49 USD) to 1,000,000 riels (245 USD; exchange rate for 12 March 2021). Moreover, Article 7 (Royal Kram 2021, NS/RKM/0321/004) stipulates that individuals who avoid quarantine or escape from isolation wards or quarantine facilities and infect others with COVID-19 will be imprisoned from six months to three years and will be fined from 2,000,000 riels (489 USD) to 10,000,000 riels (2,447 USD; exchange rate for 12 March 2021).

Article 8 stated that individuals who commit an act of avoidance, refuse medical treatment or escape from medical facilities shall be imprisoned from one to five years with a penalty ranging from 5,000,000 riels (1,223 USD) to 20,000,000 riels (4,894 USD). According to Article 9, 'an act of international transmission of COVID-19 to other people by any means shall be punished by imprisonment from 10 years to 20 years, where such an act is committed by an organized group of people or an organized entity' (Royal Kram 2021, NS/RKM/0321/004).

On 22 March, by issuing Ordinance No. 81 and Announcement No. 88, the Ministry of Health of Cambodia designated several provinces, such as Phnom Penh, Sihanoukville, Siem Reap, Kandal and Prey Veng, for the application of the mask mandate and social distancing policy (Embassy of Japan in Cambodia 2021). The cases in which individuals are required to wear face masks are quarantined persons, passengers in public transportation including taxis and persons in public places and in places where two or more people gather. Anyone without a face mask in these places is liable to pay a fine.

The precautionary measures of the second period included the execution of a law accompanied by the penal code, that is, the Law on Preventive Measures Against

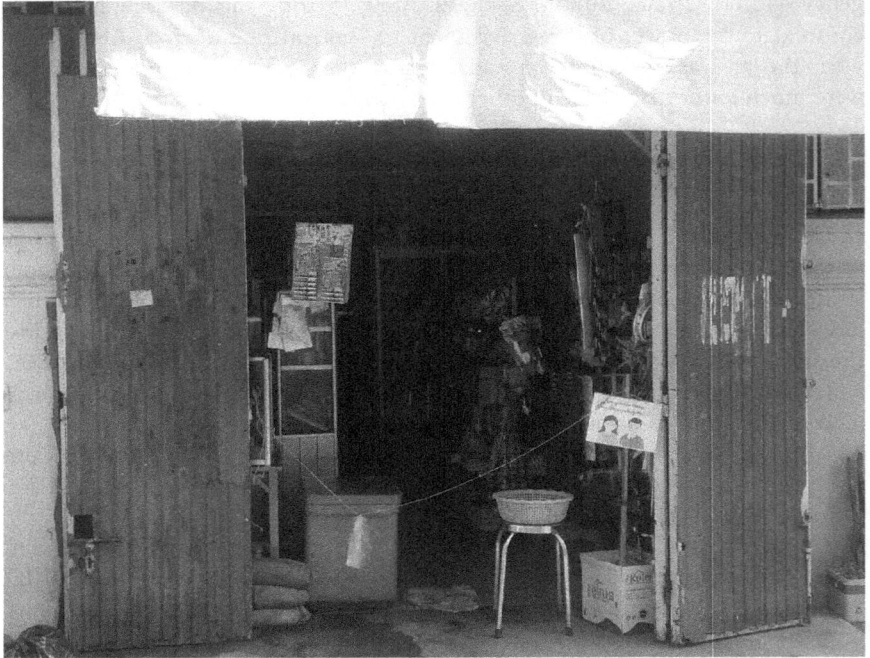

Figure 14.1 A grocery shop taking preventive measures against COVID-19
Source: Photo taken by Hiroko Oji, 18 April 2020

the Spread of COVID-19 and other Severe and Dangerous Contagious Diseases. The experts of the United Nations Human Rights Office of the High Commissioner (OHCHR) offered advice on the law because it 'undermines fundamental human rights, including freedom of movement, peaceful assembly and the right to work' (OHCHR 2021) on the ground that it was a violation of human rights.

14.4 Responses of Cambodians to the legal and administrative measures by the government

First, this section discusses the responses of the people of Cambodia to the actions taken by the government against COVID-19, access to information about COVID-19 related to governmental measures and how people used this information in daily life. In a survey on the opinions of the local people, a semi-structured interview was conducted regarding the present situation. The study selected ten key persons with access to information about the abovementioned government measures, who were capable of analysing the impacts of this information on the public and on their community regarding the present situation. These interviews of key persons were chosen according to the purpose of the survey.

Table 14.1 Respondents

ID	Sex	Age	Residence	Occupation	Education
A	male	23	Phnom Penh/originally from the rural village	student	university
B	male	20	Phnom Penh	student	university
C	female	28	Phnom Penh	dormitory mother	university graduate
D	female	35	Phnom Penh	bank employee	postgraduate
E	male	41	Phnom Penh	consultant	postgraduate
F	female	37	Phnom Penh	civil servant	postgraduate
G	female	36	a suburb of Phnom Penh/ household recipient of food distribution	selling beverages[1]	primary school (not finished)
H	female	30	a regional city/household recipient of food distribution	staff in a mobile street stall[2]	high school graduate
I	female	28	province/rural village	primary school teacher	high school graduate
J	male	23	province/rural village	primary school teacher/ farming	high school graduate

Source: Classified by author

14.4.1 Tools and sources of information

Through the interviews, the study found that mobile phones were popular tools for accessing information, where social media was one of the main sources of information. In Cambodia, mobile phones are commonly used and are currently considered one of the necessities of life, given that even secondhand cell phones are available at reasonable prices. Landline telephones are much less popular, which may be due to the lack of infrastructure.

In Cambodia, the popularity of mobile phones encourages the government and ministries to send information through their homepages and social network services (SNSs), such as Facebook. The government established the Communicable Disease Control Department (CDC), an internal special organisation under the Ministry of Health. This department releases the latest information on COVID-19 on their Facebook page and the homepage of their official website, in liaison with international organisations, such as the WHO. Many people in Cambodia have accessed the CDC website to obtain information on the current situation.

University student living in Phnom Penh mentioned that:

> The Facebook page of the Ministry of Health is really convenient to know newly confirmed cases daily, deaths and the vaccination status, which is updated every day. I think it is important to know the situation as early as

possible, because I cannot be indifferent to the current domestic situation. I sometimes check up with WHO on Facebook, which is also updated.

(A; aged 23 years)

The majority of the respondents answered that they consider information released by the Ministry of Health as reliable.

'Updating information is faster than the early days of the corona impact, and I feel the government gives close observations to domestic situations'.

'The necessary information is updated every day'.

'I want to know the domestic situation, such as the vaccination status, as soon as possible. When I visit the website of the Ministry of Health, I never fail to get the information I want to know. That is why I think they are reliable'.

In addition to the website of the Ministry of Health, the interviewees commonly accessed the Facebook page of the prime minister, the WHO and Telegram (an SNS service that relays announcements from the government). In Khmer, *Koh Santapiaph* was also popular.

The United Nations Children's Fund (UNICEF) conducted an assessment survey of behaviours for the prevention of transmission entitled Review of Risk Communication and Community Engagement Initiative for COVID-19 (UNICEF 2020).[3] The results of the review and the present study were similar, that is, people in Cambodia collect governmental information mainly from social media on a daily basis (UNICEF 2020).

Meanwhile, people living in the suburbs of Phnom Penh and other rural areas displayed a tendency to attach more importance to the human network in the community as the source of information. Although SNSs, such as Facebook, were also used, the people considered that information from the village leader or friends in the neighbourhood was more reliable. Moreover, the survey found that a few of these were high school graduates or gave up primary education before completion. For people living in rural areas, human relationships and community networks were social resources for their daily lives.

G (aged 36 years), who is living in a suburb of Phnom Penh and is certified to receive official food distribution as COVID-19 support, answered that contact with 'the village leader' was the main source of information:

'In my village, the village leader announces when something important happens, by walking around the community and visiting village members. Actually, I learned about COVID-19 from the leader'.

Similarly:

I usually gain information from the village leader and the village guard, [and that] when there is something we really have to know, the village leader walks around the community and tells us about it, as he did this time. I trust the leader, because he knows the neighborhood very well and we know him very well. What he says is reliable. (Moreover) I have had food distribution twice under the COVID-19 official support, and I was given rice, fish, soy sauce and noodles. The families whom the leader certified as ones in need were called to the distribution for poor family. My family is so needy that I can't buy enough food. That is why I appreciate the service.

(H; aged 30 years)

According to the personal details such as the places where they lived and their academic backgrounds, differences in how to collect information were created. Moreover, *H* said about the governmental policies that:

A curfew was imposed all of a sudden. I was just about to go out to the local market to buy groceries as usual. But I followed the order. If not, it would have been bothering others. There are seven of us living in the same house, so if I were infected with corona, it could be passed from me to them. I believe following the government's orders is the best way to protect ourselves against corona.

14.4.2 Governmental policies and daily life

Regarding the measures taken by the government against COVID-19, the respondents gave favourable responses overall, except for two respondents who responded with 'it depends on when and what action the government takes'. Initially, the study expected that the government may have pushed forward authoritarian policies for COVID-19, which developed heavy-handed politics. In certain cases, the people of Cambodia felt confused and displayed disapproval of the firm decisions, such as the sudden execution of laws with severe penalties, such as fines and imprisonment. Nonetheless, the people have seemingly managed to accept the mandates.

To support this view, the authors noted that the respondents behaved cautiously because of the strong fear of contracting COVID-19. The medical capacity of Cambodia remains insufficient. In rural areas, particularly, medical services are much less accessible. In rural villages, great social risks emerge when infected with COVID-19, such as financial burden for medical treatment, the surveillance system of the authorities and being placed under quarantine, because of the pressure and strict social norms, which are typical features of village life in Cambodia. Given such social risks, the study inferred that the respondents were likely to follow official instructions to avoid being infected.

From my point of view, Cambodians generally are cooperative with the government's orders. In my village, people mostly follow them, so our government mobilises us successfully. Some people do not have good access to the internet or mobile phones. In that case, the village leader visits them to let them know the official notice when issued. The leader makes an announcement once each week or two, going over to the far end of the village.

(I; aged 28 years)

I think we have to put up a united fight against the corona crisis. I usually follow the comprehensive measures and the penal regulations. In my opinion, following the government's instructions will lead to protecting each of us from being infected with coronavirus.

(J; aged 23 years)

Additionally:

Our government has done very well in conducting the preventive measures . . . the government issued instructions to reduce the financial burden in our daily lives, by distribution of food to families in need, and reduction in taxes, electricity bills and bank loans. In my village, the village leader distributed face masks and alcohol sanitizer to each household and to schools as well, once every three weeks. That I was really grateful for.

(J; aged 23 years)

In contrast to the favourable opinions about government action, criticism on these instructions also emerged, especially with the sudden execution of laws and official notices.

I think regulations like a ban on travelling between provinces from tonight and the lockdown of the cities from tonight seemed to be unreasonable. They were unrealistic. Still, I think sometimes that these regulations might have generated more disadvantages than advantages, because the sudden orders caused us to panic. But we have never had an experience like the corona crisis before, so we probably could not have thought of anything else but we had had no choice but to cope with the situation as we did.

(E; aged 41 years)

Amongst the respondents, two were school teachers, who expressed their fear of the extension of school closure and mentioned that the government should have framed more stringent rules and regulations during the lengthy school closure.

On the one hand, I appreciate some of the measures taken by the government. On the other hand, I feel worried because schools are long closed by the lockdown and movement restriction. I fear for the situation because there is not much consideration for education.

(A; aged 23 years)

Schools were closed for the first time on 16 March 2020 (through an official notice issued by MoEYS). On 18 April, the closure of all schools across Cambodia was extended (MoEYS and UNICEF 2021). Beginning 16 March, the closure of 13,482 schools across Cambodia affected 3.2 million students. Specifically, educational institutions were closed for five months in 2020 before restarting in September. At the same time, the government offered e-learning to secure educational opportunities for children when the school closure was extended. On 1 August 2020, the Ministry of Education and the Ministry of Post and Telecommunications recommended the download of an application for distance learning and released the link to the public. However, making full use of the contents on the Internet may have been, in fact, difficult according to individual Internet environments.

14.4.3 Wearing face masks and precautionary measures

In terms of wearing face masks, the respondents tended to follow this mandate as part of the necessary precautionary measures. A few of the respondents referred to their families, who are living in rural villages, as follows:

> My family members in a farming village usually buy surgical masks in a pharmacy or a clinic or a grocery shop. If no mask is available, a krama/Kroma (a traditional Cambodian scarf) can be a substitute for it.
>
> (J; aged 23 years)

According to the results of the survey conducted by UNICEF, the precautionary measures popularly employed by Cambodians were thorough cooking of food (94%), hand cleaning (75%), covering mouths when coughing (72%), safe distancing (60%), avoidance of packed places (52%), sneezing into their elbows (51%) and no touching of the face (20%). On the basis of these findings, people in Cambodia adopted various precautionary measures against COVID-19 (UNICEF 2020).

The interviews practiced various precautionary measures, such as handwashing; sterilisation, using alcohol gels and sprays; wearing face masks; maintaining social distancing; consuming a good diet to strengthen immunity; securing good sleep and vaccination. The items common to all respondents were face covers, clean hands and sterilisation. When asked what led them to take these precautions, the majority cited that they practiced these measures voluntarily to avoid contracting COVID-19.

By contrast, social norms and peer pressure urged the adoption of precautionary measures for a few cases.

> I have to follow the rules because the authorities told us to do so.
>
> (E; aged 41 years)

> I surely have some fear for the transmission, but I have to show that I follow the rules properly when the guard comes to check around the village.
>
> (G; aged 36 years)

In summary, the people of Cambodia were highly conscious of wearing face masks to prevent the spread of COVID-19. Although the respondents provided a few answers and said that the mandates were simply an instruction from the government, we conclude that the people were motivated to practise precautionary measures under the influence of various social conditions and domestic situations, such as social hygiene, fragile medical system, strict social norms and constant pressure from the community.

14.5 Conclusion

This chapter intended to illustrate the influence of a series of measures taken by the Cambodian government and the awareness of the people about such measures. The top-down political system in Cambodia enabled the government to launch policies for COVID-19 and to employ various administrative and legal measures against COVID-19. The notable mandates are the State of Emergency Law on 27 April and Ordinance No. 37 or the Law on Preventive Measures Against the Spread of COVID-19 and other Severe and Dangerous Diseases on 12 March. These stringent regulations included severe punishments and the imposition of fines for offenders. The government also took other precautionary measures, such as the wearing of face masks, social distancing and restriction on movement, which influenced the daily life of Cambodians.

Amongst the Cambodians, the measures were viewed with positive and negative feelings, especially the immediate and authoritative ones. Generally, however, these measures were seemingly followed as containment policies appropriate to the current situation on the ground that firstly, the Cambodian government exercised firm political pressure that can force the majority to side with the government. This aspect constitutes the central feature of the political system. Secondly, the healthcare capacity in Cambodia remains insufficient. Moreover, the outbreak of COVID-19 has led to various uneasy feelings and thoughts, such as the financial burden of medical expenses when infected with COVID-19, the fear for anxiety over the possibility of infecting other members, especially those in large families.

The COVID-19 situation in Cambodia reveals geographical, social and environmental differences between urban and rural areas. International support helped Cambodia to implement measures against COVID-19, such as identifying positive cases, establishing an isolation system, improving the medical system and tracing patients infected with COVID-19. With international support, such as the UN agencies, Cambodia has constructed a practical and operational system of medical health thus far. This view forms a notable feature of the modern history of Cambodia. The government organised several fact-finding surveys in cooperation with international organisations. On the basis of these results, the government has framed the measures for the control of the spread of COVID-19.

The impact of the COVID-19 crisis on rural villages and people in need remains unclear. However, this study infers that the extension of school closure has exerted a significant influence over school-aged children in many ways. For further study, conducting a thorough observation of the next direction for Cambodia in the face of this health crisis is necessary.

Acknowledgement

I would like to extend my sincere thanks to Hiroko Oji, representative of Nom Popok, for her generous cooperation in conducting the research for this paper.

Notes

1 In Cambodia, beverages are sold in a mobile wagon in the street or outside a shop. Mixed fruit juice and coffee with condensed milk are popular. When ordered, drinks are served in a plastic cup or a plastic bag. The respondent, whose ID was *G*, in the interview sold drinks outside her shop and also had an indoor drinking space.
2 Street stall snack shops are commonly seen in Cambodia, which are usually set up adjoining the local primary school. Children come and buy snacks and drinks hung at the shop front, during a break or while going to and from school. The respondent, whose interviewing ID was *H*, worked in such a shop.
3 This survey was aided by the United States Agency for International Development (USAID), the government of Japan and the Danish International Development Agency (Danida). This was also organised under the public and private partnership, joined by SMART, a Cambodian major communications company; Cellcard; Facebook, a provider of social network service; the Chief Executive of the Municipality of Phnom Penh, an administrative organisation; and local NGOs. 310 women and 444 men were surveyed (a total of 754). The results served as an assessment of precautionary measures against COVID-19 in collaboration between Cambodia and WHO.

References

Amnesty International (2019, 10 November) Cambodia: Reprieve for Kem Sokha a token gesture that should not distract from human rights crisis, (Accessed 27 July 2021), <www.amnesty.org/en/latest/press-release/2019/11/cambodia-reprieve-for-kem-sokha-a-token-gesture-that-should-not-distract-from-human-rights-crisis/>.
Chheng, N. (2020) 'Cambodian gets COVID-19', *The Phnom Penh Post*, 8 March, (Accessed 25 July 2021), <www.phnompenhpost.com/national/cambodian-gets-covid-19>.
Council for the Development of Cambodia (n.d.) FDI (Foreign Direct Investment), (Accessed 24 August 2021), <www.cambodiainvestment.gov.kh/why-invest-in-cambodia/investment-enviroment/fdi-trend.html>.
Embassy of Japan in Cambodia (2021, 28 March) The mandate of wearing a face mask and social distancing, (Accessed 3 August 2021), <www.kh.emb-japan.go.jp/itpr_ja/b_000421.html>.
Global Freedom Status (2021) Comparative and Historical Data Files: All Data, FIW 2013–2021 Freedom in the world 2013–2021 Raw Data, (Accessed 24 August 2021), <https://freedomhouse.org/explore-the-map?type=fiw&year=2021>.
Human Rights Watch (2018, 12 May) Cambodia: Release ex-radio free Asia Journalists now held for six months on politically motivated espionage charges, (Accessed 27 July 2021), <www.hrw.org/news/2018/05/12/cambodia-release-ex-radio-free-asia-journalists>.

Human Rights Watch (2020, 24 March) Cambodia: COVID-19 clampdown on free speech, cease arrests, detention of outspoken opposition activists, others, (Accessed 3 August 2021), <www.hrw.org/news/2020/03/24/cambodia-covid-19-clampdown-free-speech>.

Ministry of Education, Youth and Sport (2020) Government extends school closure to combat COVID-19 pandemic, (Accessed 25 July 2021), <www.moeys.gov.kh/index.php/en/draf/3639.html?highlight=WyJzY2hvb2wiLCJzY2hvb2wncyIsIn NjaG9vbCciLCJbG9zdXJlIiwic2Nob29sIGNsb3N1cmUiXQ==#.YRkLlYj7SUl>.

Ministry of Education, Youth and Sport and UNICEF (2021, March) Cambodia COVID-19: Joint education needs assessment, (Accessed 22 July 2021), <www.unicef.org/cambodia/media/4296/file/Cambodia%20COVID-19%20Joint%20Education%20Needs%20Assessment.pdf>.

OHCHR (United Nations Human Rights Office of the High Commissioner) (2021, April 12) UN experts urge Cambodia to review approach to COVID-19, (Accessed 15 October 2021), <www.ohchr.org/en/NewsEvents/Pages/DisplayNews.aspx?NewsID=26985&LangID=E>.

Rinith, T. (2020a) 'All Senate Members Support "State of Emergency" Law', *Khmer Times*, 17 April, (Accessed 31 July 2021), <www.khmertimeskh.com/714457/all-senate-members-support-state-of-emergency-law/>.

Rinith, T. (2020b) 'Cambodian schools to reopen in stages from August', *Khmer Times*, 4 July, (Accessed 25 August 2021), <www.khmertimeskh.com/741403/cambodian-schools-to-re-open-in-stages-from-august/>.

Royal Government of Cambodia (2020) April-9–2020.pdf, (Accessed 25 July 2021), <https://policypulse.org/wp-content/uploads/2020/04/April-9-2020.pdf>.

Royal Government Spokesperson Unit (2020, 23 March) (Accessed 25 July 2021) <www.facebook.com/rgsucambodia/photos/pcb.2978066635770588/2978066115770640/?type=3&theater>.

Royal Kram (2021, 13 March) Royal Government of Cambodia, ROYAL KRAM: Law on Preventive Measures against the Spread of COVID-19 and Other Severe and Dangerous Contagious Diseases, NS/RKM/0321/004, Royal government of Cambodia, (Accessed 3 August 2021), <https://policypulse.org/wp-content/uploads/2021/03/MOJ-4.pdf>.

Sokhean, B. (2020) 'CCC approves State of Emergency draft law', *Khmer Times*, 27 April, (Accessed 31 July 2021), <www.khmertimeskh.com/717548/ccc-approves-state-of-emergency-draft-law/>.

UNICEF (United Nations Children's Fund) (2020) Review of risk communication and community engagement initiative for COVID-19: Prevention behaviours in Cambodia, (Accessed 3 August 2021), <www.unicef.org/cambodia/media/3856/file/FinalReport.pdfs>.

WHO (2020a, January 28) Ministry of Health responds to first positive case of new coronavirus, (Accessed 25 July 2021), <www.who.int/cambodia/news/detail/28-01-2020-ministry-of-health-responds-to-first-positive-case-of-new-coronavirus>.

WHO (2020b) COVID-19 in Cambodia, (Accessed 14 April 2021), <www.who.int/cambodia/emergencies/covid-19-ewsponse-in-cambodia>.

15 Conclusion

Comparative perspectives on mask-wearing policies and public behaviours

Xavier Mellet, Noriko Suzuki and Susumu Annaka

15.1 Mask-wearing beyond culture

The generalisation of mask-wearing, as part of the global response to COVID-19, was a challenge and an opportunity for comparative politics due to the diversified implementation of its use in various contexts at a similar time. COVID-19 *emerged in all countries under study at nearly the same time*: from January 2020 in the majority of Asian countries beginning with China, followed by Thailand (Chapter 13 of this book) and several European countries, such as France (Chapter 4), Germany (Chapter 5), and Canada (Chapter 9), to February in a few European countries, such as Greece (Chapter 8) in this book. The number of cases largely increased at similar timepoints with certain specificities, such as Finland, where the cases peaked at a later time: the first wave occurred between March and May 2020 in the majority of cases, whereas the second wave was observed between February and March 2021 (Chapter 6). For contextual reasons, a few chapters focused on the first wave (Chapter 4), whereas others emphasised the evolution from the first to the second wave (Chapters 12 and 13). Within this period of time, face masks served as an indicator of common patterns and local specificities. In other words, although each chapter addressed the same object, its social impact or symbolic value was grounded on pre-existing issues and representations.

Since the beginning of the pandemic, a common assumption assumed that Asian people are more likely to wear masks than Europeans, which led to a tendency to attribute this difference to Asian culture. However, *the majority of Asian countries, except for Japan and Taiwan, lacked a strong mask-wearing culture* prior to COVID-19. For example, mask- wearing was interestingly notable as uncommon in China, whose experience with air pollution and the SARS epidemic failed to lead to a consolidated use of masks (Chapter 14), making its mask-wearing experience more similar to the one in European countries than it may look. As another example, only 19% of the Thai population as of 2016 was found to wear masks during a cold or flu (Chapter 13). These stereotypes most likely resulted from the mental expansion to all Asian countries of a strong habit grounded on specific contexts, such as the Japanese one. There is an impression that Asians wear masks, to the extent that a medical professional in the UK called

DOI: 10.4324/9781003244127-17

mask-wearing among 'a false reassurance' (Chapter 1). The situation in Canada also illustrates how the historical connection to masks is more complex than that of the East–West divide. Canadian provinces implemented mask-wearing during the Spanish flu and the SARS epidemic. However, the practice disappeared after these crises. Nevertheless, previous experiences influenced the acceptance of mask-wearing during COVID-19, which rendered it less conflictual than in Europe.

Taking the *historical perspective* helped in contextualising the emergence of mask-wearing habits worldwide and, thus, overcoming this preconception. The fact that masks were mostly used by Asians when broadly considered and created less public controversies in the majority of Asian countries contributed to the creation of an '*Asian mask culture*', which does not correspond to historical evidence. The experience of the Spanish flu in the 1910s constituted the first step in the utilisation of face masks as a solution for preventing epidemics. The case study of Hungary in Chapter 3 detailed how this innovation began in Europe and expanded into Asian countries. The historical analysis on Taiwan revealed that its mouth-covering culture was a result of the Japanese occupation during the Spanish flu in 1918 and the SARS experience in the 2000s. The fact that masks were referred to using the Japanese word *masuku*, which is derived from the English word *mask*, illustrates its intercontinental dimension. Masks continued to be recommended in Taiwan after the flu, such as in crowded places or during an encephalitis epidemic, in a manner similar to that of Japanese colonisers. However, the mask-wearing culture eventually disappeared before the emergence of SARS in the 2000s. Prior to COVID-19, only a few people wore masks on the street, especially those who were ill or wanted to protect themselves from pollution, such as in Japan and South Korea.

This conclusion will endeavour to shed light on the complexity of mask-wearing policies and behaviours and the common patterns and differences between the countries under study by *summarising their main findings* on the basis of the following questions: Who wore masks and who did not? What was the basis for the decision to wear or not wear a mask? The first misconception lies in the statement that Asian countries succeeded against COVID-19 due to their pre-pandemic mask-wearing culture, as previously mentioned. If this is the case, then how did the governments promote mask-wearing among citizens as a measure for controlling the spread of COVID-19? What were the social effects of the mask-wearing policy? The second misconception pertains to the explanation of the success of Asian countries according to their capacity to enforce mask-wearing through authoritarian measures or systems and to obtain popular obedience to collective rules. These two misconceptions were common to the news media in various countries but did not reflect the realities of the (diversified) situations. The analysis has revealed the importance of overcoming (or complexifying) the distinction between East and West (Asia and Europe) to understand mask-wearing policies and behaviours as one of the public policies against COVID-19. In summarising these discussions, we intend to draw certain conclusions (albeit limited) for this book.

15.2 Difficulty in the acceptance of masks in Europe

15.2.1 *From resistance to convergence*

The results of a large-scale statistical analysis of 400,000 mask wearers in 29 countries in 2020 demonstrate that, geographically, people in Asia were more likely to wear masks than people in Scandinavia (Chapter 2). In European countries, mask-wearing was not customary for healthy people, because the main assumption was that only sick people wore masks. However, after the World Health Organization recommended that masks were effective in preventing COVID-19 infection, governments issued instructions recommending or requiring mask-wearing. Meanwhile, in Asia, more people were wearing masks or cloth face covering and easily accepted mask-wearing compared with Europeans. Although populations highly supported mask-wearing policies in similar proportions, a major continental difference was noted in *the emergence or non-emergence of public resistance against mask-wearing and controversies related to masks*. In the majority of countries, the anti-mask population or those against anti-COVID-19 measures reached approximately around 20% of the population. Beyond this common quantitative fact, one major difference between Europe and Asia is the manner in which this minority transformed mask-wearing into public controversies, which could be observed in mass-media content or in the streets. A significant example of such a difference is the number of European countries as well as British Columbia that experienced xenophobia against Asians. In this manner, many Asians worried that mask-wearing would make them a target mainly due to the initially negative perception about covering one's face in public in many Western societies (Chapter 9).

Nevertheless, the experience of mask-wearing in various countries at similar moments revealed an international *convergence in the acceptance of masks* as an efficient means of protection against COVID-19. All countries under study presented similar high levels of mask-wearing (approximately 80%) at the end of the acceptance path, despite the fact that the time and steps taken to reach this peak varied across countries. The polls mentioned in the previous chapters illustrated this convergence in Finland in November 2020: 68% wore masks regularly, 78% in public transports, and only less than 10% did not wear masks (Chapter 6); in Greece, 78% of the population approved mask- wearing as of September 2020 (Chapter 8). A few months after the onset of COVID-19 (Spring 2020), approximately 80% of the Swedish declared a change in habits (Chapter 6). A similar situation was noted in Asia. For example, approximately 66% of the population in Thailand observed that everyone in their community properly wore face masks between June and August 2021. In broad terms, the majority of countries positively evaluated the measures, where support reached approximately 80% from various countries, such as Canada in as early as June 2020 (Chapter 9) and Germany all along the period (Chapter 5). One can be astonished by how mask-wearing, and beyond it the measures against COVID-19, were accepted by a large majority of the populations, in all the studied countries, no matter what policies were implemented. In other words, the large majority of populations accepted mask-wearing and considered it a valuable measure of protection despite high levels of political distrust, such as that in France or Greece. In addition, public support for the governments implementing the measures increased in all countries with variations among them, from a high increase (Taiwan and Finland) to a low increase or decrease (Greece and Poland), as we see in Chapters 6, 7, 8, and10.

15.2.2 Controversies on mask-wearing in Europe

Many European countries took a longer time in accepting mask-wearing measures for various reasons, such as the *inconsistency of the recommendations* provided by public authorities. At the beginning of the pandemic, many official institutions did not acknowledge the efficiency of mask-wearing. In March 2020, the French Minister of Health explained that 'masks are not useful to self-protection' when a German federal government agency proposed that evidence does not exist for its efficiency (Chapters 4 and 5). Similar doubts existed in Sweden and Finland, where it took all the year 2020 for masks to obtain scientific legitimacy, a report declaring that there was no evidence for mask efficiency, which became the government position of Finland for the first half of 2020 (Chapter 6). Moreover, a significant difference between countries can be observed in the variations of such measures over time. Many European countries were characterised by significant evolution across time, whereas China presented certain stability in its mask-wearing measures (Chapter 14). For example, measures in Greece largely varied from a general lockdown to compulsory mask-wearing in March 2020. The country lifted the majority of its measures during the summer, except for mask-wearing in closed spaces, prior to imposing stricter measures, which were lifted again in May 2021 with the same exception. The same cycle occurred three times until November 2021, when the number of vaccinated citizens reached the majority of the population (Chapter 8). Similar variations were perceived in the occurrences of the concept of mask in news media: in this book, Joachim Scharloth identified six phases in Germany, whereas Xavier Mellet identified five phases in France in 2020 (Chapters 5 and 4). Differences existed between neighbouring countries. For example, Norway and Denmark were characterised by quick political decision-making, whereas Sweden and Finland adopted a slow expertise-based path (Chapter 6). Other countries were characterised by two long phases of measures corresponding to the first two waves of the pandemic, such as Cambodia and the province of British Columbia (Chapters 12 and 9). Beyond these time differences, countries adopted similar types of measures against COVID-19.

Reaching a common course took different times and forms due to *the initial lack of domestic mask supplies.* Initially, mask-wearing was not recommended in France (February 2020) or Finland (June 2020) partially due to the impossibility of providing the population with sufficient supplies (Chapters 4 and 6). A few countries decided on regulating mask-wearing, such as Poland, which empowered an authority in charge of controlling the sales and retails of goods related to health protection on 2 March 2020 (Chapter 7). The state of emergency in Canada bestowed the province of British Columbia with a similar power to establish prices for essential goods, such as medical supplies and food (17 March 2020) (Chapter 9). Many countries in Asia experienced the same situation. For example, the Thai authorities had to control mask supplies and prices in response to the excessive demands during the first wave due to the lack of supply and the absence of the mask-wearing culture prior to COVID-19 (Chapter 13). In Cambodia, the lack of medical capacity and budget prevented the authorities from taking precautionary measures (Chapter 12). Thus, many countries created programmes that intended to nationalise mask production and distribution, which led to a certain convergence in the domestic supply of masks. In Poland, a Polish Sewing Works programme (*Polskie Szwalnie*) and an Industrial Development Agency (*Agencja Rozwoju Przemysłu*) were established, whereas the Taiwanese government promulgated a ban on exporting face masks on 24 January 2020 (Chapters 7 and 10). On 4 February, the Thai government listed face masks as regulated products for the same reason (Chapter 13). Moreover, the Japanese Prime Minister endeavoured to provide the population with free masks in spring 2020, such that a policy labialised as *Abenomask* was derived from his name.

Another factor that fed the controversies was *the emergence of scandals* related to the production, importation, or distribution of masks, like the '*mask affair*' occurring in Germany (March 2021), which pertains to politicians of ruling parties, who enriched themselves with considerable commissions (Chapter 5). Similar cases were observed in Finland and Poland, where large-scale money-laundering operations benefited politicians, ministers, and government agencies (Chapters 6 and 7). In Japan, the high cost and low efficiency of the 'Abenomask' policy led to certain levels of dissatisfaction. These cases can be seen as a detriment to the temporary strengthening of executive power in a state of emergency. However, it never transformed into public demonstrations, which is in contrast to the majority of European countries, such as Germany, which experienced demonstrations against the measures, gathering members of the far right, especially during summer 2020 (Chapter 5). Masks became topics of public issues in contexts, where their meaning resonated with social worries beyond hygiene standards. On the one hand, the news media in many countries have emphasised the radical minorities against mask-wearing, which made this measure a public controversy that divided the people into two sides, namely, for or against. These controversies occurred despite the large majority of the populations that approved mask-wearing. The Greek digital media particularly focused on celebrities, politicians or religious leaders who publicly claimed their opposition to mask-wearing measures (Chapter 8). On the other hand, many news media in Europe have seemingly adopted a single perspective by blaming those who refuse mask-wearing and highlight experts recommending it. Masks were presented as a symbol of altruism, that is, protecting others instead of the self, by public authorities and in mass media of European countries, such as France and Finland (Chapters 4 and 6). This manufacture of consent nourished the opposition of minorities who were distrustful of the political system even prior to the pandemic (Chapter 5). Arguably, *masks were a pretext to the criticism of political systems.* In Germany, criticism towards mask-wearing focused on two major aspects, namely, restrictions on fundamental rights and the opinion that COVID-19 is not dangerous and is only a mild form of influenza, or the denial of its existence. This minority did not consider masks a serious means of protection against COVID-19 but as a means for oppression and disguise, which was identified with federal political leadership. Masks became a symbol for criticising the political system due to its demagogic (lying to dominate) and dictatorship or coercive dimensions. Such a symbolic dimension of the concept of masks only seemingly occurred in European countries except for Scandinavia. Chino Yabunaga and Madoka Watanabe explained the relative absence of conflicts between citizens and governments in Finland and Sweden according to the success of the measures; the freedom granted to individuals; the open manner in which the measures were taken; and, generally, trust grounded in the welfare systems and equality (Chapter 6).

15.3 Mask-wearing behaviours beyond East and West

15.3.1 Reasons for mask-wearing choice

What is the basis for the decision to wear masks? Three types of rational attitudes towards mask-wearing were observed. Mask-wearing can be adopted as *a means of self-preservation, a result of social pressure, or a result of obedience to collective rules.* The countries under study presented significant differences in this choice. Cambodia was found to be an example of self-preservation, because the population assumed that public authorities were unable to guarantee public health. Thus, mask-wearing was necessary for survival and was directly related to the lives of the people who lacked the possibility of relying on external authorities. In Cambodia, access to medical services is difficult; thus, individuals are largely reliant on self-commitment to avoid being infected with COVID-19. Moreover, the community village life added social risks of being marginalised apart from the financial burden of medical treatment and the surveillance system of the authorities. Hence, ordinary people who are unable to afford masks covered their faces with cloth (Chapter 12). The sense of community was the main rationale behind mask-wearing in Thailand, where individuals put social pressure on people who do not wear face masks in public areas by staring at them. The weight of social pressure varied in Thailand, being lower for the youth who tended to loiter in public spaces and remove their face masks when socialising (Chapter 13). Following the rules established by public authorities became the main factor for Taiwan and France, whereas social pressure seemingly played a major role in Japan. In China, mask-wearing behaviour depended more on obedience to local authorities than belief in the efficacy of masks. This notion is in contrast to Europe, where personal preferences about mask-wearing were more important (Chapter 14). However, social pressure seemingly played a major role in Finland, that is, the fear of discrimination if one is not wearing a mask and the fear of being looked at negatively. More than 80% of the population regarded collective safety as more important than personal freedom. During the pandemic, the degree of individualism was the demarcating line between the two Scandinavian states (more individualistic in Sweden but more collectivism in Finland, explained by Chapter 6).

Do individuals rely on the *state* or the *self* in terms of responsibility? Moreover, do they trust other individuals or the state when considering the most efficient method? A comparative analysis on individual behaviours revealed a continuum between trust in public authorities as in charge and capable of guaranteeing public health and self-awareness or individual responsibility. For example, Japan presented a case of liberal self-responsibility and low levels of trust in authorities, whereas France exhibited low levels of trust in others but displayed a sense of state responsibility and adherence to collective rules (Chapters 1 and 4). The Greek mentality of 'free rider' (*tzampatzis*), which is based on distrust in authorities, partially explained the difficulty in enforcing mask-wearing as a first step (Chapter 8). Mask-wearing was also related to trust in others. Social trust may lead to social commitment without legal enforcement. Countries with high levels of distrust in government, such as France, tended to rely more on sanctions, although clearly perceiving such a direct causal relationship is impossible. The Thai people were not wearing masks at home, which is in contrast to recommendations, because they trusted family members (Chapter 13).

15.3.2 *Structural factors of mask-wearing behaviour*

Beyond personal decisions, *many factors* seemed to have impacted mask-wearing behaviour, such as education, social background, trust in others and the government, gender, and age. Each situation and individual behaviour may be determined using a unique mix of causal mechanisms, which makes the extraction of international patterns difficult. At a macro level, it has been proven that citizens of democratic countries where a high level of individual freedom is granted are less likely to wear masks (Chapter 2). Aside from political regime (discussed in section 15.4), two main structural factors have been recognised as impactful beyond national contexts for explaining mask-wearing behaviour, namely, *gender* and *economic condition* (Chapter 2). Firstly, women are more likely to wear masks than men, as well as more likely to respect rules, such as social distancing or hand-washing (Chapter 8). The reasons for this divide can vary across contexts and people. For example, it has been argued that women were more convinced of the harmfulness of masks than men were in Poland or that men are more inclined to fear being viewed as weak (Chapters 7 and 8). Secondly, citizens in prosperous countries are less inclined to wear masks than are citizens of poorer countries (Chapter 2). The primacy of the economic variable concretely appeared in the study, when individuals declared mask-wearing as a means of survival in Cambodia, where the authorities are assumed to be unable to guarantee public health (Chapter 12). In contrast, European countries were more reluctant to wear masks.

Other causal mechanisms played different roles across countries and situations. Combining all identified causes in the book, determining the ideal portrait of the perfect mask wearer is possible: a woman living in a poor country, preferably in Asia, with many cases regardless of the number of deaths. This wearer achieves a low level of education and trusts her government, is supporting the measures, and is influenced by social pressure at the same time. Susumu Annaka observed that the number of cases exerted a significant influence on mask-wearing behaviour as the key indicator for evaluating risk. The reason for this notion is that people living in affected countries tended to wear masks more frequently. Population density was also a significant causal factor for explaining mask-wearing behaviour (Chapter 2). Finally, the level of education may play a certain role in the perception of mask efficiency. In 2020, the percentage of respondents in Poland who claimed that masks are ineffective increased with the level of education and was the highest among people with the highest level, at approximately 20%. People with only primary education tended to believe that masks primarily protect those who wear them, whereas respondents with high levels of education were aware that they primarily protect those around them (Chapter 7).

15.4 Political regimes and enforcement of mask-wearing measures

15.4.1 *Mask-wearing measures: constraining or counting on citizens?*

How did the government impose mask-wearing on citizens as a measure for reducing the spread of COVID-19? Public authorities *used similar sets of policies* against the pandemic, which accompanied and were integrated with mask-wearing, such as social distancing and closure for schools, restaurants, shops and public spaces for a limited period of time. The majority of European and Asian countries imposed temporary lockdowns, which forced the citizens to stay home, except for Japan and Sweden, where a lockdown was only recommended. The nature and length of the lockdown varied. Other countries, such as Germany, used *light* and *hard* lockdowns. The first consisted of nationwide restrictions on public life and social contacts; the second one imposed mobility restrictions (Chapter 5).

Strong variations existed in the *degree of constraints over individuals* exerted by public authorities regarding mask-wearing, which became compulsory in most cases, and recommended only in a few cases. The intensity of its imposition also varied (mandatory or advised), as well as the places where it was requested: from indoor to outdoor. After a time of hesitation, masks became mandatory in Germany (from April to May 2020) and France (after the first confinement period on 10 May), with the respective governments using the specific concept of '*everyday mask*' (*Alltagsmasken*) and '*general public mask*' (*masque grand public*). The territories of mask-wearing expanded from indoor to outdoor places, which was finally imposed during the most critical moments. Mandatory masks in schools were an issue in France and Germany in September 2020 (Chapters 4 and 5). Greece imposed masks as mandatory in indoor places, such as schools, transportations and shops, in March 2020. The Ministry of Health published an official document online stating that masks should fully cover the nose and mouth and should only be touched using clean hands. Moreover, the government recommended mask-wearing for children above two years old. This rule was imposed in primary schools, but it was not the case in most countries (Chapter 8). Cambodia also made masks mandatory in the second phase of the epidemic in a large number of situations, which included occasions where two or more people were gathered (Chapter 12). Thailand took one step further and encouraged mask-wearing within private residences to prevent infection among family members. The population massively approved this measure, but it was not strongly followed for being impractical (Chapter 13).

Many European and Asian countries enforced mandatory mask-wearing, but not Japan or Sweden, where it was only recommended by authorities. In Japan, however, private places, such as shops and restaurants, could refuse anyone who did not wear a mask. Japan represents a country where the rules were the most liberal, individuals remaining free to move and not to wear masks on the streets if they did not want to (but many Japanese wear masks voluntarily in schools, shops, public places, etc.). In Sweden, masks were initially perceived as an excuse for not staying at home before being recommended for public transportation at the end of the year 2020 and from February to May 2021. The recommendation was lifted on 1 July with the decline in the number of cases, which is in contrast to Japan, where it was never lifted (Chapter 6). British Columbia followed the same path by only recommending mask-wearing (Chapter 9). However, China occupied an intermediate position, because the central government did not directly oblige citizens to wear masks but indirectly provided guidance to local governments and businesses (Chapter 14).

Apart from Sweden and Japan, most countries decided to use *a sanction system* that accompanied compulsory mask-wearing from a fine to a prison sentence. The French government enforced a fine of 135 euros (nearly 153 USD) for those found without a mask, whereas Poland fined 500 PLN (nearly 121 USD) by the end of November 2020 (Chapters 4 and 7). Taking cost of living into account, the Greek fine of 150 euros – 300 euros if in a hospital – created in summer 2020 was more severe, especially if we consider the 1,000 euros sanction for employers who fail in making employees wear masks (Chapter 8). Thailand and Cambodia had examples of severe policies in Asia. Those who violate the measures are subject to a fine of up to 20,000 baht in Thailand (600 USD) from June 2020. In Cambodia, a law passed in March 2021 included a fine ranging from 200,000 riels (49 USD) to 1,000,000 riels (245 USD), among other severe measures, such as imprisonment from six months to three years, for individuals who avoid quarantine or escape from quarantine facilities (Chapters 12 and 13).

Another notable aspect is the variations between countries in terms of *the level of political authority* in implementing the measures. France offered a very centralised decision-making process, where mask-wearing measures, among others, were directly announced by the president and decided within the extraordinary possibilities offered by the state of emergency. The French citizens were mainly reliant on the central state for being in charge of public safety. Local authorities and legislative power were following the primary definer role of the executive power (Chapter 4). In this regard, it was found that national policies in many Asian countries reach individuals more directly and forcefully through intermediate entities, such as local governments and businesses, as mentioned earlier about China. In Japan, the recommendations were issued at both national and local levels, which included many private initiatives related to mask-wearing in specific places. The case of Cambodia also reflects the importance of intermediate bodies, where guidelines were passed to the residents of the community through the village mayor (Chapter 12). Meanwhile, Canada offered a hybrid situation, where health was a responsibility shared by both levels of government. However, the delivery of health care is a local responsibility with assistance through federal money transfers (Chapter 9).

15.4.2 *Legal protections against the risk of authoritarianism*

Mask-wearing policies represented *a challenge for political studies*. Perceived as both a condition for collective freedom and a symbol of dictatorship, masks questioned the very core of democratic theory, because they symbolised political constraints over individual freedom in the name of public safety. Does the absurd severity of some sanctions reflect the authoritarian nature of certain political systems? The measures raised the question of the (right amount of) authoritarian response required during crises and, as a result, the question of the inherent *authoritarian dimension* in democratic regimes. The pandemic led to the enforcement of various measures that overlooked human rights through the temporary reduction of individual freedom, which rendered mask-wearing a symbol of dictatorship in many countries, especially in Europe and among the far-right anti-mask minorities. The majority of countries declared a *state of emergency*, which rendered possible the restraint of individual freedom inside and outside of countries and suspended economic activities and social gatherings (i.e. larger than a family-hold at home or in an open-air public area in British Columbia, as we see in Chapter 9). Can these measures and mask-wearing itself be considered authoritarian? The pandemic increased the risk of authoritarian measures in the name of security and nourished an anti-democratic risk, because all governments can use fear to impose unjustified measures that restricted human rights.

Many countries were confronted with *legal limitations* in the implementation of the extraordinary measures required by the circumstance. In Sweden, no constitutional authority existed to restrict individual movement and impose mask-wearing during the pandemic. As such, state intervention required minimisation, which led to lenient policies compared with those in Finland. The guarantee of freedom of movement, independence of public authorities and autonomy of local authorities were the three major limitations preventing authorities from imposing authoritarian, albeit more efficient (?) policies against COVID-19 (Chapter 6). At a different level, implementing mask-wearing led to a few specific legal issues in France and Canada due to past laws forbidding people to hide their faces in public. There were anti-mask laws in Canada to fight against riots and laws against radical Islamism in the name of state religious neutrality in France in 2011 and in Quebec in 2017 (Bill 62) (Chapters 4 and 9).

Many governments followed *a two-step trajectory of legal adaptation* consisting in reacting at first with the means at their disposal while preparing a new law that enables them to implement additional restrictive and consistent policies. The Cambodian government prepared a law before the second phase of the epidemics, which was initiated in February 2021. Passed in March, this law was very severe and led to major concern about individual freedom (Chapter 12). Thailand also started with recommendations before announcing the 'National Communicable Disease Committee's Regulation regarding the Violation of Disease Control Preventive Measures' in June 2021. This regulation enforced mask-wearing in response to the fourth wave (Chapter 13). Concerns rapidly emerged on the extra-legal nature of a few anti-COVID-19 decisions taken in Poland, when the government introduced regulations that interfered with the constitutional right to privacy and overcame parliamentary controls. The Polish two-step trajectory consisted of amending the Act on Preventing Infectious Diseases of 2008, which granted the possibility of imposing mask-wearing on 29 November 2020. However, the obligation was issued through an executive regulation much earlier, on 15 April (Chapter 7).

The main issues related to *the threat of a global increase of authoritarianism* due to the pandemic is related to the severity of measures and the possibility of returning to the normal situation after the disappearance of the threat. Sweden illustrated how the rule of law prevented the government from implementing extremely strict measures and how authoritarian regimes, such as Cambodia, could use legal means to better restrain individual freedom. In the end, however, the Cambodian government managed to consolidate its authority and passed bills that clearly reflected its authoritarian evolution. In this manner, accusations of dictatorship were targeting a key aspect of the extraordinary measures. The concept of dictatorship refers to the extraordinary powers granted to a general of the Roman republic by the Senate (*imperium*), which restrains the freedom of citizens for a limited amount of time to win a major war and preserve the integrity of Rome. Once again, the current pandemic revealed how the rule of law is the best guarantee for avoiding the erosion of the *liberal pillar* of democratic systems, that is, the rule of law, which guarantees individual freedom and the existence of a free public realm in the name of public security, and the *democratic pillar*, which is based on the sovereignty and representation of the people (Habermas 1998; Mouffe 2000).

Beyond conjunctural public controversies, COVID-19 exerted certain major underlying social effects, which remain difficult to clearly perceive and measure at the moment. Although *the pandemic clearly contributed to increasing inequalities*, their nature and degrees remain to be assessed. Thus, one can infer that the increasing risk of authoritarianism may be a political answer corresponding mechanically to the fragmentation of social bodies. For example, we know that COVID-19 affected more foreign-born citizens in Sweden and Finland due to the poor living conditions, which elevated the issue of *equitable health* in Sweden and elicited xenophobic reactions from the *True-Finns* against some immigrants' supposed lifestyle in Finland (Chapter 6). Beyond these specific cases, the pandemic may have contributed to the increase in social, territorial, gender and generational inequalities, which are partially evident in mask-wearing behaviour, according to who can access masks and at which cost and who accepts to wear it and for which reasons.

References

Habermas, J. (1998) *The Inclusion of the Other: Studies in Political Theory.* Cambridge, MA: MIT Press.
Mouffe, C. (2000) *The Democratic Paradox.* London: Verso.

Index

Page numbers in italics indicate a figure and page numbers in bold indicate a table on the corresponding page. Page numbers followed by "n" indicate a note.

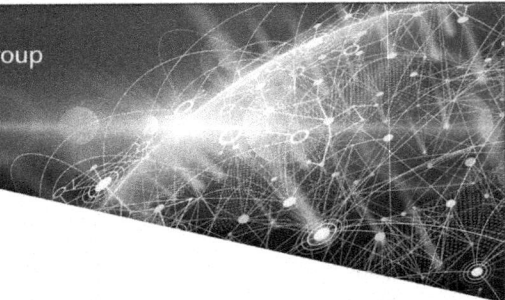

For Product Safety Concerns and Information please contact our EU
representative GPSR@taylorandfrancis.com
Taylor & Francis Verlag GmbH, Kaufingerstraße 24, 80331 München, Germany

www.ingramcontent.com/pod-product-compliance
Lightning Source LLC
Chambersburg PA
CBHW060241220326
41598CB00027B/4000

9 7 8 1 0 3 2 1 5 4 2 9 9